Implantation and Early Development

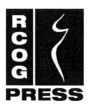

RCOG PRESS

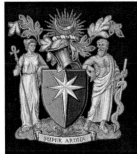

Since 1973 the Royal College of Obstetricians and Gynaecologists has regularly convened Study Groups to address important growth areas within obstetrics and gynaecology. An international group of eminent scientists and clinicians from various disciplines is invited to present the results of recent research and to take part in in-depth discussions. The resulting volume, containing the papers presented and also edited transcripts of the discussions, is published within a few months of the meeting and provides a summary of the subject that is both authoritative and up-to-date.

SOME PREVIOUS STUDY GROUP PUBLICATIONS AVAILABLE

Infertility
Edited by AA Templeton and JO Drife

Intrapartum Fetal Surveillance
Edited by JAD Spencer and RHT Ward

Early Fetal Growth and Development
Edited by RHT Ward, SK Smith
and D Donnai

Ethics in Obstetrics and Gynaecology
Edited by S Bewley and RHT Ward

The Biology of Gynaecological Cancer
Edited by R Leake, M Gore
and RHT Ward

Multiple Pregnancy
Edited by RHT Ward and M Whittle

The Prevention of Pelvic Infection
Edited by AA Templeton

Screening for Down Syndrome in the First Trimester
Edited by JG Grudzinskas and RHT Ward

Problems in Early Pregnancy: Advances in Diagnosis and Management
Edited by JG Grudzinskas and PMS O'Brien

Gene Identification, Manipulation and Treatment
Edited by SK Smith, EJ Thomas
and PMS O'Brien

Evidence-based Fertility Treatment
Edited by AA Templeton, ID Cooke
and PMS O'Brien

Fetal Programming: Influences on Development and Disease in Later Life
Edited by PMS O'Brien, T Wheeler
and DJP Barker

Hormones and Cancer
Edited by PMS O'Brien and AB MacLean

The Placenta: Basic Science and Clinical Practice
Edited by JCP Kingdom, ERM Jauniaux
and PMS O'Brien

Disorders of the Menstrual Cycle
Edited by PMS O'Brien, IT Cameron
and AB MacLean

Infection and Pregnancy
Edited by AB MacLean, L Regan
and D Carrington

Pain in Obstetrics and Gynaecology
Edited by AB MacLean, RW Stones
and S Thornton

Incontinence in Women
Edited by AB MacLean and L Cardozo

Maternal Morbidity and Mortality
Edited by AB MacLean and J Neilson

Lower Genital Tract Neoplasia
Edited by Allan B MacLean, Albert Singer
and Hilary Critchley

Pre-eclampsia
Edited by Hilary Critchley, Allan MacLean,
Lucilla Poston and James Walker

Preterm Birth
Edited by Hilary Critchley, Phillip Bennett
and Steven Thornton

Menopause and Hormone Replacement
Edited by Hilary Critchley, Ailsa Gebbie
and Valerie Beral

Implantation and Early Development

Edited by

Hilary Critchley, Iain Cameron
and Stephen Smith

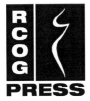

Hilary OD Critchley MD FRCOG FRANZCOG
Professor of Reproductive Medicine and Consultant Gynaecologist, Centre for Reproductive Biology,
University of Edinburgh, The Chancellor's Building, 49 Little France Crescent, Edinburgh EH16 4SB

Iain T Cameron BSc MA MD FRCOG MRANZCOG
Professor of Obstetrics and Gynaecology and Head of the School of Medicine, University of
Southampton, Level C (801), South Academic Block, Southampton General Hospital, Tremona Road,
Southampton SO16 6YD

Stephen K Smith DSc FRCOG FMedSci
Principal of the Faculty of Medicine, Imperial College London, London SW7 2AZ

Published by the RCOG Press at the Royal College of Obstetricians and Gynaecologists,
27 Sussex Place, Regent's Park, London NW1 4RG

www.rcog.org.uk

Registered charity no. 213280

First published 2005

ISBN 1-904752-16-0

RCOG Editor: Andrew Welsh
Design/typesetting by Karl Harrington, FiSH Books, London
Index by Liza Furnival
Printed by Henry Ling Ltd, The Dorchester Press, Dorchester DT1 1HD

Contents

Participants   ix

Preface   xv

SECTION 1 PREPARATION FOR IMPLANTATION – THE UTERINE ENVIRONMENT

1   **Endocrine and paracrine signalling in the human endometrium: potential role for the prostanoid family in implantation**
Henry N Jabbour, Kurt J Sales and Hilary OD Critchley   3

2   **Immunology of implantation**
Anita Trundley, Susan Hiby, Lucy Gardner, Andrew Sharkey, Charlie Loke and Ashley Moffett   16

3   **Progestin-induced decidualisation promotes human endometrial haemostasis and vascular stability**
Frederick Schatz, Graciela Krikun, Se-Te Huang, Edmund Funai, Lynn Buchwalder, Mizanur Rahman, Rebeca Caze, Caroline Tang and Charles J Lockwood   32

4   **Adhesion molecules and implantation**
John D Aplin   49

5   **Vascular growth and modelling in the endometrium**
D Stephen Charnock-Jones   61

6   **Tissue remodelling at the fetal–maternal interface: the regulation of matrix metalloproteinase 9 transcription**
Marie Cohen and Paul Bischof   70

7   **Embryo interactions in human implantation**
Francisco Domínguez, Jose A Horcajadas, Ana Cervero, Antonio Pellicer and Carlos Simón   79

8   **Experimental models of implantation of the human embryo: reconstructing the endometrial–embryo dialogue *in vitro***
Helen Mardon   90

SECTION 2 THE EMBRYO

9   **What makes a good egg?**
Alison A Murray and Norah Spears   103

10   **What makes 'good sperm'?**
Allan Pacey   119

11   **Morphogenesis of the early mammalian embryo:**
cell lineage heterogeneity and developmental potential
Tom P Fleming, Judith J Eckert, Fay C Thomas and
Bhavwanti Sheth   129

12   **Epigenetics in development and cloning by nuclear transfer:**
alternative approaches to nuclear reprogramming
Keith HS Campbell and Ramiro Alberio   141

13   **Risks associated with assisted reproduction: insights**
from animal studies
Kevin D Sinclair and Ravinder Singh   155

14   **Pre-implantation genetic testing**
Peter Braude, Jan Grace and Tarek El Toukhy   169

SECTION 3 LESSONS FROM ANIMAL MODELS (TRANSGENICS) AND NOVEL TECHNOLOGIES

15   **To implant or not to implant: the role of leukaemia**
inhibitory factor
Susan J Kimber, Ali A Fouladi-Nashta, Lisa Mohamet,
Carolyn JP Jones and Gemma Schofield   185

16   **Are gene arrays useful for the study of implantation?**
Andrew Sharkey, Rob Catalano and Jane Borthwick   203

SECTION 4 CLINICAL SEQUELAE

17   **Sporadic early pregnancy loss: aetiology and management**
Siobhan Quenby   219

18   **Recurrent miscarriage – the role of prothrombotic disorders**
Arvind Vashisht and Lesley Regan   229

19   **Reproductive disorders and pregnancy outcome**
Jan J Brosens, Luca Fusi, Robert Pijnenborg and Ivo A Brosens   240

20   **Risk factors for first-trimester miscarriage:**
summary of results from the National Women's Health Study
Noreen Maconochie and Pat Doyle   253

21   **Single-embryo transfer**
Siladitya Bhattacharya and Zabeena Pandian   256

22   **Paediatric outcome after assisted reproductive technology**
Alastair G Sutcliffe   268

SECTION 5 CONSENSUS VIEWS

23   Consensus views arising from the 48th Study Group:
Implantation and Early Development   283

Index   287

DECLARATION OF INTEREST

All contributors to the Study Group were invited to make a specific Declaration of Interest in relation to the subject of the Study Group. This was undertaken and all contributors complied with this request. Henry Jabbour is associated with several patent applications on prostaglandin receptors and their signalling pathways in the endometrium (but the patents are not in relation to implantation). D Stephen Charnock-Jones is an inventor on a patent relating to the basic technology of gene transfer to the endometrium. This has already been licensed by the University of Cambridge and no additional income will be derived from it. He is also an inventor on two patents relating to the transcript profile (i.e. gene array data) in endothelial cells after treatment with angiogenic and other stimuli. There are of an extremely basic nature and are of marginal relevance to the topic of vascular remodelling. He is a founder of and consultant to a biotechnology company, Gene Networks International, which uses computer modelling to identify the gene regulatory networks in endothelial cells. Allan Pacey is associated with a patent application (0403611.7, 'Analysis of cell morphology and motility') filed in February 2004. This patent describes a method to obtain the morphological characteristics of motile sperm. Peter Braude has undertaken paid work for BMJ Books. He is associated with patents on pre-eclampsia testing and tests for cholestasis. Keith Campbell is a member of the Scientific Board for ACT Advanced Cell Technologies, MA, USA and receives a consultancy. Andrew Sharkey has a patent pending on endometrial gene transfer filed in 1997: US patent number 08/860,047; European application number 95941229.7. This patent (pending) describes a method to transfect DNA into endometrium in vivo, to alter function. It was licensed in 1997 to Ares-Serono. The status of the application is unknown. Lesley Regan is a trustee for Save the Baby and a medical adviser for the Miscarriage Association.

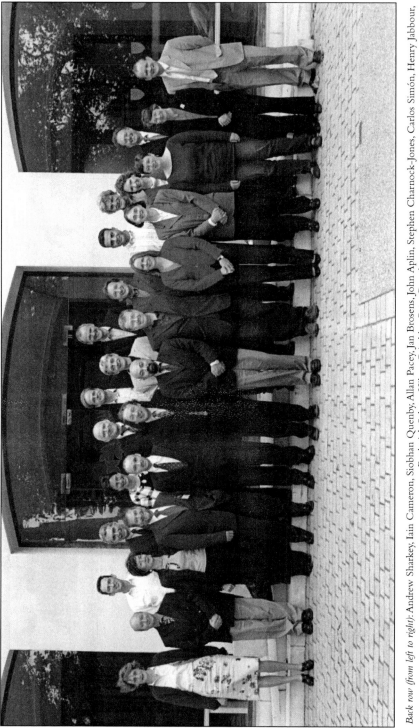

Back row (from left to right): Andrew Sharkey, Iain Cameron, Siobhan Quenby, Allan Pacey, Jan Brosens, John Aplin, Stephen Charnock-Jones, Carlos Simón, Henry Jabbour, Frederick Schatz, Hilary Critchley, Peter Braude

Front row (from left to right): Ashley Moffett, Stephen Pennington, Lesley Regan, Paul Bischof, Kevin Sinclair, Keith Campbell, Siladitya Bhattacharya, Tom Fleming, Helen Mardon, Susan Kimber, Norah Spears, Ruth Bender Atik, Alastair Sutcliffe

Participants

John D Aplin
Professor of Reproductive Biomedicine, Division of Human Development,
The Medical School, University of Manchester, Research Floor, St Mary's Hospital,
Manchester M13 0JH, UK.

Siladitya Bhattacharya
Senior Lecturer and Honorary Consultant, Department of Obstetrics and
Gynaecology, Foresterhill, Aberdeen AB25 2ZD, UK.

Paul Bischof
Professor, University of Geneva, Laboratoire d'Hormonologie, Maternité,
Bd de la Cluse, 1211 Geneva 14, Switzerland.

Peter Braude
Professor of Obstetrics and Gynaecology, Centre for Preimplantation Genetic
Diagnosis, Guy's and St Thomas' NHS Trust and GKT School of Medicine, London
SE1 9RT, UK.

Jan J Brosens
Professor of Reproductive Sciences and Honorary Consultant Gynaecologist
Obstetrician, Institute of Reproductive and Developmental Biology,
Imperial College London, Hammersmith Hospital, Du Cane Road,
London W12 ONN, UK.

Iain T Cameron
Professor of Obstetrics and Gynaecology and Head of the School of Medicine,
University of Southampton, Level C (801), South Academic Block,
Southampton General Hospital, Tremona Road, Southampton SO16 6YD, UK.

Keith HS Campbell
Professor of Animal Development, Division of Animal Physiology, School of
Biosciences, University of Nottingham, Sutton Bonington Campus,
Loughborough, UK.

David Stephen Charnock-Jones
University Reader, Department of Obstetrics and Gynaecology,
University of Cambridge, The Rosie Hospital, Cambridge CB2 2SW, UK.

Hilary OD Critchley
Professor of Reproductive Medicine and Consultant Gynaecologist,
Centre for Reproductive Biology, University of Edinburgh,
The Chancellor's Building, 49 Little France Crescent, Edinburgh EH16 4SB, UK.

Pat Doyle
Reader in Epidemiology, London School of Hygiene and Tropical Medicine,
Keppel Street, London WC1E 7HT, UK.

Tom P Fleming
Professor Developmental Biology, School of Biological Sciences,
University of Southampton, Bassett Crescent East, Southampton SO16 7PX, UK.

Henry N Jabbour
Senior Scientist, MRC Human Reproductive Sciences Unit,
Centre for Reproductive Biology, The University of Edinburgh Academic Centre,
49 Little France Crescent, Edinburgh EH16 4SB, UK.

Susan J Kimber
Reader, Faculty of Life Sciences, New University of Manchester, Stepford Building,
Oxford Road, Manchester M13 9PT, UK.

Helen Mardon
Professor of Reproductive Science, Nuffield Department of Obstetrics and
Gynaecology, Division of Medical Sciences, University of Oxford Women's Centre,
Level 3, John Radcliffe Hospital, Headington, Oxford OX3 9DU, UK.

Ashley Moffett
Fellow in Medical Sciences and Director of Clinical Studies,
King's College, Cambridge, and Associate Lecturer, Department of Pathology,
University of Cambridge, Tennis Court Road, Cambridge CB2 1QP, UK.

Allan Pacey
Senior Lecturer, Academic Unit of Reproductive and Developmental Medicine,
Level 4, The Jessop Wing, Royal Hallamshire Hospital, Tree Root Walk,
Sheffield S10 2SF, UK.

Stephen Pennington
Conway Institute of Biomolecular and Biomedical Research,
University College Dublin, Benfield, Dublin 4, Ireland.

Siobhan Quenby
Senior Lecturer and Honorary Consultant, 1st Floor, Liverpool Women's Hospital,
Crown Street, Liverpool L8 7SJ, UK.

Lesley Regan
Professor and Head of Department of Obstetrics and Gynaecology,
Imperial College at St Mary's Hospital, Mint Wing, South Wharf Road,
London W2 1NY, UK.

Frederick Schatz
Research Scientist, Department of Obstetrics, Gynecology and Reproductive
Sciences, Yale University School of Medicine, Room 335 FMB, 333 Cedar Street,
PO Box 208063, New Haven, CT 06520-2083, USA.

Andrew M Sharkey
Senior Research Associate, Department of Pathology, University of Cambridge,
Tennis Court Road, Cambridge CB2 1QP, UK.

Carlos Simón
Research Director, Fundacion Instituto Valenciano de Infertilidad, Guadassuar,
1 Majo, Valencia 46015, Spain.

Kevin D Sinclair
Senior Lecturer, School of Biosciences, University of Nottingham,
Sutton Bonington Campus, Loughborough LE12 5RD, UK.

Stephen K Smith
Principal, Faculty of Medicine, Imperial College London, London SW7 2AZ, UK.

Norah Spears
Reader, University of Edinburgh, SBCLS, Hugh Robson Building, George Square,
Edinburgh EH8 9XD, UK.

Alastair G Sutcliffe
Senior Lecturer in Paediatrics and Honorary Consultant, Academic Department of
Child Health, Royal Free Campus, Royal Free and University College Medical
School, Rowland Hill Street, London NW3 2PF, UK.

Additional contributors

Ramiro Alberio
RCUK Research Fellow, Division of Animal Physiology, School of Biosciences,
University of Nottingham, Sutton Bonington Campus, Loughborough, UK.

Jane M Borthwick
Department of Pathology, University of Cambridge, Tennis Court Road,
Cambridge CB2 1QP, UK.

Ivo A Brosens
Emeritus Professor, Leuven Institute for Fertility and Embryology, Leuven,
Belgium.

Lynn Buchwalder
Research Associate, Department of Obstetrics, Gynecology and Reproductive
Sciences, Yale University School of Medicine, LCI Room 810, 333 Cedar Street,
New Haven, CT 06510, USA.

Rob Catalano
Postdoctoral Research Associate, Department of Pathology,
University of Cambridge, Tennis Court Road, Cambridge CB2 1QP, UK.

Rebeca Caze
Research Associate, Department of Obstetrics, Gynecology and Reproductive Sciences, Yale University School of Medicine, LCI Room 803, 333 Cedar Street, New Haven, CT 06520, USA.

Ana Cervero
Implantation Research, Fundacion Instituto Valenciano de Infertilidad, Guadassuar, 1 Majo, Valencia 46015, Spain.

Marie Cohen
Post-doctoral Fellow, University of Geneva, Laboratoire d'Hormonologie, Maternité, Bd de la Cluse, 1211 Geneva 14, Switzerland.

Francisco Domínguez
Research Leader: Implantation, Fundacion Instituto Valenciano de Infertilidad, Guadassuar, 1 Majo, Valencia 46015, Spain.

Judith J Eckert
Lecturer, University of Southampton, Developmental Origins of Health and Disease (DoHaD) Division, Princess Anne Hospital, Coxford Road, Southampton SO16 5YA, UK.

Tarek El Toukhy
Specialist Registrar in Obstetrics and Gynaecology, Centre for Preimplantation Genetic Diagnosis, Guy's and St Thomas' NHS Trust and GKT School of Medicine, London SE1 9RT, UK.

Ali A Fouladi-Nashta
Research Associate, University of Nottingham, School of Biosciences, Sutton Bonington Campus, Loughborough LE12 5RD, UK.

Edmund Funai
Associate Professor, Department of Obstetrics, Gynecology and Reproductive Sciences, Yale University School of Medicine, 333 Cedar Street, PO Box 208063, New Haven, CT 06520-2083, USA.

Luca Fusi
Senior Lecturer, Institute of Reproductive and Developmental Biology, Wolfson & Weston Research Centre for Family Health, Imperial College London, Faculty of Medicine, Hammersmith Hospital, London W12 0NN, UK.

Lucy Gardner
Technician, Department of Pathology, University of Cambridge, Tennis Court Road, Cambridge CB2 1QP, UK.

Jan Grace
Subspecialty Trainee in Reproductive Medicine, Centre for Preimplantation Genetic Diagnosis, Guy's and St Thomas' NHS Trust and GKT School of Medicine, London SE1 9RT, UK.

Susan Hiby
Senior Research Associate, Department of Pathology, University of Cambridge, Tennis Court Road, Cambridge CB2 1QP, UK.

Jose A Horcajadas
Molecular Biology Group Leader, Fundacion Instituto Valenciano de Infertilidad, Guadassuar, 1 Majo, Valencia 46015, Spain.

Se-Te Huang
Associate Research Scientist, Department of Obstetrics, Gynecology and Reproductive Sciences, Yale University School of Medicine, LCI Room 801A, 333 Cedar Street, New Haven, CT 06510, USA.

Carolyn JP Jones
Research Fellow, Department of Obstetrics and Gynaecology, Research Floor, St Mary's Hospital, Hathersage Road, Manchester M13 0JH, UK.

Graciela Krikun
Research Scientist, Department of Obstetrics, Gynecology and Reproductive Sciences, Yale University School of Medicine, LCI Room 803, 333 Cedar Street, New Haven, CT 06520, USA.

Charles J Lockwood
The Anita O'Keefe Young Professor of Women's Health and Chair, Department of Obstetrics, Gynecology and Reproductive Sciences, Yale University School of Medicine, Room 333 FMB, 333 Cedar Street, PO Box 208063, New Haven, CT 06520-2083, USA.

Charlie Loke
Professor of Reproductive Immunology and Fellow, King's College, Cambridge CB2 1ST, UK.

Noreen Maconochie
Senior Lecturer in Epidemiology, London School of Hygiene and Tropical Medicine, Keppel Street, London WC1E 7HT, UK.

Lisa Mohamet
Faculty of Life Sciences, University of Manchester, Stopford Building, Oxford Road, Manchester M13 9PT, UK.

Alison A Murray
Research Associate, Reader, University of Edinburgh, SBCLS, Hugh Robson Building, George Square, Edinburgh EH8 9XD, UK.

Zabeena Pandian
Specialist Registrar, Department of Obstetrics and Gynaecology, Foresterhill, Aberdeen AB25 2ZD, UK.

Antonio Pellicer
Director, Instituto Valenciano de Infertilidad, Plaza de la Policía Local, 3, Valencia 46015, Spain.

Robert Pijnenborg
Professor, Department of Obstetrics and Gynaecology, Catholic University of Leuven, Leuven, Belgium.

Mizanur Rahman
Research Associate, Department of Obstetrics, Gynecology and Reproductive
Sciences, Yale University School of Medicine, LCI Room 810, 333 Cedar Street,
New Haven, CT 06520, USA.

Kurt J Sales
Investigator Scientist, MRC Human Reproductive Sciences Unit,
Centre for Reproductive Biology, The University of Edinburgh Academic Centre,
49 Little France Crescent, Edinburgh EH16 4SB, UK.

Gemma Schofield
Research Associate, Institute of Human Genetics, Central Parkway,
Newcastle upon Tyne NE1 3BZ, UK

Bhavwanti Sheth
Experimental Officer, School of Biological Sciences, University of Southampton,
Bassett Crescent East, Southampton SO16 7PX, UK.

Ravinder Singh
Research Fellow, School of Biosciences, University of Nottingham,
Sutton Bonington Campus, Loughborough LE12 5RD, UK.

Caroline Tang
Research Associate, Department of Obstetrics, Gynecology and Reproductive
Sciences, Yale University School of Medicine, 333 Cedar Street, New Haven, CT
06520, USA.

Fay C Thomas
Senior Scientist, Capsant Neurotechnologies, Biomedical Sciences Building,
Bassett Crescent East, Southampton SO16 7PX, UK.

Anita Trundley
Research Associate, Department of Pathology, University of Cambridge, Tennis
Court Road, Cambridge CB2 1QP, UK.

Arvind Vashisht
Department of Obstetrics and Gynaecology, Imperial College at St Mary's Hospital,
Mint Wing, South Wharf Road, London W2 1NY, UK.

Discussant

Ruth Bender Atik
National Director, The Miscarriage Association, c/o Clayton Hospital, Northgate,
Wakefield WF1 3JS, UK.

Preface

Successful implantation and early development require a union of healthy gametes and subsequent growth and development within an optimal uterine environment. The 48th RCOG Study Group comprised a national and international multidisciplinary expert forum that considered factors involved in preparation for implantation within the uterus, what makes a good egg and good sperm and hence a good embryo. Lessons from animal models and transgenic and genomic technologies received consideration. Attention was given to both sporadic and recurrent early pregnancy loss and to the scale of these distressing events. New treatment options were critically discussed and empirical approaches to management, without evidence of identifiable aetiological factors and rigorous evaluation, were cautioned against.

Assisted reproductive technologies have had a huge impact on the management of fertility problems over the past 25 years. Discussion included the arguments for single-embryo transfer and the developmental consequences of assisted reproductive technologies. The Group emphasised the need to continue to extend and refine the evidence base available for investigation and treatment options across the spectrum of early pregnancy management.

The 'consensus views' contained within this publication are not formal recommendations, but the conclusions of independent experts. Areas where future research is much needed have been identified. Emphasis is given to the multidisciplinary approach required if there is to be a substantial impact on our knowledge base, whether biological or clinical. The chapters herein have provided the authors with the opportunity to express further their individual views and to discuss issues in more detail and depth. We hope that this publication will provide a valuable resource for gynaecologists, specialist nurses, embryologists, basic scientists and all those with an interest in early pregnancy and development.

Hilary Critchley
Iain Cameron
Stephen Smith

SECTION 1

PREPARATION FOR IMPLANTATION – THE UTERINE ENVIRONMENT

Chapter 1

Endocrine and paracrine signalling in the human endometrium: potential role for the prostanoid family in implantation

Henry N Jabbour, Kurt J Sales and Hilary OD Critchley

Introduction

The endometrium undergoes morphological and functional differentiation during the mid–late secretory phase of the menstrual cycle in preparation for implantation. Successful implantation is dependent on appropriate embryo development and uterine receptivity. The latter consists of differentiation and secretory transformation of the glandular epithelial cells followed by decidualisation of the stromal compartment during the mid–late secretory phase of the menstrual cycle. This period is also characterised by extensive tissue remodelling in the superficial layer of the endometrium in preparation for the invasion and implantation of the proliferating trophoblast cells. These changes are orchestrated by endocrine factors such as ovarian steroid hormones. However, local autocrine/paracrine signalling is also crucial in the preparation of the endometrium for successful establishment of pregnancy. A host of local factors are known to play a role in the implantation process. Some of these factors have been identified following null mutation of individual genes. Others have been implicated in the implantation process following observational studies of temporal and spatial gene expression during the window of implantation. More recent technological advances, such as application of cDNA array and proteomic technology, will outline valuable clues as to the hierarchy of molecular changes and events that culminate in the preparation of a receptive endometrium. A better understanding of the mechanisms that govern successful implantation is of clinical relevance as it will assist in the development of improved strategies to correct for pathologies associated with impaired implantation, early pregnancy development and uteroplacental function.

Endocrine regulation of morphological and functional changes in endometrium during implantation

The endometrium undergoes well-described morphological and functional changes during each menstrual cycle in preparation for implantation.[1] The cyclical features of endometrial proliferation and differentiation are the consequence of sequential exposure to oestradiol and progesterone from the developing ovarian follicle and corpus luteum, respectively.

Progesterone is essential for the transformation of an oestrogen-primed endometrium in preparation for implantation. Much remains poorly understood about the molecular and cellular mechanisms by which the sex steroid hormones promote uterine receptivity. It is, however, recognised that sex steroids, acting via their cognate receptors, initiate a pattern of gene expression essential for implantation and the early stages of pregnancy. Consequently, if specific steroid-induced molecules can be identified there is the potential for their use as markers of uterine receptivity or targets for early pregnancy interruption. Many studies have examined the temporal and spatial expression of presumed progesterone-regulated genes across the menstrual cycle. Studies involving a candidate gene approach and those utilising data-driven microarray technologies have contributed to the body of knowledge concerning genes and their products likely to play a key role in human implantation. For example, expression of calcitonin mRNA has been demonstrated to be progesterone-dependent and temporally restricted to the mid-secretory phase of the cycle (maximal expression during days 19–21), a period that coincides with the putative window of implantation.[2] Evidence for regulation of this gene by progesterone was derived from examination of endometrium collected from women treated with a progesterone antagonist, mifepristone. Calcitonin expression in the glandular epithelium was reduced in women exposed to acute administration of mifepristone in the early luteal phase.

Further examples of local candidate endometrial molecules that are regulated by progesterone include glandular secretion of glycodelin (PP14)[3] and the enzymes 15-hydroxyprostaglandin dehydrogenase (PGDH)[4–6] and 17β-hydroxysteroid dehydrogenase (17β-HSD type 2).[7]

Decidualisation is a crucial step in the initiation and establishment of pregnancy and is a feature of those species that have an invasive haemochorial placentation. In the human, decidualisation is independent of the blastocyst and signs of predecidual changes are first observed in stromal cells close to vascular structures in the mid–late secretory phase. These same stromal cells express progesterone receptor throughout the luteal phase. *In vivo*, decidualisation is controlled most effectively by progesterone action on an oestrogen-primed uterus. This process can, however, be induced *in vitro* and a central role for cyclic adenosine 3′-5′-monophosphate (cAMP) has also been demonstrated as a decidualisation stimulus.[8,9]

The cellular interactions and progesterone target genes involved in decidualisation are complex. Multiple growth factors, cytokines and hormones have been recognised as important signals for initiation and maintenance of decidualisation.[10,11] The use of methods for screening large numbers of activated genes in human tissues, by 'high-density oligonucleotide microarray technology',[12,13] may result in the identification of genes, gene families and signalling pathways that are essential for the molecular mechanisms underlying the process of embryo implantation.

In the absence of pregnancy, the withdrawal of progesterone that occurs with luteal regression is the initiating factor for breakdown of the endometrium at menstruation. The molecular mechanisms by which sex steroids induce these events within the endometrium involve complex interactions between the endocrine and immune system.[14]

The morphological and functional changes that take place within the endometrium across the cycle and during implantation are thus the consequence of steroid interaction with target cells via specific nuclear receptors. The expression of endometrial sex steroid receptors (progesterone receptor, PR; oestrogen receptor, ER; androgen receptor, AR) varies temporally and spatially across the cycle.[15–18] The expression of ER and PR are under dual control of oestradiol and progesterone. Both endometrial ER and PR are upregulated during the follicular phase by ovarian oestradiol and subsequently downregulated in the luteal phase by progesterone acting at both the transcriptional and post-transcriptional level.[19] The presence of PR is considered evidence of a functional ER-mediated pathway. There are two distinct subtypes of the human PR, PR-A ($M_r = 81\,000$) and PR-B ($M_r = 116\,000$), that arise from a single gene and function as transcriptional regulators of progestin-responsive genes.[20] PR-A is the shorter subtype, missing 164 amino acids present at the N-terminus of the B subtype. It is otherwise identical.[21] There is a significant decline in PR expression in the glands of the functional layer of the endometrium (that region which is shed at menstruation) with the transition from the proliferative to the secretory phase of the cycle. In contrast, PR expression persists in the stroma in the functional layer, being particularly highly expressed in stromal cells in close proximity to the uterine vasculature. The basal layer is differentially regulated as the glands and stroma of the deeper zones express PR throughout the cycle. These differences between the superficial and basal layers of the endometrium are likely to be functionally important. Localisation studies utilising antibodies that recognise both PR subtypes have described differential regulation of PR in the endometrial epithelium and stromal cells. For example, during the luteal phase the PR-B subtype appears to decline in the stroma and PR-A becomes the predominant form at this time in the cycle.[22,23]

There are two forms of ER, alpha (ERα) and beta (ERβ).[24,25] ERβ, like ERα, is encoded by eight exons, with the highest levels of homology between ERα and ERβ present in the DNA and ligand binding domains.[26] The function of ERβ in the uterus remains unknown. In the functional layer, ERα expression increases in both glandular and stromal cells in the proliferative phase and declines in the secretory phase owing to suppression by progesterone. In the basal layer, ERα is present in glandular and stromal cells throughout the cycle.[16] In both the human and non-human primate endometrium, ERβ, like ERα, is expressed in the nuclei of glandular epithelial and stromal cells and has been observed to decline in the late secretory phase in the functional layer.[15] However, unlike ERα, ERβ is detected in the nuclei of vascular endothelial cells. The presence of ERβ in endometrial endothelial cells indicates for the first time that oestrogen may act directly on endometrial blood vessels. Such direct effects of oestrogen may be involved in endometrial angiogenesis and vascular permeability changes during the cycle. PR is absent from the vascular endothelium of the spiral arteries, which suggests that the effects of progesterone withdrawal on these vessels, which play such a key role in menstrual induction, are indirectly mediated by the PR-positive perivascular stromal cells.[15,27]

The endometrium is also a target for androgen action. During all stages of the menstrual cycle, AR is expressed in the endometrial stroma, and there is considerably higher intensity of AR immunostaining during the follicular as compared with the luteal phase.[18] Although the physiological role of endometrial AR is not known, androgen treatments can suppress oestrogen action in the endometrium, and this effect is presumed to be mediated by endometrial AR. Any role for AR in implantation or menstruation remains to be ascertained.

Genes involved in implantation

Gene-targeting experiments in mice have identified a host of genes whose deletion results in a phenotype of implantation or placentation defect. These genes are diverse in their known functions and include steroid receptors such as the ER[28] and PR,[29] cell surface and cell adhesion molecules such as basigin[30] and integrin $\beta1$,[31] homeobox genes such as *HoxA10*[32] and *HoxA11*,[33] inflammatory genes such as cytosolic phospholipase $A_{2\alpha}$[34] and cyclooxygenase 2 (COX2),[35] cytokines such as leukaemia inhibitory factor (LIF)[36] and cell surface receptors such as the epidermal growth factor receptor (EGFR),[37] interleukin 11 receptor[38] and gp130[STAT].[39]

With the advent of cDNA array technology, several researchers have applied this methodology to identify the various classes of genes that are upregulated during the window of implantation, both in animal models and human endometrium. These studies have recently been reviewed and a degree of overlap in the identity of implantation-regulated genes exists between species.[40] In this review, Dey *et al.*[40] emphasise that, despite the wealth of knowledge that has been accumulated on the role of various steroid hormones, growth factors, cytokines, transcription factors, inflammatory and homopoietic genes in implantation, their hierarchical blueprint in directing uterine and embryonic function during the implantation process remains to be fully elucidated. Here we address some of the aspects of the cyclooxygenase (COX)/prostaglandin (PG) biosynthetic pathway as potential regulators of implantation.

Prostaglandins as potential regulators of the implantation process

Prostaglandins are COX metabolites of arachidonic acid (AA). Following activation of phospholipase A_2 (PLA$_2$), AA is released from plasma membrane phospholipids or dietary fats and is cyclised, oxygenated and reduced to the intermediary prostaglandin H_2 (PGH$_2$) by COX enzymes. This intermediate serves as the substrate for terminal prostanoid synthase enzymes. These are named according to the prostaglandin they produce such that prostaglandin D_2 (PGD$_2$) is synthesised by prostaglandin D synthase (PGDS), prostaglandin E_2 (PGE$_2$) by prostaglandin E synthase (PGES), prostaglandin $F_{2\alpha}$ (PGF$_{2\alpha}$) by prostaglandin F synthase (PGFS), prostacyclin (PGI$_2$) by prostaglandin I synthase (PGIS) and thromboxane (TXA$_2$) by thromboxane synthase (TXS)[41] (Figure 1.1). Two isoforms of COX enzyme (COX1 and COX2) have been reported to catalyse the committed step in prostanoid biosynthesis.[42,43] COX1 has long been considered a constitutive enzyme involved in performing normal physiological functions, whereas COX2 is an immediate early gene that is rapidly induced by growth factors, oncogenes, carcinogens and tumour-promoting phorbol esters, and a role has been ascertained for COX2 in rheumatic disease, inflammation and tumorigenesis.[44–46]

Following biosynthesis, prostanoids are rapidly transported out of the cell by means of a prostaglandin transporter (PGT) and act in an autocrine/paracrine manner on their cognate heptahelical transmembrane G-protein-coupled receptors (GPCRs) in the vicinity of their sites of production. PGD$_2$, PGE$_2$, PGF$_{2\alpha}$, PGI$_2$ and TXA$_2$ exert their biological function through interactions with DP, EP, FP, IP and TP GPCRs, respectively.[41] Ligand–receptor coupling dissociates the heterotrimeric G-protein complex from the GPCR and activates second messenger systems such as the cAMP and inositol 1,4,5-trisphosphate (IP$_3$). In turn, these second messenger systems initiate a cascade of intracellular signal transduction, such as activation of the mitogen-activated protein kinase (MAPK) pathway. In addition, prostaglandins can interact with nuclear prostanoid receptors located within the nuclear envelope as well as with peroxisome proliferator-activated receptors (PPARs), which belong to the nuclear

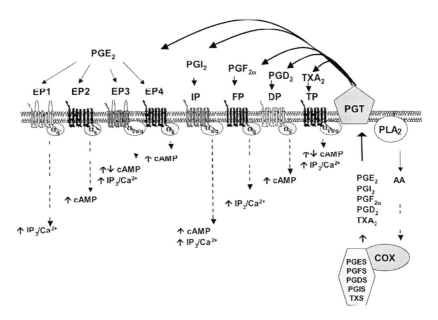

Figure 1.1. A schematic representation of the cyclooxygenase (COX)/prostanoid biosynthetic and signalling pathways; in this cartoon, arachidonic acid (AA) is released from plasma membrane phospholipids by phospholipase A_2 (PLA$_2$) and utilised by cyclooxygenases and specific synthase enzymes, such as prostaglandin (PG) D synthase (PGDS), PGES, PGFS, PGIS and thromboxane synthase (TXS), to form PGD$_2$, PGE$_2$, PGF$_{2\alpha}$, PGI$_2$ and TXA$_2$; these are actively transported out of the cell by means of a prostaglandin transporter (PGT), where they exert an autocrine/paracrine effect by coupling to heptahelical transmembrane receptors to activate second messenger systems, such as cyclic adenosine 3′,5′-monophosphate (cAMP) and inositol 1,4,5-trisphosphate (IP$_3$), and intracellular signalling cascades; in addition, prostanoids such as PGI$_2$ can also act as ligands for peroxisome proliferator-activated receptor delta (PPARδ) or nuclear EP receptors to directly promote target gene transcription

hormone receptor superfamily.[47] In the mouse, three PPARs have been cloned, PPARα, PPARβ and PPARδ. PGI$_2$ has been identified as a ligand for PPARδ and has been shown to play a crucial role in the decidualisation and implantation processes in the mouse.[48] The cellular effects of PGI$_2$–PPARδ interaction remain to be unravelled although a potential role in cell proliferation and angiogenesis at the implantation site has been suggested.[47]

Role for paracrine regulation of implantation by COX2 and prostanoids

Recent advances using transgenic animals have boosted our understanding of the roles of the COX enzymes, prostanoids and prostanoid receptors in the reproductive tract.[49,50] Gene ablation studies in rodents have demonstrated that COX1 is dispensable for most reproductive functions, including ovulation, implantation and decidualisation, however, in certain genetic strains of mice, a compensatory mechanism by COX2 has been reported to occur during the pre-implantation period.[51] Inactivation of COX1, however, causes parturition failure and closer examination of the COX1 knockout phenotype has shown the lack of production of $PGF_{2\alpha}$ to be the main cause of the parturition failure, and normal labour can be initiated in COX1-deficient animals by administration of exogenous $PGF_{2\alpha}$.[52,53] These findings have implicated $PGF_{2\alpha}$ as a major product of COX1 for the initiation of labour; an observation confirmed by ablation of the FP receptor gene in mice, which also manifest loss of parturition but display normal ovulation and implantation.[54]

In contrast to the findings of the COX1 knockout, disruption of COX2 either by gene ablation or chemical inhibition results in several reproductive failures, including impaired ovulation, implantation and decidualisation.[35] In certain genetic strains of mice, ablation of COX2 causes a compensatory upregulation of COX1 to rescue this phenotype, giving rise to live young, although the litter size is reduced[55] because decidual growth is restricted.[56]

Until recently, the relative paracrine signalling of the individual prostanoids acting via their receptors to facilitate reproductive processes, such as implantation, has been largely unexplored. Mice lacking each respective prostanoid receptor subtype have now been produced.[49] Interestingly, of all the prostanoid receptor ablations performed, only the EP2 and FP receptor-deficient mice are known to manifest a reproductive phenotype. Ablation of the EP2 receptor in mice manifests similar reproductive pathologies associated with COX2-null mice, namely impaired ovulation and fertilisation, whereas deletion of the FP receptor, as mentioned earlier, manifests failed parturition.[57,58] However, since more than 95% of the EP4 receptor knockout mice die within the first 24 hours after birth, it is not known whether ablation of EP4 receptor in these animals promotes a reproductive pathology. Similarly, it is not reported whether there is any aberrant reproductive function in IP receptor or DP receptor knockout mice.

Paracrine signalling of COX2 in implantation

Several studies have now been carried out to ascertain the cause of the implantation defect in COX2 knockout mice (whether it is due to the disruption of paracrine signalling at the level of the blastocyst or the endometrium). One such study involved blastocyst transfer from wild-type mice into COX2-deficient mice.[35] The data from this study showed complete implantation failure in the COX2-null mice receiving the wild-type blastocysts, indicating a defect in local uterine environment of COX2-null mice for the failed implantation. Since the EP2 receptor-null animals manifest similar reproductive phenotype to that observed with the COX2-deficient animals, a similar blastocyst transfer was conducted on the EP2 receptor-null mouse to determine the role of the EP2 receptor during implantation. These studies showed no difference between the ability of the EP2 receptor knockout mice and that of the wild-type mice to support implantation and raised a few interesting issues.[57] Since there was no difference between the EP2 knockout and wild-type animals to support an implanting embryo, it appeared that either the EP2 receptor did not play a critical role in implantation, or EP4 receptor could fulfil the role of the EP2 receptor following ligand–receptor activation. Another possible explanation for these differences arose from the redundancy of the prostanoid biosynthetic pathway brought about by the fact that many members of the prostanoid receptor superfamily activate convergent intracellular signalling pathways, such as the MAPK pathway, suggesting that a compensatory mechanism brought about by another prostanoid receptor may be at play to counteract effects due to ablation of EP2 receptor.[59,60] Furthermore it is also possible that PGE_2 plays a minor role in implantation compared with other prostanoids produced by COX2. Recent data have shown that PGI_2, followed by PGE_2, is the most abundant prostanoid produced at the site of implantation in mice.[48] Moreover, administration of a PGI_2 analogue to COX2-null mice can rescue blastocyst implantation via activation of PPARδ.[61]

The role of COX2 and prostanoids in blastocyst adhesion and invasion

Implantation begins with apposition, where the trophectoderm of the free-floating blastocyst lies adjacent to the uterine epithelium. Soon thereafter, direct contact between the plasma membrane of the endometrial epithelial cells and trophectoderm occurs and blastocyst adhesion to the uterine wall is stabilised. The dynamics of this process rely on the endocrine and paracrine ligand–receptor interaction by effector molecules such as prostaglandins, integrins, mucins and pro-angiogenic/vascular permeability factors, etc., which may be hormonally regulated.[62] Following adhesion of the blastocyst to the endometrium, the embryonic trophoblast penetrates the basal membrane and invades the stroma up to the uterine blood vessels (Figure 1.2). This environment creates a dialogue between the different trophoblast lineages and the various endometrial cell types, such as the stromal cells, endothelial cells and immune cells. The exact endocrine and local factors involved in implantation at the site of blastocyst attachment are still unclear but may involve the downregulation of anti-adhesion molecules, such as MUC1,[62] and the upregulation of adhesion molecules, such as integrins.[31,40]

In an *in vitro* model system, elevated COX2 expression in epithelial cells promotes cell adhesion to extracellular matrix.[63] Since COX2 levels are elevated in the surface epithelial cells of the blastocyst at the time of implantation, the paracrine sequelae brought about by elevated prostanoid biosynthesis may facilitate adhesion of the blastocyst to the uterine epithelium during the attachment period.[40] Although many of the observations elucidating the role of COX2 in promoting an alteration in cell behaviour are derived from cancer model systems, tumour invasion and trophoblast invasion share many of the same biochemical mediators. Following initial attachment of the blastocyst to the endometrial epithelium, matrix metalloproteinases (MMPs) are released to digest the host tissues. Human cytotrophoblast cells produce MMPs and are known to be constitutively invasive.[64,65] Although the regulatory processes governing their invasion during implantation remain to be fully elucidated, the paracrine signals mediating these effects may be brought about by cytokines and growth factors either from the invading trophectoderm or by the endometrial epithelial cells or stroma and these may be in turn regulated by the COX2/prostanoid biosynthetic pathway. These factors may also modulate the expression of proteins involved in cell–cell adhesion, such as E-cadherin. COX2 has been shown to increase the expression of MMPs, especially MMP2, in epithelial cells, and downregulate E-cadherin,[63] to promote a wave of invasion through extracellular matrix. COX2 may act similarly in the endometrium to upregulate MMPs and downregulate cell adhesion molecules, such as E-cadherin, to facilitate invasion of the trophoblast (Figure 1.2).[66]

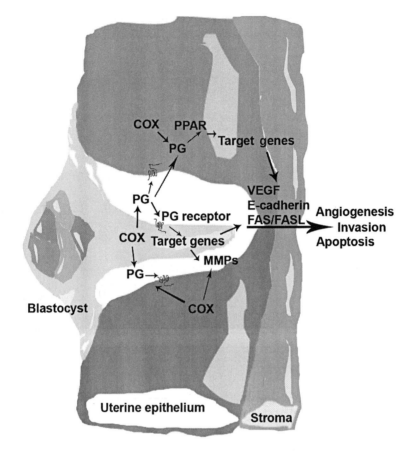

Figure 1.2. Endocrine/paracrine regulation of implantation by the cyclooxygenase (COX)/prostaglandin (PG) biosynthetic pathway; this cartoon shows a schematic representation of the paracrine sequelae between the invading trophectoderm (blastocyst) and the endometrial epithelium; prostaglandins produced by the trophectoderm and endometrial epithelia can act on prostanoid G-protein-coupled-receptors or peroxisome proliferator-activated receptors (PPARs) in the vicinity of their sites of production to promote the release of matrix metalloproteinases (MMPs) to facilitate degradation of the extracellular matrix and transcription of target genes, such as vascular endothelial growth factor (VEGF), E-cadherin and FAS/FASL to promote angiogenesis, invasion and apoptosis

Angiogenesis is regulated by the COX/PG biosynthetic pathway during implantation

One of the prerequisites for implantation is increased vascular permeability and angiogenesis at the site of blastocyst apposition.[67] In the absence of COX2, the local factors required for neovascularisation and vascular permeability are dysregulated, giving rise to defects in implantation.[61] Vascular permeability and angiogenesis are profoundly influenced by the paracrine actions of vascular endothelial growth factor

(VEGF) (Figure 1.2).[68] VEGF exerts its angiogenic function by coupling to two transmembrane tyrosine kinase receptors VEGFR1 (FLT1) and VEGFR2 (KDR).[68,69] There is now mounting evidence for a role for COX2, prostaglandins and prostanoid receptors in the regulation of VEGF expression. In *in vitro* model systems, upregulation of COX2 and consequent elevation in prostanoid biosynthesis promotes the upregulation of pro-angiogenic factors such as VEGF, which in turn can act on endothelial cells to promote endothelial cell branching and sprouting for neovascularisation.[70] In addition to the upregulation of pro-angiogenic factors, COX2 can also mediate the downregulation of anti-angiogenic factors to promote vascularisation.[71] Moreover, recent studies have shown that prostanoids can mediate their angiogenic function by coupling with specific target receptors. In endometrial epithelial cells, PGE_2 promotes the expression and secretion of VEGF following coupling to and activation of the EP2 receptor.[56] Several model systems have now demonstrated a role for EP2 receptor in the regulation of VEGF expression and secretion.[59,72,73] Thus, even though the EP2 receptor knockout mouse model shows that EP2 receptor is not critical for blastocyst implantation,[57] it may play a role in preparing the uterus to receive the conceptus by regulating the expression of pro-angiogenic genes. Alternatively, other prostanoid receptors acting via the same signalling pathways may similarly promote the transcription of target angiogenic genes. As outlined above, PGI_2 is the most abundant prostanoid at the site of implantation in the mouse.[48,62] Remodelling of blood vessels during blastocyst implantation may thus be regulated by the paracrine signals directed by the actions of COX2-derived prostaglandins, such as PGI_2. Whether PGI_2 exerts a synergistic action with PGE_2 or other prostanoids in the local environment to facilitate implantation remains to be elucidated (Figure 1.2).

Programmed cell death is necessary for blastocyst implantation

During adhesion of the implanting blastocyst to the endometrium, locally regulated uterine apoptosis is necessary to promote tissue remodelling and invasion of the epithelium. This process of programmed cell death is seen in rodents, where a progressive, continuous wave of induction of apoptosis is observed in the maternal tissues surrounding the conceptus in the rat.[74] Similar evidence of controlled apoptosis in the uterine epithelium during implantation is seen in the mouse.[75] In the human, the blastocyst is observed to rescue the endometrial epithelial layer from apoptosis during the apposition phase.[75,76] Since the expression of COX2 is high in the epithelial cells surrounding the blastocyst, the rescue of the endometrial epithelial cells from apoptosis may be brought about by the paracrine actions of COX2-derived prostaglandins on target prostanoid receptors present in the endometrium. COX2 has been known to promote the inhibition of apoptosis in epithelial cells by promoting the synthesis and release of PGE_2.[70] Upon adhesion of the blastocyst to the endometrial epithelium, however, a wave of apoptosis is triggered in a paracrine fashion specifically at the site of attachment.[76] Although, the biochemical effector molecules mediating this wave of apoptosis during blastocyst implantation remain to be fully elucidated, neutralising adhesion assays have revealed that the FAS/FAS ligand (FASL) death system is involved and may be activated by direct contact of the blastocyst with the endometrial epithelium (Figure 1.2).[76] The breach of the endometrial epithelial barrier only at the site of blastocyst adhesion is thus a well-coordinated series of events, which may be orchestrated to prevent invasion of the epithelial layer by pathogen.

Conclusion

Over the past few years a great deal of progress has been made towards identifying the endocrine and local factors involved in implantation. Much of this knowledge is derived from studies of transgenic mouse models, embryo transfer and *in vitro* culture. The challenge for the future is to unravel the exact nature of the molecules, the cross-talk that may exist between them and the signalling pathways they activate in order to culminate in successful implantation. Only with this knowledge will we be able to apply novel therapeutic intervention strategies in pathologies that are associated with implantation defects such as recurrent miscarriage, pre-eclampsia and intrauterine growth restriction.

References

1. Noyes RW, Hertig AT, Rock J. Dating the endometrial biopsy. *Fertil Steril* 1950;1:3–25.
2. Kumar S, Zhu LJ, Polihronis M, Cameron ST, Baird DT, Schatz FDA, *et al*. Progesterone induces calcitonin gene expression in human endometrium within the putative window of implantation. *J Clin Endocrinol Metab* 1998;83:4443–50.
3. Chard T, Olajide F. Endometrial protein PP14: a new test of endometrial function. *Reprod Med Rev* 1994;3:43–52.
4. Casey ML, Hemsell DL, MacDonald PC, Johnston JM. NAD+- dependent 15-hydroxyprostaglandin dehydrogenase activity in human endometrium. *Prostaglandins* 1980;19:115–22.
5. Cameron ST, Critchley HOD, Buckley CH, Chard T, Kelly RW, Baird DT. The effects of post-ovulatory administration of onapristone on the development of a secretory endometrium. *Hum Reprod* 1996;11:40–9.
6. Greenland KJ, Jantke I, Jennatschke S, Bracken KE, Vinson C, Gellerson B. The human NAD+ dependent 15-hydroxyprostaglandin dehydrogenase gene promoter is controlled by Ets and activating protein-1 transcription factors and progesterone. *Endocrinology* 2000;141:581–97.
7. Maentausta O, Svalander P, Gemzell-Danielsson K, Bygdeman M, Vihko R. The effects of an antiprogestin, mifepristone, and an anti-estrogen, tamoxifen, on endometrial 17beta hydroxysteroid dehydrogenase and progestin and estrogen receptors during the luteal phase of the menstrual cycle: an immunohistochemical study. *J Clin Endocrinol Metab* 1993;77:913–18.
8. Tang B, Guller S, Gurpide E. Mechanism of human endometrial stromal cell decidualization. *Ann N Y Acad Sci* 1994;734:19–25.
9. Brosens JJ, Takeda S, Acevedo CH, Lewis MP, Kirby PL, Symes EK, *et al*. Human endometrial fibroblasts immortalized by simian virus 40 large T antigen differentiate in response to a decidualization stimulus. *Endocrinology* 1996;137:2225–31.
10. Osteen KG. The endocrinology of uterine decidualisation. In: *Endocrinology of Pregnancy*. Bazer FW, editor. New Jersey: Human Press Inc; 1999. p. 541–53.
11. Jabbour HN, Critchley HOD. Potential roles of decidual prolactin in early pregnancy. *Reproduction* 2001;121:197–205.
12. Kao LC, Tulac S, Lobo S, Imani B, Yang JP, Germeyer A, *et al*. Global gene profiling in human implantation during the window of implantation. *Endocrinology* 2002;143:2119–38.
13. Riesewijk A, Martin J, van Os R, Horcajadas JA, Polman J, Pellicer A, *et al*. Gene expression profiling of human endometrial receptivity on days LH+2 versus LH+7 by microarray technology. *Mol Hum Reprod* 2003;9:253–64.
14. Critchley HOD, Kelly RW, Brenner RM, Baird DT. The endocrinology of menstruation – a role for the immune system. *Clin Endocrinol* 2001;55:701–10.
15. Critchley HOD, Brenner RM, Drudy TA, Williams K, Nayak NR, Slayden OD, *et al*. Estrogen receptor beta, but not estrogen receptor alpha, is present in vascular endothelium of the human and nonhuman primate endometrium. *J Clin Endocrinol Metab* 2001;86:1370–8.
16. Garcia E, Bouchard P, DeBrux J, Berdah J, Frydman R, Schaison G, *et al*. Use of immunocytochemistry of progesterone and estrogen receptors for endometrial dating. *J Clin Endocrinol Metab* 1988;67:80–7.
17. Lessey BA, Killam AP, Metzger DA, Haney AF, Greene GL, McCarty KS. Immunohistochemical analysis of human uterine estrogen and progesterone receptors throughout the menstrual cycle. *J Clin Endocrinol Metab* 1988;67:334–40.

18. Slayden OD, Nayak NR, Burton KA, Chwalisz K, Cameron ST, Critchley HOD, *et al.* Progesterone antagonists increase androgen receptor expression in the rhesus macaque and human endometrium. *J Clin Endocrinol Metab* 2001;86:2668–79.
19. Chauchereau A, Savouret JF, Milgrom E. Control of biosynthesis and post-transcriptional modification of progesterone receptor. *Biol Reprod* 1992;46:174–7.
20. Conneely OM, Lydon JP. Progesterone receptors in reproduction: functional impact of the A and B isoforms. *Steroids* 2000;65:571–7.
21. Tung L, Mohamed MK, Hoeffler JP, Takimoto GS, Horwitz KB. Antagonist occupied human progesterone B receptors activate transcription without binding to progesterone response elements and are dominantly inhibited by A-receptors. *Mol Endocrinol* 1993;7:1256–65.
22. Wang H, Critchley HOD, Kelly RW, Shen D, Baird DT. Progesterone receptor subtype B is differentially regulated in human endometrial stroma. *Mol Hum Reprod* 1998;4:407–12.
23. Brosens JJ, Hayashi N, White JO. Progesterone receptor regulates decidual prolactin expression in differentiating human endometrial stromal cells. *Endocrinology* 1999;140:4809–20.
24. Green S, Walter P, Kumar V, Krust A, Bornert JM, Argos P, *et al.* Human oestrogen receptor cDNA: sequence, expression and homology to v-erb-A. *Nature* 1986;320:134–9.
25. Kuiper GGJM, Enmark E, Pelto-Hukko M, Nilsson S, Gustafsson JA. Cloning of a novel estrogen receptor expressed in rat prostate and ovary. *Proc Natl Acad Sci U S A* 1996;93:5925–30.
26. Enmark E, Pelto-Huikko M, Grandien K, Lagercrantz S, Lagercrantz J, Fried G, *et al.* Human estrogen receptor beta gene structure, chromosomal localization, and expression pattern. *J Clin Endocrinol Metab* 1997;82:4258–65.
27. Perrot-Applanat M, Deng M, Fernandez H, Lelaidier C, Meduri G, Bouchard P. Immunohistochemical localisation of estradiol and progesterone receptors in human uterus throughout pregnancy: expression in endometrial blood vessels. *J Clin Endocrinol Metab* 1994;78:216–24.
28. Lubahn DB, Moyer JS, Golding TS, Couse JF, Korach KS, Smithies O. Alteration of reproductive function but not prenatal sexual development after insertional disruption of the mouse estrogen receptor gene. *Proc Natl Acad Sci U S A* 1993;90:11162–6.
29. Lydon JP, DeMayo FJ, Funk CR, Mani SK, Hughes AR, Montgomery CA, *et al.* Mice lacking progesterone receptor exhibit pleiotropic reproductive abnormalities. *Genes Dev* 1995;9:2266–78.
30. Igakura T, Kadomatsu K, Kaname T, Muramatsu H, Fan QW, Miyauchi T, *et al.* A null mutation in basigin, an immunoglobulin superfamily member, indicates its important roles in peri-implantation development and spermatogenesis. *Dev Biol* 1998;194:152–65.
31. Stephens LE, Sutherland AE, Klimanskaya IV, Andrieux A, Meneses J, Pedersen RA, *et al.* Deletion of beta 1 integrins in mice results in inner cell mass failure and peri-implantation lethality. *Genes Dev* 1995;9:1883–95.
32. Satokata I, Benson G, Maas R. Sexually dimorphic sterility phenotypes in Hoxa10-deficient mice. *Nature* 1995;374:460–3.
33. Hsieh-Li HM, Witte DP, Weinstein M, Branford W, Li H, Small, K, *et al.* Hoxa 11 structure, extensive antisense transcription, and function in male and female fertility. *Development* 1995;121:1373–85.
34. Song H, Lim H, Paria BC, Matsumoto H, Swift LL, Morrow J, *et al.* Cytosolic phospholipase A2alpha is crucial [correction of A2alpha deficiency is crucial] for 'on-time' embryo implantation that directs subsequent development. *Development* 2002;129:2879–89. Erratum in: *Development* 2002;129:3761.
35. Lim H, Paria BC, Das SK, Dinchuk JE, Langenbach R, Trzaskos JM, *et al.* Multiple female reproductive failures in cyclooxygenase 2-deficient mice. *Cell* 1997;91:197–208.
36. Stewart CL, Kaspar P, Brunet LJ, Bhatt H, Gadi I, Kontgen F, *et al.* Blastocyst implantation depends on maternal expression of leukaemia inhibitory factor. *Nature* 1992;359:76–9.
37. Threadgill DW, Dlugosz AA, Hansen LA, Tennenbaum T, Lichti U, Yee D, *et al.* Targeted disruption of mouse EGF receptor: effect of genetic background on mutant phenotype. *Science* 1995;269:230–4.
38. Robb L, Li R, Hartley L, Nandurkar HH, Koentgen F, Begley CG. Infertility in female mice lacking the receptor for interleukin 11 is due to a defective uterine response to implantation. *Nat Med* 1998;4:303–8.
39. Ernst M, Inglese M, Waring P, Campbell IK, Bao S, Clay FJ, *et al.* Defective gp130-mediated signal transducer and activator of transcription (STAT) signaling results in degenerative joint disease, gastrointestinal ulceration, and failure of uterine implantation. *J Exp Med* 2001;194:189–203.
40. Dey SK, Lim H, Das SK, Reese J, Paria BC, Daikoku T, *et al.* Molecular cues to implantation. *Endocr Rev* 2004;25:341–73.

41. Narumiya S, Sugimoto Y, Ushikubi F. Prostanoid receptors: structures, properties, and functions. *Physiol Rev* 1999;79:1193–226.

42. Morita I. Distinct functions of COX-1 and COX-2. *Prostaglandins Other Lipid Mediat* 2002;68–69:165–75.

43. Chandrasekharan NV, Dai H, Roos KL, Evanson NK, Tomsik J, Elton TS, *et al*. COX-3, a cyclooxygenase-1 variant inhibited by acetaminophen and other analgesic/antipyretic drugs: Cloning, structure, and expression. *Proc Natl Acad Sci U S A* 2002;99:13926–31.

44. Narko K, Ristimaki A, MacPhee M, Smith E, Haudenschild CC, Hla T. Tumorigenic transformation of immortalized ECV endothelial cells by cyclooxygenase-1 overexpression. *J Biol Chem* 1997;272:21455–60.

45. Chulada PC, Thompson MB, Mahler JF, Doyle CM, Gaul BW, Lee C, *et al*. Genetic disruption of Ptgs-1, as well as Ptgs-2, reduces intestinal tumorigenesis in Min mice. *Cancer Res* 2000;60:4705–8.

46. Kitamura T, Kawamori T, Uchiya N, Itoh M, Noda T, Matsuura M, *et al*. Inhibitory effects of mofezolac, a cyclooxygenase-1 selective inhibitor, on intestinal carcinogenesis. *Carcinogenesis* 2002;23:1463–6.

47. Lim H, Dey SK. PPAR delta functions as a prostacyclin receptor in blastocyst implantation. *Trends Endocrinol Metab* 2000;11:137–42.

48. Lim H, Gupta RA, Ma WG, Paria BC, Moller DE, Morrow JD, *et al*. Cyclo-oxygenase-2-derived prostacyclin mediates embryo implantation in the mouse via PPARdelta. *Genes Dev* 1999;13:1561–74.

49. Kobayashi T, Narumiya S. Function of prostanoid receptors: studies on knockout mice. *Prostaglandins Other Lipid Mediat* 2002;68–9:557-73.

50. Murakami M, Kudo I. Recent advances in molecular biology and physiology of the prostaglandin E2-biosynthetic pathway. *Prog Lipid Res* 2004;43:3–35.

51. Reese J, Brown N, Paria BC, Morrow J, Dey SK. COX-2 compensation in the uterus of COX-1 deficient mice during the pre-implantation period. *Mol Cell Endocrinol* 1999;150:23–31.

52. Langenbach R, Loftin C, Lee C, Tiano H. Cyclooxygenase knockout mice: models for elucidating isoform-specific functions. *Biochem Pharmacol* 1999;58:1237–46.

53. Langenbach R, Loftin CD, Lee C, Tiano H. Cyclooxygenase-deficient mice. A summary of their characteristics and susceptibilities to inflammation and carcinogenesis. *Ann N Y Acad Sci* 1999;889:52–61.

54. Sugimoto Y, Yamasaki A, Segi E, Tsuboi K, Aze Y, Nishimura T, *et al*. Failure of parturition in mice lacking the prostaglandin F receptor. *Science* 1997;277:681–4.

55. Wang H, Ma WG, Tejada L, Zhang H, Morrow J, Das SK, *et al*. Rescue of female infertility from the loss of cyclooxygenase-2 by compensatory up-regulation of cyclooxygenase-1 is a function of genetic makeup. *J Biol Chem* 2004;279:10649–58.

56. Cheng JG, Stewart CL. Loss of cyclooxygenase-2 retards decidual growth but does not inhibit embryo implantation or development to term. *Biol Reprod* 2003;68:401–4.

57. Hizaki H, Segi E, Sugimoto Y, Hirose M, Saji T, Ushikubi F, *et al*. Abortive expansion of the cumulus and impaired fertility in mice lacking the prostaglandin E receptor subtype EP2. *Proc Natl Acad Sci U S A* 1999;96:10501–6.

58. Kennedy CR, Zhang Y, Brandon S, Guan Y, Coffee K, Funk CD, *et al*. Salt-sensitive hypertension and reduced fertility in mice lacking the prostaglandin EP2 receptor. *Nat Med* 1999;5:217–20.

59. Sales KJ, Maudsley S, Jabbour HN. Elevated prostaglandin EP2 receptor in endometrial adenocarcinoma cells promotes vascular endothelial growth factor expression via cyclic 3',5'-adenosine monophosphate-mediated transactivation of the epidermal growth factor receptor and extracellular signal-regulated kinase 1/2 signaling pathways. *Mol Endocrinol* 2004;18:1533–45.

60. Sales KJ, Milne SA, Williams AR, Anderson RA, Jabbour HN. Expression, localization, and signaling of prostaglandin F2 alpha receptor in human endometrial adenocarcinoma: regulation of proliferation by activation of the epidermal growth factor receptor and mitogen-activated protein kinase signaling pathways. *J Clin Endocrinol Metab* 2004;89:986–93.

61. Matsumoto H, Ma WG, Daikoku, T, Zhao X, Paria BC, Das SK, *et al*. Cyclooxygenase-2 differentially directs uterine angiogenesis during implantation in mice. *J Biol Chem* 2002;277:29260–7.

62. Dominguez F, Remohi J, Pellicer A, Simon C. Paracrine interactions during human implantation. *Rev Endocr Metab Disord* 2002;3:97–105.

63. Tsujii M, DuBois RN. Alterations in cellular adhesion and apoptosis in epithelial cells overexpressing prostaglandin endoperoxide synthase 2. *Cell* 1995;83:493–501.

64. Bischof P, Campana A. Molecular mediators of implantation. *Baillieres Best Pract Res Clin Obstet Gynaecol* 2000;14:801–14.

65. Bischof P and Campana A. A putative role for oncogenes in trophoblast invasion? *Hum Reprod* 2000;15 Suppl 6:51–8.
66. Tsujii M, Kawano S, DuBois RN. Cyclooxygenase-2 expression in human colon cancer cells increases metastatic potential. *Proc Natl Acad Sci U S A* 1997;94:3336–40.
67. Psychoyos A. Hormonal control of ovoimplantation. *Vitam Horm* 1973;31:201–56.
68. Ferrara N, Davis-Smyth T. The biology of vascular endothelial growth factor. *Endocr Rev* 1997;18:4–25.
69. Peters KG, De Vries C, Williams LT. Vascular endothelial growth factor receptor expression during embryogenesis and tissue repair suggests a role in endothelial differentiation and blood vessel growth. *Proc Natl Acad Sci U S A* 1993;90:8915–19.
70. Tsujii M, Kawano S, Tsuji S, Sawaoka H, Hori M, DuBois RN. Cyclooxygenase regulates angiogenesis induced by colon cancer cells. *Cell* 1998;93:705–16.
71. Perchick GB, Jabbour HN. COX-2 overexpression inhibits cathepsin D mediated cleavage of plasminogen to the potent anti-angiogenic factor angiostatin. *Endocrinology* 2003;144:5322–8.
72. Sonoshita M, Takaku K, Sasaki N, Sugimoto Y, Ushikubi F, Narumiya S, *et al.* Acceleration of intestinal polyposis through prostaglandin receptor EP2 in Apc(Delta 716) knockout mice. *Nat Med* 2001;7:1048–51.
73. Eibl G, Bruemmer D, Okada Y, Duffy JP, Law RE, Reber HA, *et al.* PGE(2) is generated by specific COX-2 activity and increases VEGF production in COX-2-expressing human pancreatic cancer cells. *Biochem Biophys Res Commun* 2003;306:887–97.
74. Piacentini M, Autuori F. Immunohistochemical localization of tissue transglutaminase and Bcl-2 in rat uterine tissues during embryo implantation and post-partum involution. *Differentiation* 1994;57:51–61.
75. Kamijo T, Rajabi MR, Mizunuma H, Ibuki Y. Biochemical evidence for autocrine/paracrine regulation of apoptosis in cultured uterine epithelial cells during mouse embryo implantation *in vitro*. *Mol Hum Reprod* 1998;4:990–8.
76. Galan A, O'Connor JE, Valbuena D, Herrer R, Remohi J, Pampfer S, *et al.* The human blastocyst regulates endometrial epithelial apoptosis in embryonic adhesion. *Biol Reprod* 2000;63:430–9.

Chapter 2
Immunology of implantation

Anita Trundley, Susan Hiby, Lucy Gardner, Andrew Sharkey, Charlie Loke and Ashley Moffett

Introduction

Implantation of the developing embryo into the wall of the maternal uterus with subsequent development of the placenta is a critical stage of human pregnancy. The close apposition of placental and uterine tissues creates an immunological dilemma. The placenta, being a hybrid between paternal and maternal genomes, has the potential to express paternal antigens and thus could potentially be recognised as nonself by the maternal immune system. In transplantation, such recognition of nonself results in rejection of the grafted tissue. If similar mechanisms operate in the uterus then reproductive success must rely on some form of immunological accommodation of the mother to placental tissue. The subject of this review is to consider the unique immunological environment of the human uterus, which permits this accommodation.

Immunological models

The classical self/nonself model formulated by Burnet and Medawar proposed that each lymphocyte expresses a single receptor for a foreign antigen and signalling through this triggers an immune response (Figure 2.1).[1] Lymphocytes with receptors for nonself in the form of pathogens and allogeneic cells will be present and, if these are encountered, elimination of the infectious agent or rejection of the allograft results.[2] The random generation of these clonally distributed receptors by gene rearrangement during fetal development means that the T and B lymphocytes, which acquire receptors reactive to antigens present in the fetal thymus, need to be deleted. In this way, tolerance to self and infectious or other stimuli encountered before birth is acquired.

The revelation that it is not only T and B cells that have receptors for nonself has now changed our views of self/nonself recognition. Medzhitov and Janeway[3,4] have shown that microbes can be detected by the conserved molecular patterns that are essential to their physiology but not a part of their vertebrate hosts. These are known as pathogen-associated molecular patterns (PAMPs). The receptors for PAMPs are mainly found on antigen-presenting cells (APCs) – dendritic cells and macrophages.

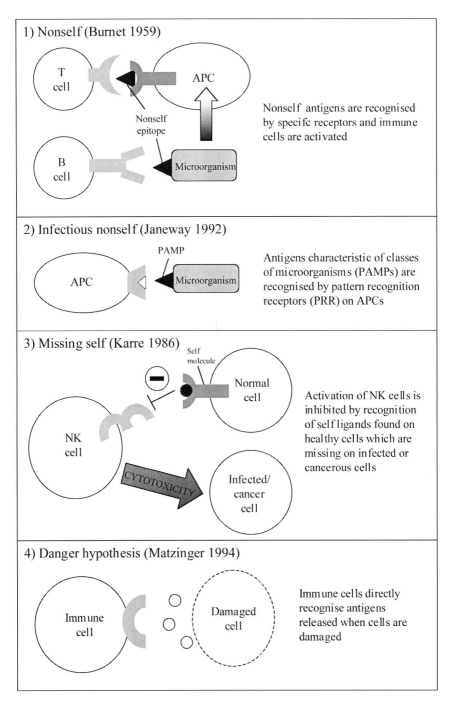

Figure 2.1. Simplified models of immunological recognition; APC = antigen-presenting cells; NK = natural killer

Upon recognition of PAMPs, the APC is induced to mature, process the microbial antigen and upregulate co-stimulatory ligands for presentation to T cells. It is, thus, the APC and not a lymphocyte that initially detects the microbial nonself. However, this model does not consider the nature of the immune response to allografts, auto-antigens or transformed cells.

Another way of detecting self depends on self-receptors, which on binding to normal host cells provide an inhibitory signal preventing leucocyte activation. If self-molecules are missing, the lack of inhibition allows dominance of activating receptors which can drive leucocytes to kill or phagocytose. This 'missing self' hypothesis was proposed by Kärre in relation to natural killer (NK) cells which are prevented from cytotoxicity by binding to self major histocompatibility complex (MHC) class I molecules on target cells.[5] NK cells survey the levels of class I molecules on a host's cell and downregulation of these class I molecules (for example by viral infection) will lead to killing. In this way the host can therefore perceive something as foreign by both the presence of difference (T cells) as well as the absence of similarity (NK cells).

Matzinger has introduced a broader model to understand how the immune system discerns any unhealthy cell and this has moved away from the concept of entities such as self/nonself, foreign or microbial. The danger model proposes that the host is alerted by the presence of alarm signals released by damaged cells and tissues.[6,7] The insult may be exogenous (e.g. microbial, poison) or endogenous (e.g. viral, necrosis) but will not emanate from healthy tissue. This proposal is attractive in its simplicity as it turns around the problem of defining all the agents and situations to which the immune system will react towards the concept that normal healthy cells and tissues will *not* stimulate leucocyte activation.

It is worth reflecting on the fact that the proponents of these models came from the field of classical immunology where response to pathogens and transplants is a dominant preoccupation. Reproductive immunologists have always followed main-stream immunology and tried to fit the immunology of the maternal–fetal relationship into the paradigms of the day. Can this be done with any of these models? Much is known about the immunology of the maternal–fetal interaction in human and this will form the basis of this chapter.

HLA class I genes expressed by normal somatic cells:

<u>A</u>   <u>B</u>   <u>C</u>   E   (F?)

HLA class I genes expressed by extravillous trophoblast:

      E

Figure 2.2.   HLA genes and trophoblast; classical, polymorphic class I genes are underlined

Anatomy of early placentation

In order to understand the immunological interactions at the implantation site it is necessary to understand its anatomy. Attachment of the blastocyst to the uterine lining is thought to trigger the differentiation of the trophectoderm into two layers: an inner cytotrophoblast layer and an outer syncytium of syncytiotrophoblast. It is initially the syncytiotrophoblast that invades into the decidua and the blastocyst quickly becomes submerged in the maternal tissue.

Erosion of maternal capillaries by the invading trophoblast causes spaces within the syncytium to fill with maternal blood. Eventually, fusion of these lacunae allows the formation of a sponge-like network through which maternal blood circulates, bathing the blastocyst in nutrients and allowing gaseous exchange. This primitive network eventually becomes the intervillous space.

Two weeks after attachment, the underlying cytotrophoblast proliferates into buds, which will protrude through the syncytium. Subsequently, the cytotrophoblast will have two cell fates, known as villous trophoblast and extravillous trophoblast. These two cell populations make different contributions in establishing efficient transport between the maternal and fetal circulations. Villous trophoblast covers the chorionic villi providing the barrier through which metabolic exchange between mother and fetus occurs and it interacts with maternal blood in the intervillous space.

The primary role of extravillous cytotrophoblast is thought to be to regulate maternal blood flow into the intervillous space by their invasion and transformation of decidual arteries. Initially, a population of extravillous trophoblast migrates into the decidua and comes to surround the maternal spiral arteries. Where this occurs the muscular walls of the arteries are destroyed and the endothelial cells swell. A second subtype of extravillous cytotrophoblast, known as endovascular trophoblast, invades into these altered arteries. Endovascular trophoblast cells migrate down the luminal walls of these arteries and eventually replace the maternal endothelial cells.[8] The consequence of these adaptations is to convert the arteries from muscular vessels to low-resistance channels that are incapable of responding to vasoactive stimuli.

In healthy pregnancies, extravillous trophoblast cells invade as far as the inner third of the myometrium. The health of both the fetus and mother are contingent upon regulating the extent of trophoblast invasion. Inadequate tapping of the maternal arteries has been associated with pre-eclampsia (PE) and intrauterine growth restriction (IUGR).[9] However, excessive invasion can also occur. In human pregnancy this aggressive invasion by trophoblast can be witnessed when the blastocyst implants either ectopically, for example in the fallopian tube, or in a site devoid of decidua, for example into scar tissue left by a previous caesarean section.

Immunology of trophoblast

Trophoblast is an unusual cell type. It is extra-embryonic and invasive and has several distinctive properties such as the expression of endogenous retrovirus products, oncofetal proteins and imprinted genes.[10] In addition, the DNA in trophoblast is relatively unmethylated. All these properties could have some relevance in interactions with the maternal immune system in terms of PAMP recognition.

However, the most obvious genes of interest are *MHC* and *MHC*-like genes as these are known to be important for self/nonself recognition. Although the fetus proper expresses the full array of its paternally inherited *MHC* genes, trophoblast cells only express a select few of the MHC antigens at their disposal (Figure 2.2).[10] Trophoblast does not express MHC class II molecules even after stimulation with interferon γ (IFN-γ). Nor does it express the two main classical MHC class I antigens, human leucocyte antigen A (HLA-A) and HLA-B, which are expressed by the majority of cells in the adult soma. Only three MHC class I subtypes have been detected on certain subsets of human trophoblast. They are HLA-C, HLA-G and HLA-E. A report in 2003 that HLA-F is present awaits confirmation.[11]

HLA-C is a classical MHC class I molecule and its expression is widespread in somatic cells but it is expressed at about 10% of the levels of HLA-A and HLA-B and is less polymorphic. Trophoblast has been shown to express mRNA from both the maternal and paternal alleles of HLA-C.[12]

The *HLA-G* locus is relatively nonpolymorphic but a number of potential isoforms, generated by alternative splicing, have been identified, including a putative soluble variant.[11,13] HLA-G also appears to be unusual in that high molecular weight forms can be detected at the cell surface.[14] Another novel feature among class I molecules is the nature of the carbohydrate structure. HLA-G carries *N*-acetyl galactosamine when expressed by trophoblast but this is not a feature of HLA-G transfectants.[15] Despite many studies, the function of HLA-G in pregnancy is not known. Adults homozygous for a highly truncated 'null' allele of *HLA-G* have been identified.[16] The birth of these individuals suggests that the expression of full-length, membrane-associated HLA-G in trophoblast is not an obligate requirement for pregnancy.

The third HLA antigen to be discovered on trophoblast was HLA-E, which, like HLA-G, is a nonclassical class I molecule with limited sequence polymorphism.[17] The cell surface expression of HLA-E is dependent on its binding of signal peptides cleaved from other class I molecules. Signal peptides from both HLA-G and HLA-C have been shown to bind to HLA-E. Even the null allele of *HLA-G* could potentially provide peptide and thus cause an upregulation of HLA-E expression.

Differential expression of MHC proteins on trophoblast subpopulations

The various trophoblast populations differ with respect to both their expression of MHC and which maternal immune cells they encounter. These subdivisions result in three different interfaces existing between mother and placenta. Villous syncytio-trophoblast lines the intervillous space and is thus in contact with immune cells in the maternal blood. This syncytium does not express any MHC class I antigens and thus is presumably immunologically inert to T cell-mediated responses. The absence of MHC class I does not cause cytolytic activation of blood NK cells, which are generally inhibited by MHC molecules expressed on a cell's surface. This could be because of both a lack of activating ligands and protection of the surface by high levels of glycosylation.

Endovascular trophoblast lines the maternal spiral arteries and so it is also in contact with maternal blood. This population expresses HLA-C, HLA-G and HLA-E.[10,18] The expression of HLA-G and HLA-E in this population may confer protection from blood NK cells. Interstitial trophoblast invades into the decidua and thus may interact with the mucosal immune cells that densely infiltrate the implantation site. Like the endovascular trophoblast, these cells express HLA-C, HLA-G and HLA-E.[10,18] Owing to the high number of uterine NK (uNK) cells at the implantation site, there has been a lot of interest in potential interactions between receptors on these NK cells and MHC ligands on the interstitial trophoblast.

Decidualisation

The human uterine mucosa (endometrium) is unlike other mucosal surfaces in that it undergoes cyclic rounds of breakdown and regeneration throughout reproductive life.[19] Post-ovulation, the oestrogen-primed endometrium is seen to undergo differentiation in the so-called secretory phase. It is during this phase that preparations for implantation can be seen, primarily in the glands and stroma of the functional layer: the glands begin their secretion into the uterine cavity and the stromal cells, especially around the spiral arteries, change from fibroblastic to epithelioid in appearance. This morphological change is known as pre-decidualisation and in humans it occurs even in the absence of fertilisation. The secretory phase is also characterised by the appearance in the endometrium of a large number of leucocytes.[10]

In the event of pregnancy, decidualisation of the stroma becomes more extensive. Leucocytic infiltration persists and is a particularly striking feature of the decidua basalis where the placenta is implanting. Therefore, the invading trophoblast will potentially interact not only with the glands and stroma but also with maternal immune cells. Leucocytes in the uterine mucosa make intimate contact with the semi-allogeneic placenta and potentially regulate the trophoblast invasion.

Uterine mucosal lymphocytes

Immunohistology using an antibody against CD45 (leucocyte common antigen) has shown that during the first trimester of pregnancy up to 40% of cells in the decidua are leucocytes. Detailed phenotyping of this population has revealed a unique composition of immune cells, which is unlike that seen in other tissues or mucosal surfaces.[10]

Only a few B cells can be detected in endometrium and decidua in small lymphoid aggregates found in the basal layer. Their number does not vary during the menstrual cycle or pregnancy. Uterine B cells can respond to antigenic challenge – in the event of intrauterine infection germinal centres form and plasma cells can be found, but these are not features of normal pregnancy.[20]

NKT cells are a subset of T cells that also express NK cell markers. They have been found to have an immunomodulatory role in infection, cancer and transplantation through the production of cytokines.[21] Boyson *et al.*[22] and Tsuda *et al.*[23] reported that the percentages of NKT cells were increased in decidua compared with the peripheral blood. The former group also described the expression of CD1d on extravillous trophoblast, which may form part of the NKT cell ligand. These results raise the possibility that NKT cells might have an immunomodulatory role in pregnancy.

Dendritic cells are thought to be critical to the generation of tolerance and immunity at mucosal sites.[24] Studies in our laboratory by fluorescence-activated cell sorting (FACS) and immunohistology have identified a small population of dendritic cells (< 1% of total cells) in first-trimester decidua. These cells have the phenotype of immature myeloid dendritic cells but their function is, as yet, unknown.[25]

Endometrial macrophages express the CD14 macrophage differentiation antigen and class II MHC antigens.[26] *In vitro*, decidual macrophages are adherent and phagocytic. Immunohistology reveals that approximately 20% of leucocytes in endometrium are macrophages. This percentage is relatively invariant throughout the menstrual cycle and also in pregnancy. However, the distribution of macrophages in the pregnant uterus is striking. There is enrichment of these cells at the implantation site but in the decidua parietalis, where no trophoblast invasion occurs, macrophages are sparse. Interestingly, the immune receptor ILT2, which may recognise HLA-G (see below), is expressed by all decidual macrophages.[17] Decidual macrophages, though not as numerous as uNK, are found in close association with the invading trophoblast, making it possible that they can respond to placental HLA-G.

T cells account for around 10% of leucocytes in decidua. They are found scattered throughout the stroma, within epithelia and also in the basal lymphoid aggregates. As with B cells, their number is static during the menstrual cycle and they do not accumulate at the implantation site.[27]

In the transplant situation, the responding T cells can respond *directly* or *indirectly* to the polymorphic antigens of the donor (Figure 2.3). As extravillous trophoblast cells only express one polymorphic HLA class I molecule, HLA-C, and never express HLA class II molecules (see below), direct presentation is unlikely to be very important. In *indirect* presentation, allogeneic molecules are taken up and processed by recipient APC so the processed peptides are presented to recipient T cells in the context of self-MHC. In the decidua, maternal dendritic cells and HLA-DR⁺ macrophages could fulfil this role. To generate an immune response these cells would have to mature and migrate to regional lymph nodes where trophoblast-specific lymphoid cells would be generated, and then migrate back to the implantation site. Whether other polymorphic molecules on the surface of trophoblast could act as minor histocompatibility antigens is as yet unknown.

The nature of systemic T cell responses appears to be different during pregnancy, with a shift towards Th2 differentiation.[28] The severity of autoimmune diseases such as systemic lupus erythematosus (SLE), multiple sclerosis and rheumatoid arthritis can vary in pregnancy, with either an improvement in or an exacerbation of symptoms. Some experimental studies on circulating T cells during normal pregnancy have suggested that a shift towards Th2 cell differentiation does occur, although not all aspects of Th2/Th1 responses are affected. For example, interleukin 12 (IL12) production by monocytes was found to be unaltered.[29] Thus, the nature of maternal T cell responses to *all* antigens (infections, self or fetal) may deviate towards Th2 differentiation, probably owing to the dramatic changes in hormonal stimuli during pregnancy.[30]

Interestingly, the CD3⁺ cells found in decidua differ phenotypically from resting T cells in blood. Some groups have described a downregulation of the CD3 T cell receptor (TCR) expression on T cells in decidua.[31,32] The expression by decidual T cells of activation markers such as CD69, HLA-DR and CD45RO has also been reported.[32,33] This raises the possibility that activated T cells could influence trophoblast invasion. Other evidence indicates that decidual T cells may be anergic as is seen with their counterparts in the gut: when decidual lymphocytes, including T cells, were mixed *in vitro* either with trophoblast or allogeneic peripheral blood lymphocytes (PBL), they did not proliferate as would be seen in a mixed lymphocyte reaction.[34]

It seems that local decidual T cells, whether activated or not, do not produce a detrimental response against extravillous trophoblast. The reasons for this are, as yet, unknown but there are likely to be several overlapping mechanisms to prevent decidual T cell activation. For example, the type of dendritic cells present in decidua

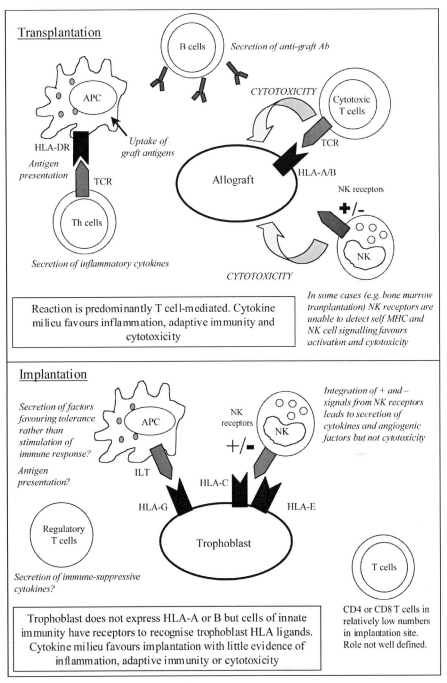

Figure 2.3. Comparison of simplified models of immune responses in transplantation and pregnancy; APC = antigen-presenting cells; HLA = human leucocyte antigen; ILT = immunoglobulin-like transcripts; NK = natural killer; TCR = T cell receptor; Th cells = T helper cells

and the microenvironment rich in hormones are likely to induce a tolerogenic rather than an immunogenic signal to the T cells.[25] Furthermore, CD4[+]CD25[+] T regulatory (Treg) cells have been described in first-trimester decidua and these may suppress T cell responses to trophoblast antigens.[35] The potential role of other mechanisms to suppress T cell activity, such as tryptophan metabolism, are reviewed elsewhere.[36]

Uterine NK cells

The most distinctive feature of the uterine mucosa during reproductive life is the presence of a large population of NK cells. Up to 70% of decidual leucocytes are CD56[+].[37] Ultrastructurally, a typical uterine CD56[+] cell is a large lymphocyte with a reniform eccentric nucleus and short cytoplasmic projections. They also possess varying numbers of membrane-bound cytoplasmic granules that contain cytolytic molecules such as granzyme and perforin.[38,39]

In early pregnancy, decidual NK cells make up around 30% of the stromal compartment. They are particularly populous at the implantation site, where they are found scattered throughout the stroma and thickly clustered around glands and spiral arteries. Their high-level infiltration puts them in close apposition to the invading trophoblast. The stimulus for the presence of so many NK cells in the uterus is not completely understood. In humans, uNK cells are present before implantation and in nonpregnant cycles where the number of uNK cells changes during the course of the menstrual cycle.[40] CD56[+] cells are rare in the proliferative phase but increase in number from the mid-secretory phase onwards, an increase that is sustained into early pregnancy.

Functions of uNK cells

As yet there is no convincing demonstration of a fundamental role of uNK cells in human reproduction. Uterine NK cells may be important in the renewal, different-iation and breakdown of the endometrium during the menstrual cycle and preg-nancy. The close encirclement of spiral arteries by uNK cells suggests that they may influence mucosal vascularisation. Secretory-phase endometrial NK cells have been shown by *in situ* hybridisation to express mRNA for vascular endothelial growth factor C (VEGF C), placental growth factor (PGF) and angiopoietin 2 (ANG2), all these factors could influence arterial stability.[41] NKG5, an NK cell derived soluble factor, was isolated from decidua and is mitogenic for endothelial cells.[42] Future investigations should address what influence these NK cells might have on processes such as decidualisation, angiogenesis and menstrual breakdown.

It is possible that the function of uNK cells is modified after ligation of uNK receptors with ligands expressed by extravillous trophoblast and that this modification could influence trophoblast invasion. It is therefore relevant to ask how uNK cells could recognise trophoblast antigens.

NK cell receptors

NK activity is controlled by the integration of both activating and inhibitory signals. The most studied NK receptors are the killer immunoglobulin receptors (KIR), the immunoglobulin-like transcripts (ILT) and the CD94/NKG2 proteins (Figure 2.4).[43]

KIR are immunoglobulin-superfamily (Ig-SF) receptors, which are expressed mainly by NK cells but also by certain T cell subsets. These genes are classified by the number of extracellular Ig-like domains they encode (two domains, 2D, or three domains, 3D) and by whether they have a long or short cytoplasmic domain (L or S). In general, the long-tailed KIR are inhibitory receptors while the short-tailed KIR transduce activating signals to the NK cell by associating with the adaptor protein DAP12.

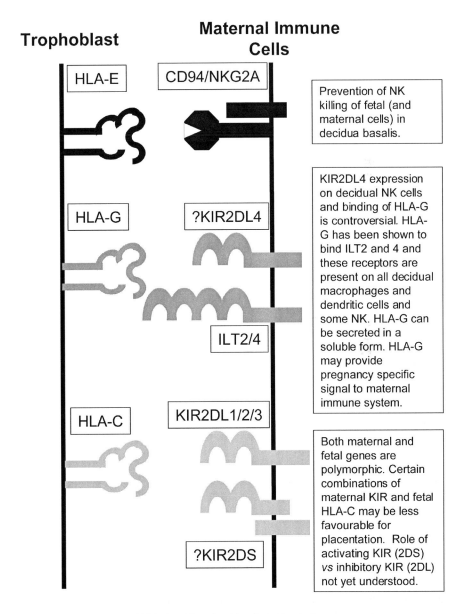

Figure 2.4. Interactions of HLA class I ligands with maternal innate immune receptors

Certain loci have been found in all human haplotypes that have been genotyped or sequenced so far.[44] They are *KIR3DL3*, *KIR3DL2*, and *KIR2DL4*. These loci form a framework with regions of variable gene content in between. Unrelated individuals are unlikely to share the same *KIR* genotype owing to haplotypic differences in *KIR* gene number and also intragenic polymorphism.[45]

Unlike the allele specificity of the TCR, KIR recognise groups of *HLA* alleles that have certain amino acids in common. For example, NK cells that express KIR2DL1 recognise HLA-C allotypes with lysine at position 80 of the γ1 domain while KIR2DL2 and KIR2DL3 have been shown to recognise HLA-C molecules with asparagine at position 80.

The *ILT* genes, also known as *LLIR*, *LIR*, *MIR* and *CD85*, have many similarities to the *KIR* genes. They also encode Ig-SF receptors, which can also be either inhibitory or activating when binding their MHC class I ligands. However, unlike KIR they are expressed on a broad variety of immune cell types such as monocytes/macrophages, dendritic cells, B cells and T cells.[46]

CD94 is an invariant protein encoded by a single gene. It forms disulphide-linked heterodimers with members of the NKG2 glycoprotein family and it is the NKG2 partner that determines whether the heterodimer is activating or inhibitory in response to binding of class I MHC proteins. The *NKG2* family in humans consists of five genes (*NKG2A*, *C*, *E* and *F*), which produce seven products (NKG2B and NKG2H being splice variants of NKG2A and E respectively). NKG2A/B inhibits NK cell function upon ligand binding and CD94/NKG2A has been shown to bind HLA-E.[47] NKG2C, E, F and H encode stimulatory proteins, which, like the activating KIR, associate with DAP12. NKG2D is a rogue in this family in that it does not pair with CD94 but instead forms homodimers and it is thought to recognise MHC-like proteins.[43]

Uterine NK cell recognition of trophoblast HLA

In blood NK cells most NK receptors are clonally expressed, apart from KIR2DL4, whose mRNA is expressed by all NK cells in most individuals tested.[44] Importantly, each NK cell expresses at least one inhibitory receptor for a self-MHC class I molecule, be it a KIR or CD94/NKG2A. Surprisingly, not all the HLA allotypes of an individual will have a matching KIR and conversely some of the KIRs expressed may not have a cognate HLA ligand in a particular individual. Pregnancy is the only physiological situation where KIR specific for nonself HLA allotypes may meet their cognate ligands.

Owing to the trophoblast-specific expression and nonpolymorphism of HLA-G, there has been a great deal of work done on whether uNK cells express receptors for HLA-G. Soluble KIR2DL4-Ig has been reported to bind several HLA class I molecules, notably HLA-G.[48,49] However, surface expression of 2DL4 is minimal, both in the blood and decidua. Two common alleles of *KIR2DL4* exist, 9A and 10A, which differ in the number of adenine residues at the end of the transmembrane exon. Only the 10A allele is expressed at the cell surface and then only on the minor CD56[bright] subset in blood.[50] Some individuals could express 2DL4 as a soluble isoform but the functional significance of this observation for pregnancy is not known. It has been shown that KIR2DL4 is not essential for pregnancy, as a woman has been described who is homozygous for a genotypic deletion of *KIR2DL4* – she has no severe health problems and has had several children.[51]

Fusion proteins of ILT2 demonstrate promiscuous binding to many HLA types including HLA-G and binding occurs with greater avidity to the HLA-G oligomers leading to enhanced inhibition of NK cytotoxicity. However, as ILT2 is only expressed by 20% of uNK cells the significance of this observation to the *in vivo* situation in pregnancy is not known.[17]

In contrast to blood where only approximately 50% of NK cells express CD94/NKG2A, all decidual NK cells are characterised by expression of high levels of CD94/NKG2A. The activating heterodimer NKG2C is transcribed by uNK cells but the protein is not expressed at high level by decidual NK cells.[52] Both maternal decidual cells and trophoblast express HLA-E and thus have the ability to interact with uNK cells. An added level of complexity results from the expression of HLA-G by trophoblast. HLA-E in complex with the HLA-G leader peptide has particularly high affinity for both the activating and inhibitory CD94/NKG2 receptors.[53] Decidual NK cells may thus be able to respond differentially to HLA-G+ trophoblast and maternal somatic cells expressing all the HLA class I proteins.

Interestingly, studies comparing, in parallel, the blood and decidua of pregnant women show that blood NK cells and uNK differ in their expression of some class I receptors. A greater proportion of decidual NK cells than blood NK cells express KIR specific for HLA-C.[54,55] These data are suggestive of a decidual-specific bias of the NK receptor repertoire toward recognition of HLA-C. HLA-C, unlike HLA-E or HLA-G, is polymorphic. This means that maternal NK cells may potentially encounter nonself paternal HLA-C alleles on trophoblast. Since KIR are also polymorphic in the population, each pregnancy may present a different combination of KIR and HLA-C. Studies are currently underway to see whether some combinations of maternal KIR genes and fetal HLA-allotypes are less favourable for healthy pregnancy than others.

Immunology of pre-eclampsia

Inadequate placentation and poor placental perfusion are features of PE, a specific disorder of human pregnancy that is associated with a significant maternal mortality and morbidity.[56] PE develops in stages, with the maternal systemic illness being a late manifestation of the placental ischaemia that is secondary to the reduced uteroplacental blood flow.[57] The primary pathological defect in this disease is the failure of transformation of the uterine spiral arteries.[9,58] Genetic studies of PE have implicated a contribution from both maternal and paternal genotypes. A family history in maternal relatives is associated with a four-fold increase in risk.[59] Despite this, no concordance is found in monozygotic twins.[60] In population-based studies a contribution of paternal as well as maternal factors in the development of the disease is apparent.[61] That immune recognition is involved is suggested by the increased risk in first pregnancies and in multiparae, but only after changing partners.[62] Importantly, there is also a greatly increased risk in women who have received donated oocytes (approximately 30%).[63] In this scenario the fetus will share neither maternal haploid gene set with the recipient mother.

Control of the fetal supply line may depend on the allogeneic interaction between maternal KIR on uNK cells and paternal HLA-C expressed by trophoblast. Therefore, uNK cell function during one pregnancy is likely to be influenced by a combination of two polymorphic sets of genes – the maternal *KIR* genotype as well as the trophoblast (fetal) *HLA-C* allotypes. Using DNA typing, we analysed how maternal *KIR* and fetal *HLA-C* genes combine to influence the risk of PE and reproductive success.[64] Striking differences were observed when these polymorphic ligand–receptor pairs were considered in combination. Mothers lacking most or all activating KIR (*AA* genotype) when the fetus possessed *HLA-C* belonging to the *HLA-C2* group were at greatly increased risk of PE. This was true even if the mother herself also had *HLA-C2*, indicating that neither nonself nor missing self discrimination is operative. Different human populations have a reciprocal relationship between *AA* frequency and *HLA-C2* frequency, suggesting selection against this combination.

The outcome of recognition of trophoblast HLA by uNK cells

The potential does exist for uNK class I receptor engagement by trophoblast HLA, however the outcome of such an interaction is incompletely understood. Drawing inspiration from the missing self hypothesis, early speculation was that expression of class I molecules by trophoblast was necessary to prevent NK cell attack.[65] Trophoblast cells had previously been shown to be resistant to lysis by NK cells. However, trophoblast cell lines were still protected from lysis by NK cells even in the presence of blocking antibodies against HLA class I molecules, CD94, ILT or KIR.[17,66]

An alternative hypothesis is that recognition of trophoblast causes the uNK cells to change their cytokine production profile. Factors such as trophoblast metallo-proteinase and integrin expression could be influenced by the cytokine milieu at the implantation site, thus altering their invasive behaviour. Isolated decidual NK cells produce cytokines such as granulocyte-macrophage colony-stimulating factor (GM-CSF), CSF-1 and IFN-γ for which trophoblast has receptors.[67]

Conclusions

Pregnancy is a unique situation that has intrigued immunologists for more than half a century. The growing fetus requires maternal blood for its nutrition but direct interaction of maternal leucocytes with allogeneic fetal cells would be unfavourable. Instead the fetus surrounds itself with a specialised extra-embryonic tissue with which it can tap into the maternal blood without provoking a detrimental immune response. The cells of the placenta have an unusual surface phenotype, especially in terms of the complement of MHC proteins they present.

The mother prepares for and responds to pregnancy with both systemic and local adaptations. Locally within the uterus the highly invasive nature of trophoblast is kept in check by a specialised layer, the decidua, but exactly how the decidua functions in this capacity is not completely understood. What is known is that the immunological response to the trophoblast is not like that seen in transplantation and that the populations of maternal leucocytes present in the uterus are unique. Most work has been performed on decidual T cells and NK cells. The other cells present at the implantation site, such as macrophages, dendritic cells and NKT cells, will doubtless have roles to play but these are less well studied.

Systemically, maternal T cell responses are apparently altered in pregnancy but at the level of the uterus overt signs of decidual T cell recognition of trophoblast such as proliferation do not occur. Whether this is due to inability of the decidual T cells to recognise trophoblast antigens or due to active suppression mechanisms has not been unravelled.

Much about decidual NK cells also remains mysterious. They are very numerous at the site of trophoblast invasion and can be seen in close proximity to trophoblast. However, although they are potentially cytolytic, they do not kill trophoblast in normal pregnancy. Decidual NK cells have been shown to have receptors that could respond to trophoblast MHC or cytokines. However, how decidual NK cells respond to trophoblast and what purpose this serves are unanswered questions. Decidual NK cells may exert control over trophoblast through production of cytokines or they may be necessary for maintenance of the decidua.

Future studies should result in a more integrated understanding of how the different cell types in the decidua interact with one another and with trophoblast to create the correct environment for implantation to be a success from both the maternal and fetal perspectives. Overall, the conclusion is that the interaction between maternal immune cells and the trophoblast may have a physiological function in regulating the development of the placenta rather than the idea that there is a maternal immunological defence against her allogeneic fetus. This would be a new perspective on an old problem.

References

1. Burnet FM. *The Clonal Selection Theory of Acquired Immunity*. Nashville: Vanderbilt University Press; 1959.
2. Billingham RE, Brent L, Medawar PB. 'Actively acquired tolerance' of foreign cells. *Nature* 1953;172:603–6.
3. Janeway CA. The immune system evolved to discriminate infectious nonself from noninfectious self. *Immunol Today* 1992;13:11–16.
4. Medzhitov R, Janeway CA. Decoding the patterns of self and nonself by the innate immune system. *Science* 2002;296:298–300.
5. Kärre K, Ljunggren HG, Piontek G, Kiessling R. Selective rejection of H-2-deficient lymphoma variants suggests alternative immune defence strategy. *Nature* 1986;319:675–8.
6. Matzinger P. Tolerance, danger and the extended family. *Annu Rev Immunol* 1994;12:991–1045.
7. Matzinger P. The danger model: a renewed sense of self. *Science* 2002;296:301–5.
8. Zhou Y, Genbacev O, Fisher SJ. The human placenta remodels the uterus by using a combination of molecules that govern vasculogenesis or leukocyte extravasation. *Ann NY Acad Sci* 2003;995:73–83.
9. Pijnenborg R, Vercruysse L, Hanssens M, van Assche A. Incomplete trophoblast invasion: the evidence. In: Critchley H, MacLean A, Poston L, Walker J, editors. *Pre-eclampsia*. London: RCOG Press; 2003. p. 15–26.
10. Loke YW, King A. *Human Implantation: Cell Biology and Immunology*. Cambridge: Cambridge University Press; 1995.
11. Ishitani A, Sageshima N, Lee N, Dorofeeva N, Hatake K, Marquardt H, et al. Protein expression and peptide binding suggest unique and interacting functional roles for HLA-E, F, and G in maternal–placental immune recognition. *J Immunol* 2003;171:1376–84.
12. King A, Burrows TD, Hiby SE, Bowen JM, Joseph S, Verma S, et al. Surface expression of HLA-C antigen by human extravillous trophoblast. *Placenta* 2000;21:376–87.
13. Hiby SE, King A, Sharkey A, Loke YW. Molecular studies of trophoblast HLA-G: polymorphism, isoforms, imprinting and expression in preimplantation embryo. *Tissue Antigens* 1999;53:1–13.
14. Boyson JE, Erskine R, Whitman MC, Chiu M, Lau JM, Koopman LA, et al. Disulfide bond-mediated dimerization of HLA-G on the cell surface. *Proc Natl Acad Sci U S A* 2002;99:16180–5.
15. McMaster M, Zhou Y, Shorter S, Kapasi K, Geraghty D, Lim KH, et al. HLA-G isoforms produced by placental cytotrophoblasts and found in amniotic fluid are due to unusual glycosylation. *J Immunol* 1998;160:5922–8.
16. Ober C, Aldrich C, Rosinsky B, Robertson A, Walker MA, Willadsen S, et al. HLA-G1 protein expression is not essential for fetal survival. *Placenta* 1998;19:127–32.
17. King A, Allan DS, Bowen M, Powis SJ, Joseph S, Verma S, et al. HLA-E is expressed on trophoblast and interacts with CD94/NKG2 receptors on decidual NK cells. *Eur J Immunol* 2000;30:1623–31.
18. Blaschitz A, Hutter H, Dohr G. HLA Class I protein expression in the human placenta. *Early Pregnancy* 2001;5:67–9.

19. Noyes RW, Hertig AT, Rock J. Dating of the endometrial biopsy. *Fertil Steril* 1950;1:3–25.

20. More IAR. The normal human endometrium. In: Haines M, editor. *Haines & Taylor Obstetrical and Gynaecological Pathology*. Edinburgh: Churchill Livingstone; 1987. vol. 1, p. 302–19.

21. Godfrey DI, Hammond KJ, Poulton LD, Smyth MJ, Baxter AG. NKT cells: facts, functions and fallacies. *Immunol Today* 2000;21:573–83.

22. Boyson JE, Rybalov B, Koopman LA, Exley M, Balk SP, Racke FK, *et al.* CD1d and invariant NKT cells at the human maternal–fetal interface. *Proc Natl Acad Sci U S A* 2002;99:13741–6.

23. Tsuda H, Sakai M, Michimata T, Tanebe K, Hayakawa S, Saito S. Characterization of NKT cells in human peripheral blood and decidual lymphocytes. *Am J Reprod Immunol* 2001;45:295–302.

24. Nagler-Anderson C. Man the barrier! Strategic defences in the intestinal mucosa. *Nat Rev Immunol* 2001;1:59–67.

25. Gardner L, Moffett A. Dendritic cells in the human decidua. *Biol Reprod* 2003;69:1438–46.

26. Bulmer JN, Morrison L, Smith JC. Expression of class II MHC gene products by macrophages in human uteroplacental tissue. *Immunology* 1988;63:707–14.

27. Starkey PM, Clover LM, Rees MC. Variation during the menstrual cycle of immune cell populations in human endometrium. *Eur J Obstet Gynecol Reprod Biol* 1991;39:203–7.

28. Piccinni MP, Beloni L, Livi C, Maggi E, Scarselli G, Romagnani, S. Defective production of both leukemia inhibitory factor and type 2 T-helper cytokines by decidual T cells in unexplained recurrent abortions. *Nat Med* 1998;9:1020–4.

29. Sacks GP, Redman CW, Sargent IL. Monocytes are primed to produce the Th1 type cytokine IL-12 in normal human pregnancy: an intracellular flow cytometric analysis of peripheral blood mononuclear cells. *Clin Exp Immunol* 2003;131:490–7.

30. Ostensen M. Sex hormones and pregnancy in rheumatoid arthritis and systemic lupus erythematosus. *Ann N Y Acad Sci* 1999;876:131–43.

31. Morii T, Nishikawa K, Saito S, Enomoto M, Ito A, Kurai N, et al. T-cell receptors are expressed but down-regulated on intradecidual T lymphocytes. *Am J Reprod Immunol* 1993;29:1–4.

32. Saito S, Nishikawa K, Morii T, Narita N, Enomoto M, Ichijo M. Expression of activation antigens CD69, HLA-DR, interleukin-2 receptor-alpha (IL-2R alpha) and IL-2R beta on T cells of human decidua at an early stage of pregnancy. *Immunology* 1992;75:710–2.

33. Saito S, Nishikawa K, Morii T, Narita N, Enomoto M, Ito A, et al. A study of CD45RO, CD45RA and CD29 antigen expression on human decidual T cells in an early stage of pregnancy. *Immunol Lett* 1994;40:193–7.

34. King A, Gardner L, Loke YW. Human decidual leukocytes do not proliferate in response to either extravillous trophoblast or allogeneic peripheral blood lymphocytes. *J Reprod Immunol* 1996;30:67–74.

35. Sasaki Y, Sakai M, Miyazaki S, Higuma S, Shiozaki A, Saito S. Decidual and peripheral blood CD4+CD25+ regulatory T cells in early pregnancy subjects and spontaneous abortion cases. *Mol Hum Reprod* 2004;10:347–53.

36. Mellor AL, Munn DH. Immunology at the maternal–fetal interface: lessons for T cell tolerance and suppression. *Annu Rev Immunol* 2000;18:367–91.

37. Bulmer JN, Morrison L, Longfellow M, Ritson A, Pace D. Granulated lymphocytes in human endometrium: histochemical and immunohistochemical studies. *Hum Reprod* 1991;6:791–8.

38. King A, Balendran N, Wooding P, Carter NP, Loke YW. CD3- leukocytes present in the human uterus during early placentation: phenotypic and morphologic characterization of the CD56++ population. *Dev Immunol* 1991;1:169–90.

39. King A, Wooding P, Gardner L, Loke YW. Expression of perforin, granzyme A and TIA-1 by human uterine CD56+ NK cells implies they are activated and capable of effector functions. *Hum Reprod* 1993;8:2061–7.

40. King A, Wellings V, Gardner L, Loke YW. Immunocytochemical characterization of the unusual large granular lymphocytes in human endometrium throughout the menstrual cycle. Hum *Immunol* 1989;24:195–205.

41. Li XF, Charnock-Jones DS, Zhang E, Hiby S, Malik S, Day K, *et al.* Angiogenic growth factor messenger ribonucleic acids in uterine natural killer cells. *J Clin Endocrinol Metab* 2001;86:1823–34.

42. Langer N, Beach D, Lindenbaum ES. Novel hyperactive mitogen to endothelial cells: human decidual NKG5. *Am J Reprod Immunol* 1999;42:263–72.

43. Borrego F, Kabat J, Kim DK, Lieto L, Maasho K, Pena J, *et al.* Structure and function of major histocompatibility complex (MHC) class I specific receptors expressed on human natural killer (NK) cells. *Mol Immunol* 2002;38:637–60.

44. Vilches C, Parham P. KIR: diverse, rapidly evolving receptors of innate and adaptive immunity. *Annu Rev Immunol* 2002;20:217–51.

45. Shilling HG, Guethlein LA, Cheng NW, Gardiner CM, Rodriguez R, Tyan D, et al. Allelic polymorphism synergizes with variable gene content to individualize human KIR genotype. *J Immunol* 2002;168:2307–15.

46. Colonna M, Nakajima H, Navarro F, Lopez-Botet M. A novel family of Ig-like receptors for HLA class I molecules that modulate function of lymphoid and myeloid cells. *J Leukoc Biol* 1999;66:375–81.

47. Braud VM, Allan DS, O'Callaghan CA, Soderstrom K, D'Andrea A, Ogg GS, et al. HLA-E binds to natural killer cell receptors CD94/NKG2A, B and C. *Nature* 1998;391:795–9.

48. Rajagopalan S, Long EO. A human histocompatibility leukocyte antigen (HLA)-G-specific receptor expressed on all natural killer cells. *J Exp Med* 1999;189:1093–100.

49. Cantoni C, Verdiani S, Falco M, Pessino A, Cilli M, Conte R, *et al*. p49, a putative HLA class I-specific inhibitory NK receptor belonging to the immunoglobulin superfamily. *Eur J Immunol* 1998;28:1980–90. Erratum in: *Eur J Immunol* 1998;28:3398.

50. Goodridge JP, Witt CS, Christiansen FT, Warren HS. KIR2DL4 (CD158d) genotype influences expression and function in NK cells. *J Immunol* 2003;171:1768–74.

51. Gomez-Lozano N, de Pablo R, Puente S, Vilches C. Recognition of HLA-G by the NK cell receptor KIR2DL4 is not essential for human reproduction. *Eur J Immunol* 2003;33:639–44.

52. Trundley A, Moffett A. Unpublished data.

53. Vales-Gomez M, Reyburn HT, Erskine RA, Lopez-Botet M, Strominger JL. Kinetics and peptide dependency of the binding of the inhibitory NK receptor CD94/NKG2-A and the activating receptor CD94/NKG2-C to HLA-E. *EMBO J* 1999;18:4250–60.

54. Verma S, King A, Loke YW. Expression of killer cell inhibitory receptors on human uterine natural killer cells. *Eur J Immunol* 1997;27:979–83.

55. Hiby SE, King A, Sharkey AM, Loke YW. Human uterine NK cells have a similar repertoire of killer inhibitory and activatory receptors to those found in blood, as demonstrated by RT-PCR and sequencing. *Mol Immunol* 1997;34:419–30.

56. Roberts JM. Pre-eclampsia: a two-stage disorder. In: Critchley H, MacLean A, Poston L, Walker J, editors. *Pre-eclampsia*. London: RCOG Press 2003; p. 66–78.

57. Redman CW. Current topic: pre-eclampsia and the placenta. *Placenta* 1991;12:301–8.

58. Moffett-King A. Natural killer cells and pregnancy. *Nat Rev Immunol* 2002;2:656–63.

59. Cincotta RB, Brennecke SP. Family history of pre-eclampsia as a predictor for pre-eclampsia in primigravidas. *Int J Gynaecol Obstet* 1998;60:23–7.

60. Treloar SA, Cooper DW, Brennecke SP, Grehan MM, Martin NG. An Australian twin study of the genetic basis of preeclampsia and eclampsia. *Am J Obstet Gynecol* 2001;184:374–81.

61. Esplin MS, Fausett MB, Fraser A, Kerber R, Mineau G, Carrillo J, *et al*. Paternal and maternal components of the predisposition to preeclampsia. *N Engl J Med* 2001;344:867–72.

62. Trupin LS, Simon LP, Eskenazi B. Change in paternity: a risk factor for preeclampsia in multiparas. *Epidemiology* 1996;7:240–4.

63. Soderstrom-Anttila V, Tiitinen A, Foudila T, Hovatta O. Obstetric and perinatal outcome after oocyte donation: comparing with in vitro fertilisation pregnancies. *Hum Reprod* 1998;13:483–90.

64. Hiby SE, Walker JJ, O'shaughnessy KM, Redman CW, Carrington M, Trowsdale J, *et al*. Combinations of maternal KIR and fetal HLA-C genes influence the risk of preeclampsia and reproductive success. *J Exp Med* 2004;200:957–65.

65. King A, Loke YW. On the nature and function of human uterine granular lymphocytes. *Immunol Today* 1991;12:432–5.

66. Avril T, Jarousseau AC, Watier H, Boucraut J, Le Bouteiller P, Bardos P, *et al*. Trophoblast cell line resistance to NK lysis mainly involves an HLA class I-independent mechanism. *J Immunol* 1999;162:5902–9.

67. Saito S, Nishikawa K, Morii T, Enomoto M, Narita N, Motoyoshi K, *et al*. Cytokine production by CD16-CD56bright natural killer cells in the human early pregnancy decidua. *Int Immunol* 1993;5:559–63.

68. Moffett A, Loke YW. The immunological paradox of pregnancy: a reappraisal. *Placenta* 2004;25:1–8

Chapter 3
Progestin-induced decidualisation promotes human endometrial haemostasis and vascular stability

Frederick Schatz, Graciela Krikun, Se-Te Huang,
Edmund Funai, Lynn Buchwalder, Mizanur Rahman,
Rebeca Caze, Caroline Tang and Charles J Lockwood

Overview

During human implantation, endovascular trophoblast invasion occurs within a matrix of decidualised stromal cells that are ideally positioned to mitigate the associated threat of pregnancy-terminating local haemorrhage. Observations made by *in situ* hybridisation and immunohistochemistry of endometrial sections, together with *in vitro* studies of human endometrial stromal cells (HESCs), indicate that progestin-induced decidualisation creates a pro-haemostatic, vascular-stabilising milieu that resists bleeding. Thus, decidualisation is associated with coordinated upregulation in the expression of:

- tissue factor (TF), which promotes haemostasis by enhancing fibrin deposition via thrombin generation
- plasminogen activator inhibitor 1 (PAI-1), the fast inactivator of the primary fibrinolytic agent, tissue plasminogen activator (tPA).

Coincidently, the peridecidual cell extracellular matrix (ECM) becomes enriched in basal laminar-type proteins, which reflects the reciprocal synthesis of new ECM proteins and inhibition in their degradation. ECM degradation is initiated by surface receptor-bound urokinase (urokinase plasminogen activator, uPA). However, the plasmin-forming activity of this uPA is inhibited by elevated levels of PAI-1 stemming from progesterone-regulated decidualisation. Plasmin can degrade several ECM proteins and activates the zymogenic form of matrix metalloproteinases (MMPs), which degrade the bulk ECM components. Therefore, lower plasmin output results in a profound inhibition of ECM-degrading activity, which is complemented by direct progestin inhibition of the synthesis by HESCs of at least two members of the MMP family, MMP1 and MMP3. This coordinated inhibition of proteolysis strengthens the perivascular ECM support scaffolding. The resulting stabilisation of the endometrial vasculature in a pro-haemostatic milieu protects against bleeding during endovascular trophoblast invasion.

Introduction

Human implantation is initiated by adhesion of the blastocyst to the luminal surface of the endometrial epithelium. Blastocyst-derived syncytiotrophoblasts then intercalate between adjacent epithelial cells and invade the underlying stroma where they breach blood vessels enmeshed in a decidualised stromal cell matrix. This process is vital to the development, growth and survival of the embryo as it provides entrance of oxygen and nutrients and egress of waste products prior to placentation.[1] That it also risks pregnancy-terminating local haemorrhage is evident from the occurrence of 'chemical pregnancy', in which trophoblast-derived human chorionic gonadotrophin (hCG) is detected briefly in maternal blood followed by 'spotting' in the decidua.[2,3]

Several lines of evidence stress the important role played by decidualisation in successful implantation and subsequent placentation. The occurrence of decidualisation is limited to species in which the trophoblast invades the stroma. Among species with a haemochorial placenta, the extent of decidualisation correlates positively with the degree of trophoblast invasion. Both processes reach their greatest expression in the human, which exhibits the most widespread decidualisation reaction and the most invasive trophoblast.[4] Following endovascular trophoblast invasion, extravillous trophoblasts breach and remodel uterine spiral arteries. Consequently, small-bore, high-resistance vessels are converted to large-bore, low-resistance vessels that meet the demands of the growing fetoplacental unit by increasing maternal blood flow.[5,6] Decidual haemorrhage during this period is associated with miscarriage, abruption and preterm birth.[7–9]

Decidualised HESCs are positioned to prevent bleeding during invasion and remodelling of endometrial vessels

The nonfertile human menstrual cycle terminates in sloughing of the functional endometrial layer, which is then restored in the next cycle. In the follicular phase, rising circulating oestradiol (E$_2$) levels initiate endometrial cell mitosis. Following ovulation, rising circulating progesterone acts on the E$_2$-primed cells in concert with a second peak of E$_2$ to block further proliferation and to initiate differentiation. During decidualisation, the fibroblast-like stromal cells of the follicular-phase endometrium differentiate into cuboidal, epithelioid decidual cells of the luteal phase. The decidualisation reaction is initiated around the blood vessels and under the glands and then spreads throughout the luteal and gestational endometrium. It involves a profound transformation in biochemical phenotype that includes expression of proteins that promote haemostasis and enhance vascular stability. Because they are concentrated at sites of endovascular trophoblast invasion, decidual cells are positioned to counteract the onset of bleeding during this process.[10,11]

Decidualised HESCs mediate haemostasis

The role of TF in promoting haemostasis

In successful human pregnancies, implantation, placentation and delivery require significant enhancement in haemostasis,[12] which is accomplished by augmented thrombin and fibrin generation across gestation as measured by elevated circulating levels of thrombin–antithrombin (TAT) complexes.[13] Thrombin is formed as a result of binding of factor VII from the circulation to tissue factor (TF), a 46 kDa cell membrane-bound glycoprotein member of the class 2 cytokine receptor family. The TF molecule comprises a cytoplasmic tail and a transmembrane domain, each of about 20 amino acids, and a longer hydrophilic extracellular domain, which acts as the receptor for factor VII or its active form, factor VIIa.[14] TF-bound VIIa initiates a series of changes that culminates in the proteolytic cleavage of prothrombin to thrombin, which promotes haemostasis by generating fibrin.[14–16]

The crucial role that TF plays in preventing bleeding during gestation was demonstrated in TF knockout mice, which develop fragile vessels and die of haemorrhage *in utero*.[17] However, incorporation of a human minigene expressing TF at only 1% of wild-type level rescued the knockout mice and produced liveborn pups. In contrast, about 40% of pregnancies in which both mother and fetus were homozygous low TF expressors were complicated by multiple intrauterine haemorrhages and intraplacental 'blood pools' in the labyrinth.[18,19]

Studies of TF expression in human endometrium

In situ hybridisation and immunohistochemistry have localised TF mRNA and protein to decidualised stromal cells of luteal-phase and gestational endometrium.[20–22] Regulation of TF expression was then evaluated during *in vitro* decidualisation of HESCs isolated from predecidualised tissues. Figure 3.1 demonstrates that medroxyprogesterone acetate (MPA), but not E_2, enhances cell-associated levels of TF protein as determined by enzyme-linked immunosorbent assay (ELISA) (a), and TF activity as determined by a clotting assay (b).[23] Co-incubation with E_2 plus MPA produced a greater than additive increase in TF levels by both measurements, thus mimicking E_2 priming of the stromal cells *in vivo* for the decidualising effects of progesterone.[24,25] Although MPA can exert glucocorticoid effects in some cell systems,[26] dexamethasone did not affect TF expression in cultured HESCs. Moreover, the antiprogestin/antiglucocorticoid mifepristone acted as a pure antiprogestin by blocking E_2 plus MPA-induced TF levels while exerting no agonist effects. Consistent with its greater susceptibility to metabolism by HESCs,[27] progesterone was less effective than MPA in elevating TF levels. Immunoblotting determined that the TF expressed by *in vitro* decidualised HESCs conformed to the expected 46 kDa of authentic TF.[20]

Incubation of HESCs with E_2 plus MPA enhanced both immunoreactive and functionally active TF levels for at least three weeks,[28] thereby attesting to the relevance of the *in vitro* decidualisation model for studying the chronic upregulation of TF expression by decidual cells of luteal-phase and gestational endometrium. The Northern blot depicted in Figure 3.2 indicates that MPA and E_2 plus MPA upregulated steady-state TF mRNA levels for 10 days in cultured HESCs.[28] Unlike the prolonged progestin induction of TF mRNA and protein levels in HESCs, growth factors, cytokines and glucocorticoids transiently enhance TF expression in other cell types. Thus, TF mRNA levels are increased for only a few hours, whereas TF protein levels are rarely elevated for longer than 24 hours.[29–34] Transcriptional regulation of TF can be mediated by activator protein 1 (AP1), nuclear factor kappa B (NFκB), early growth response 1 (EGR-1) or the Sp transcription family on the TF gene promoter.[35] In cultured HESCs, we found that specificity protein 1 (SP1) mediates basal as well as progestin-enhanced TF transcriptional activity.[36] This

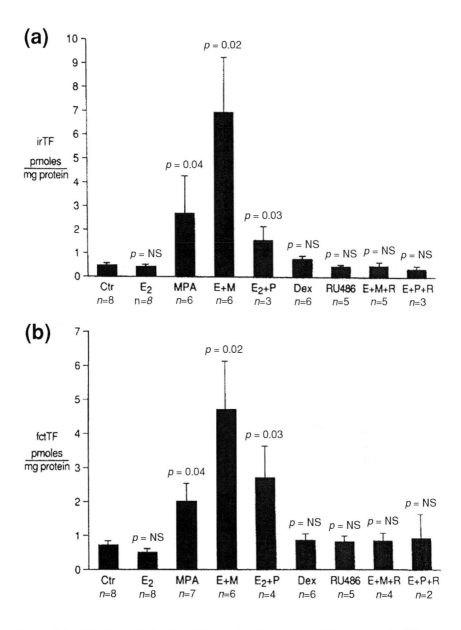

Figure 3.1. Steroid-regulated endometrial stromal cell TF expression: (a) immunoreactive TF by ELISA; (b) functional TF by two-step clotting assay. Confluent HESCs were incubated with vehicle control (Ctr), 10^{-8} M E_2, 10^{-7} M MPA, 10^{-6} M dexamethasone (Dex), E_2 + MPA, or E_2 + 10^{-6} M progesterone (P), and either 10^{-6} M mifepristone (RU486) alone or with E_2 + M, or E_2 + P for 3–4 days; TF levels in cell lysates are normalised to cell protein; mean ± SEM for n experiments; statistical comparisons by Wilcoxon signed rank test; reproduced with permission from Lockwood *et al.*[23] (*The Journal of Clinical Endocrinology & Metabolism*, © The Endocrine Society 1994)

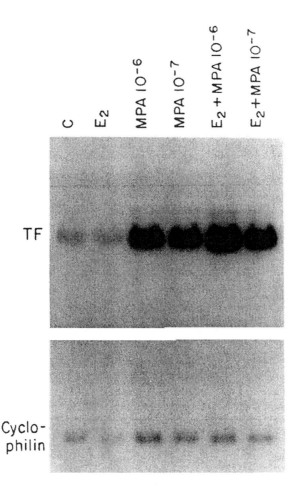

Figure 3.2. Northern blot of endometrial stromal cell TF mRNA expression. Confluent HESCs were incubated for 10 days with vehicle control (C), 10^{-8} M E_2, 10^{-7} or 10^{-6} M MPA, or E_2 + MPA; to adjust for differences in loading, the blot was stripped and reprobed for the presence of mRNA levels for the cyclophilin housekeeping gene; reproduced with permission from Lockwood *et al.*[28] (*The Journal of Clinical Endocrinology & Metabolism*, © The Endocrine Society 1993)

conclusion was drawn from the results of transient transfections of HESCs with TF promoter constructs containing overlapping SP and EGR-1 binding sites, or with these sites systematically inactivated by site-directed mutagenesis, or with SP1 over-expressing vectors alone and with a specific blocker of SP1 binding. Moreover, immunostaining of HESC monolayers and endometrial sections demonstrated that progestin-regulated decidualisation *in vitro* and *in vivo* involves an increase in the ratio of SP1 to its SP3 antagonist.[37]

Tissue-type plasminogen activator (tPA) and the type one plasminogen activator inhibitor (PAI-1) promote endometrial haemostasis

The model depicted in Figure 3.3 underscores the importance of TF–tPA interactions in establishing a local haemostatic milieu. As noted above, TF expressed by the decidualised stromal cell membrane binds to circulating factor VII to generate thrombin and promote fibrin formation. However, Figure 3.3 indicates that tPA, the primary fibrinolytic agent, opposes this pro-haemostatic action of TF. Specifically, tPA binds to fibrin where it forms plasmin by cleaving Arg^{560}-Val^{561} in its preferred substrate, plasminogen.[38] Plasmin is a broad-spectrum serine protease that efficiently degrades fibrin.[39] Figure 3.3 also introduces PAI-1, the fast inactivator of tPA, which plays a critical role in determining the haemostatic balance.[40]

Studies of tPA and PAI-1 expression in human endometrium

In endometrial biopsies evaluated across the menstrual cycle, tPA antigen and activity levels were significantly higher in the late luteal phase than in either the follicular or early luteal phases. However levels of the potent tPA inhibitor PAI-1 were also higher in late luteal-phase endometrial biopsies compared with biopsies obtained earlier in the menstrual cycle.[41] Using immunohistochemical staining, our laboratory confirmed that PAI-1 levels are elevated in the luteal-phase endometrium.[21]

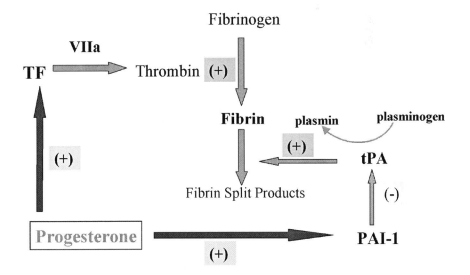

Figure 3.3. Progesterone (P4)-induced decidualisation regulates endometrial haemostasis via TF–PAI-1 interactions

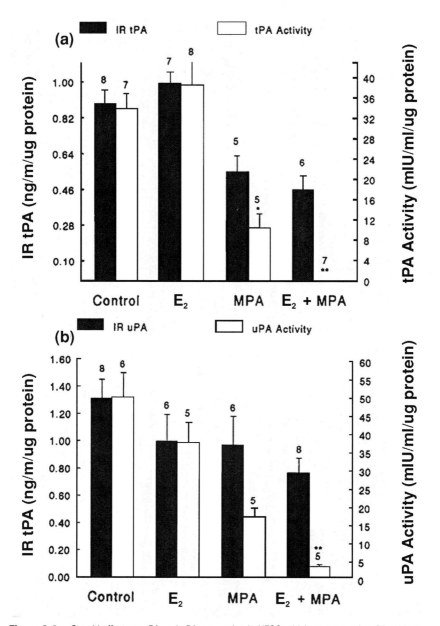

Figure 3.4. Steroid effects on tPA and uPA expression in HESCs: (a) immunoreactive tPA – black bars; tPA activity – white bars; (b) immunoreactive uPA – black bars; uPA activity – white bars. Confluent HESCs were incubated for 3 days in vehicle control, 10^{-8} M E_2, 10^{-7} M MPA, or E_2 + MPA; specific ELISAs measured immunoreactive tPA and uPA levels, and a chromogenic assay measured tPA and uPA catalytic activities; the results are normalised to cell protein; statistical significance was determined by one-way ANOVA. * $P < 0.05$; ** $P < 0.005$ (compared with control in n experiments); reproduced with permission from Schatz *et al.*[42] (*The Journal of Clinical Endocrinology & Metabolism*, © The Endocrine Society 1995)

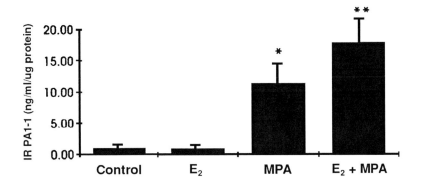

Figure 3.5. Steroid effects on PAI-1 expression in HESCs. Confluent cultures from eight specimens were incubated for 3 days in vehicle control, 10^{-8} M E$_2$, 10^{-7} M MPA, or E$_2$ + MPA; immunoreactive PAI-1 levels in the conditioned medium were measured by ELISA and normalised to cell protein; statistical significance was determined by one-way ANOVA; * $P < 0.05$; ** $P < 0.005$ (compared with control); reproduced with permission from Schatz et al.[42] (*The Journal of Clinical Endocrinology & Metabolism*, © The Endocrine Society 1995)

The effects of ovarian steroids were assessed on tPA and PAI-1 expression in HESC monolayers; Figures 3.4(a) and 3.5, respectively. Figure 3.4(a) indicates that tPA expression is inhibited in a decidualisation-dependent manner. Thus, MPA lowered HESC-secreted tPA levels as determined by ELISA (black bars) and confirmed by immunoblotting.[42] Although the cultures were refractory to E$_2$ alone, co-incubation with E$_2$ plus MPA augmented this inhibition. In addition, Figure 3.4(a) indicates that MPA preferentially reduced levels of tPA catalytic activity in parallel aliquots of HESC-conditioned medium (white bars) compared with tPA protein levels. This differential inhibitory effect was most pronounced during incubations with E$_2$ plus MPA with the conditioned medium containing significant immunoreactive tPA levels but tPA activity was barely detectable.

The potent inhibition that PAI-1 exerts on tPA activity prompted measurements of PAI-1 levels in aliquots of the HESC-conditioned medium. Figure 3.5 indicates that E$_2$ did not affect PAI-1 output, whereas PAI-1 output was enhanced by MPA and synergistically enhanced by E$_2$ plus MPA. During incubations with E$_2$ plus MPA, the reciprocal downregulation of tPA and upregulation of PAI-1 output resulted in a marked molar excess of the latter versus the former in the conditioned medium. Therefore, preferential inhibition of tPA activity primarily reflects elevated PAI-1 output. This progestin-mediated inhibition was confirmed by immunoblotting.[42] It proved to be specific for PAI-1 since the potent PA inhibitor PAI-2, was present in only minute quantities in HESC-conditioned medium, and was unaffected by the presence of steroids.[42] In correspondence with changes in immunoreactive PAI-1 levels, Northern blotting revealed that steady-state PAI-1 mRNA levels were also increased by MPA and further increased by E$_2$ plus MPA in cultured HESCs.[43]

Decidualised HESCs promote endometrial vascular stability

The basal laminar protein-enriched peridecidual ECM mediates vascular stability

During decidualisation of human endometrium, the interstitial-type ECM of the follicular phase, which is enriched in fibronectin and collagen types I, III, V and VI, is converted to a mixture of residual interstitial proteins and new peridecidual basal laminar-type components.[44] The latter includes laminin, heparin sulphate proteoglycan and collagen type IV.[45–47] The resulting peridecidual cell ECM plays an integral role in implantation by modulating migration of the invading trophoblast and in counteracting the threat of local haemorrhage during endovascular trophoblast invasion by serving as a vascular support and stabilising scaffolding structure. Transformation of the peridecidual ECM involves synthesis of new proteins, but is augmented by the reciprocal inhibition of proteases that degrade these proteins.

uPA/PAI-1/MMP interactions regulate endometrial ECM turnover

Urokinase-type plasminogen activator (uPA) is secreted as a single-chain pro-uPA zymogen that binds to the uPA receptor (uPAR) on the cell surface of cancer cells[48–50] and trophoblasts,[51] as well as stromal and decidual cells from cycling and gestational endometrium.[52,53] Binding of pro-uPA to the uPAR initiates its conversion to catalytically active double-chain uPA,[40] which mediates the cleavage of plasminogen to plasmin as described above for tPA. Plasmin can degrade several ECM proteins,[54–56] but exerts its primary impact on ECM degradation by activating the secreted, zymogenic form of matrix metalloproteinases (MMPs), which degrade the bulk of ECM components.[57]

The MMPs are classified on the basis of substrate specificity as:

1. collagenases, which degrade fibrillar collagens
2. gelatinases, which degrade basement membrane-associated collagens as well as denatured fibrillar collagens (gelatins)
3. stromelysins, which can degrade the broadest array of ECM components, including proteoglycans, glycoproteins, fibronectin, laminin, type IV and V collagen, both the non-helical amino- and carboxyl-terminal peptides of type II collagen as well as the globular, but not the triple helical regions, of interstitial collagens.[57,58] Furthermore, stromelysin 1 (MMP3) can activate zymogenic forms of other MMPs such as interstitial collagenase (pro-MMP1), gelatinase B (pro-MMP9) and collagenase 3 (pro-MMP13).[58–61] This versatility enables MMP3 to regulate an ECM-degrading proteolytic cascade.

The interaction between MMP1 and MMP3 is integral to the degradation of fibrillar collagens. Mediation of a specific cleavage in the helical region of these collagens by MMP1 promotes denaturation to gelatins, which are then processed further by MMP3 and MMP3-activated MMP9.[58,62] Coordinated changes in the expression of the *MMP1* and *MMP3* genes reflect the presence of similar response elements on their promoters.[58,63] By contrast, the gene promoter of the collagenase MMP2 is essentially devoid of such response elements.[64] The tissue inhibitors of matrix metalloproteinases (TIMPs) are a family of natural MMP inhibitors present in most tissues and body fluids that regulate MMP activity *in vivo*.[65]

Studies in human endometrium

Rodgers *et al.*[66] localised mRNAs for several MMPs and for TIMP1 in the functional endometrial layer by *in situ* hybridisation. In specimens obtained across the menstrual cycle, they found that MMP1 and MMP3 mRNA levels were lower in the progesterone-dominated luteal phase compared with the E_2-dominated follicular phase and then rose in the progesterone withdrawal-initiated menstrual phase. By contrast, mRNA levels for the 72 kDa gelatinase (MMP2) and TIMP1 were relatively unchanged throughout the menstrual cycle.

Our initial *in vitro* studies of ovarian steroid effects on ECM-degrading protease expression in HESCs focused on uPA. Figure 3.4(b) shows that E_2 and progestin elicited effects on uPA protein expression in cultured HESCs that corresponded to those observed for tPA in Figure 3.4(a). Thus, MPA preferentially inhibited secreted levels of catalytically active uPA (white bars) compared with immunoreactive uPA (black bars). Moreover, there was greater inhibition in cultures incubated with E_2 plus MPA versus MPA despite the lack of response to E_2. Similar to tPA, the preferential inhibition in uPA activity is attributable to reciprocal upregulation of PAI-1 levels. Casslen and colleagues also observed reciprocal progestin upregulation of PAI-1[67] and downregulation of uPA[68] expression in HESC monolayers.

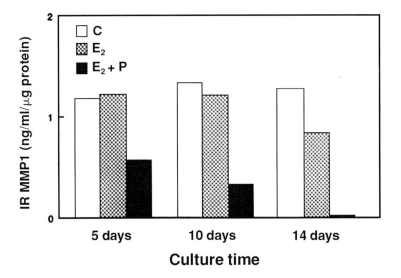

Figure 3.6. Time course of steroid modulated pro-MMP1 secretion by HESCs. Confluent HESCs were incubated in vehicle control (C), or 10^{-8} M E_2, or $E_2 + 10^{-7}$ M medroxyprogesterone acetate (P) for three consecutive 4- to 5-day intervals; the x-axis indicates pro-MMP1 levels in each collection interval measured by specific ELISA and corrected for cell protein; reproduced with permission from Lockwood *et al.*[69] (*Endocrinology*, © The Endocrine Society 1998)

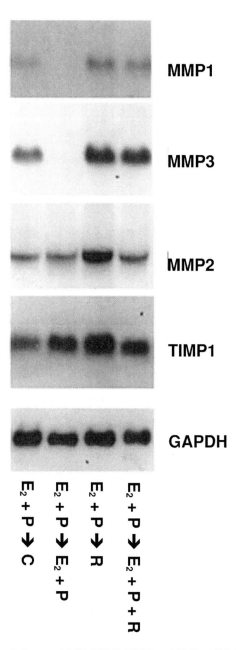

Figure 3.7. Steroid withdrawal effects on MMP1, MMP3, MMP2, and TIMP1 mRNA levels. Confluent primary HESCs were incubated with 10^{-8} M E_2 + 10^{-7} M medroxyprogesterone acetate (P) for 10 days then switched to new medium containing either vehicle control (C), or E_2 + P, or 10^{-6} M mifepristone (R), or E_2 + P + R for 8 days; to normalise for differences in RNA loading, the blot was stripped and reprobed for the *GAPDH* housekeeping gene; reproduced with permission from Lockwood *et al.*[69] (*Endocrinology*, © The Endocrine Society 1998)

Consistent with the differential steroid regulation of uPA expression depicted by Figure 3.4(b), Figure 3.6 indicates that E_2 alone did not alter HESC-secreted MMP1 levels, whereas E_2 plus MPA lowered MMP1 levels in a time-dependent fashion.[69] Progestin inhibition of MMP3 as well as MMP1 protein expression in HESCs has also been reported.[70–72] Figure 3.7 indicates that steady-state mRNA levels for MMP1 and MMP3 are inhibited by incubation with E_2 plus MPA and that this inhibition requires continuous progestin exposure. Thus, withdrawal of progestin stimulation either by switching to steroid-free medium or by exposure to the antiprogestin mifepristone reversed inhibition of MMP1 and MMP3 mRNA levels. By contrast, MMP2 and TIMP-1 mRNA levels were refractory to added progestin or progestin withdrawal. In HESCs, Salamonsen *et al.*[73] extended the absence of a progestin response to include other TIMP family members.

Discussion

The results from the *in vivo* and *in vitro* studies cited above demonstrate that progesterone-induced decidualisation of HESCs promotes haemostasis and strengthens the perivascular ECM support structure. These changes counteract the risk of pregnancy-terminating local haemorrhage during endovascular trophoblast invasion.

As illustrated in the model depicted in Figure 3.3, progesterone augmentation of endometrial haemostasis during decidualisation stems from the induction of TF expression. The consequent generation of thrombin promotes fibrin formation. The latter is enhanced by the reciprocal decrease in tPA expression and the dominant increase in PAI-1 expression. The consequent inhibition of tPA-mediated fibrinolysis complements enhanced TF expression to provide a potent pro-haemostatic signal.

The model depicted in Figure 3.8 demonstrates that progesterone-induced decidualisation of HESCs inhibits a stromal ECM-degrading proteolytic cascade. Specifically, progestin reduction in uPA activity is primarily a reflection of PAI-1 synthesis. The consequent decrease in plasmin generation curtails activation of pro-MMP1 and pro-MMP3. The reduction in MMP3 levels specifically limits positive feedback activation of pro-MMP1 and other MMP zymogens. Finally, progesterone directly inhibits the synthesis of pro-MMP1 and MMP3. This coordinated inhibition in protease activity bolsters the perivascular ECM scaffolding support structure. The resulting stabilisation of endometrial blood vessels increases resistance to local bleeding during endovascular trophoblast invasion.

This chapter has focused on the role of steroid-induced decidualisation in regulating endometrial haemostasis and vascular stability. Recent reviews by Christian *et al.*[74] and by Dunn *et al.*[75] summarised convincing evidence that other factors play key roles in modulating the decidualisation reaction *in vivo* and *in vitro*. Therefore, these factors deserve to be investigated for their potential role in directly affecting or in modulating ovarian steroid effects on the expression of regulators of haemostasis (i.e. TF and PAI-1) and of vascular stability (i.e. uPA, PAI-1, MMP1 and MMP3) during decidualisation of HESCs. Such factors include potential interactions between stromal cells and the resident leucocytes of the functional endometrial layer. Chief among these are uterine natural killer (NK) cells whose numbers increase in the peri-implantation period and represent the major leucocyte subtype at the implantation site.[76] Uterine NK cells have been implicated in maintaining decidualisation,[77] in limiting trophoblast invasion, and are a source of cytokines that could affect decidualisation.[76] The recent demonstration by Koopman *et al.*[78] that uterine NK cells

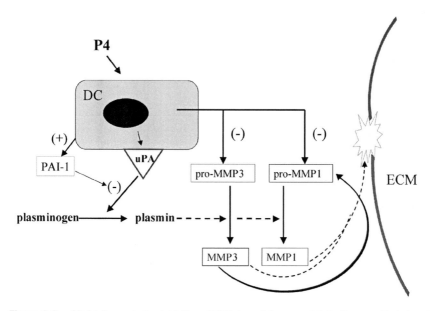

Figure 3.8. Model demonstrating inhibition of ECM degradation associated with progestin-induced decidualisation

overexpress a multitude of genes compared with their circulating CD56[bright] counterparts suggests a different origin for each.[78]

Interleukin 11 (IL11) and cyclic adenosine monophosphate (cAMP) merit particular consideration as potential modulators of decidualisation-related expression of regulators of endometrial haemostasis and vascular stability. Thus, IL11 promotes decidualisation and is produced by decidualised HESCs,[79] whereas intracellular cAMP is essential in mediating progesterone-induced decidualisation. Candidate ligands implicated in elevating intracellular cAMP levels in HESCs include prostaglandin E2, relaxin, corticotrophin-releasing hormone (CRH), luteinising hormone (LH) and follicle-stimulating hormone (FSH).[74] Intracellular cAMP activation of the protein kinase A pathway initiates a complex series of intracellular changes that account for the regulation of prolactin (PRL) expression during decidualisation.[80] To explain the paradox that elevated progesterone receptor (PR) levels act as negative regulator, whereas prolonged progestin treatment enhances decidual PRL expression, Brosens and colleagues[74] proposed a model in which 'activated PR is incorporated in a stoichiometric transcriptional active complex that contains other decidua-specific transcription factors and co-activators,' whereas 'suprastoichiometric PR levels sequester essential cofactors thereby inhibiting decidual PRL-promoter activity.' Although the PR-B isoform has generally been shown to be a stronger activator of progestin-induced transcription than the PR-A isoform, and PR-A can act as a dominant repressor of PR-B function,[81] in the model proposed by Christian *et al.*[74] PR-A but not PR-B plays a key transcriptional role.[82] Whether this model also applies to the regulation of markers of endometrial haemostasis and vascular stability in HESCs remains to be shown.

References

1. Moore KL. *The Developing Human*. 4th ed. Philadelphia: WB Saunders Company; 1988. p. 40.
2. Levy T, Dicker D, Ashkenazi J, Feldberg D, Shelef M, Goldman JA. The prognostic value and significance of preclinical abortions in *in vitro* fertilization-embryo transfer programs. *Fertil Steril* 1991;56:71–4.
3. Oka C, Makino T, Itakura I, Hara T, Nozawa S, Iizuka R. Chemical abortion in patients with recurrent fetal loss. *Nippon Sanka Fujinka Gakkai Zasshi* 1991;43:239–40.
4. Ramsey EM, Houston ML, Harris JW. Interactions of the trophoblast and maternal tissues in three closely related primate species. *Am J Obstet Gynecol* 1976;124:647–52.
5. De Wolf F, De Wolf-Peeters C, Brosens I. Ultrastructure of the spiral arteries in the human placental bed at the end of normal pregnancy. *Am J Obstet Gynecol* 1973;117:833–48.
6. Damsky CH, Fisher SJ. Trophoblast pseudo-vasculogenesis: faking it with endothelial adhesion receptors. *Curr Opin Cell Biol* 1998;10:660–6.
7. Shanklin DR, Scott JS. Massive subchorial thrombohaematoma (Breus' mole). *Br J Obstet Gynaecol* 1975;82:476–87.
8. Miller JF, Williamson E, Glue J, Gordon YB, Grudzinskas JG, Stykes A. Fetal loss after implantation. A prospective study. *Lancet* 1980;2:554–6.
9. Edmonds DK, Lindsay KS, Miller JF, Williamson E, Wood PJ. Early embryonic mortality in women. *Fertil Steril* 1982;38:447–53.
10. Bell SC. Decidualization and relevance to menstruation. In: D'Arcangues C, Fraser IS, Newton JR, Odlind V, editors. *Contraception and Mechanisms of Endometrial Bleeding*. Cambridge: Cambridge University Press; 1990. p. 188.
11. Lockwood CJ, Schatz F. A biological model for the regulation of peri-implantational hemostasis and menstruation. *J Soc Gynecol Investig* 1996;3:159–65.
12. Clark P. Changes of hemostasis variables during pregnancy. *Semin Vasc Med* 2003;3:13–24.
13. Bremme K, Ostlund E, Almqvist I, Heinonen K, Blomback M. Enhanced thrombin generation and fibrinolytic activity in normal pregnancy and the puerperium. *Obstet Gynecol* 1992;80:132–7.
14. Nemerson Y. Tissue factor and hemostasis. *Blood* 1988;71:1–8.
15. Guha A, Bach R, Konigsberg W, Nemerson Y. Affinity purification of human tissue factor: interaction of factor VII and tissue factor in detergent micelles. *Proc Natl Acad Sci U S A* 1986;83:299–302.
16. Bach RR. Initiation of coagulation by tissue factor. *CRC Crit Rev Biochem* 1988;23:339–68.
17. Carmeliet P, Mackman N, Moons L, Luther T, Gressens P, Van Vlaenderen I, et al. Role of tissue factor in embryonic blood vessel development. *Nature* 1996;383:73–5.
18. Parry GC, Erlich JH, Carmeliet P, Luther T, Mackman N. Low levels of tissue factor are compatible with development and hemostasis in mice. *J Clin Invest* 1998;101:560–9.
19. Erlich JH, Parry GC, Fearns C, Muller M, Carmeliet P, Luther T, et al. Tissue factor is required for uterine hemostasis and maintenance of the placental labyrinth during gestation. *Proc Natl Acad Sci U S A* 1999;96:8138–43.
20. Lockwood CJ, Nemerson Y, Guller S, Krikun G, Alvarez M, Hausknecht V, et al. Progestational regulation of human endometrial stromal cell tissue factor expression during decidualization. *J Clin Endocrinol Metab* 1993;76:231–6.
21. Lockwood CJ, Krikun G, Papp C, Toth-Pal E, Markiewicz L, Wang EY, et al. The role of progestationally regulated stromal cell tissue factor and type-1 plasminogen activator inhibitor (PAI-1) in endometrial hemostasis and menstruation. *Ann N Y Acad Sci* 1994;734:57–79.
22. Runic R, Schatz F, Krey L, Demopoulos R, Thung S, Wan L, et al. Alterations in endometrial stromal cell tissue factor protein and messenger ribonucleic acid expression in patients experiencing abnormal uterine bleeding while using NORPLANT-2 contraception. *J Clin Endocrinol Metab* 1997;82:1983–8.
23. Lockwood CJ, Krikun G, Papp C, Aigner S, Nemerson Y, Schatz F. Biological mechanisms underlying RU 486 clinical effects: Inhibition of endometrial stromal cell tissue factor content. *J Clin Endocrinol Metab* 1994;79:786–90.
24. Eckert RL, Katzenellenbogen BS. Human endometrial cells in primary tissue culture: modulation of the progesterone receptor level by natural and synthetic estrogens in vitro. *J Clin Endocrinol Metab* 1981;52:699–708.
25. Lubbert H, Pollow K, Rommler A, Hammerstein J. Estradiol and progesterone receptor concentrations and 17beta-hydroxysteroid-dehydrogenase activity in estrogen-progestin stimulated endometrium of women with gonadal dysgenesis. *J Steroid Biochem* 1982;17:143–8.
26. Guller S, LaCroix NC, Krikun G, Wozniak R, Markiewicz L, Wang E-Y, et al. Steroid regulation of

oncofetal fibronectin expression in human cytotrophoblasts. *J Steroid Biochem Mol Biol* 1993;46:1–10.

27. Arici A, Marshburn PB, MacDonald PC, Dombrowski RA. Progesterone metabolism in human endometrial stromal and gland cells in culture. *Steroids* 1999;64:530–4.

28. Lockwood CJ, Nemerson Y, Krikun G, Hausknecht V, Markiewicz L, Alvarez, *et al.* Steroid-modulated stromal cell tissue factor expression: A model for the regulation of endometrial hemostasis and menstruation. *J Clin Endocrinol Metab* 1993;77:1014–19.

29. Galdal KS, Lyberg T, Evensen SA, Nilsen E, Prydz H. Thrombin induces thromboplastin synthesis in cultured vascular endothelial cells. *Thromb Haemost* 1985;54:373–6.

30. Bartha K, Brisson C, Archipoff G, de la Salle C, Lanza F, Cazenave JP, *et al.* Thrombin regulates tissue factor and thrombomodulin mRNA level and activities in human saphenous vein endothelial cells by distinct mechanisms. *J Biol Chem* 1993;268:421–9.

31. Donovan-Peluso M, George LD, Hasset AC. Lipopolysaccharide induction of tissue factor expression in THP-1 monocytic cells, protein–DNA interactions with the promoter. *J Biol Chem* 1994;269:1361–9.

32. Oeth PA, Parry GCN, Kunsch C, Nantermet P, Rosen C, Mackman N. Lipopolysaccharide induction of tissue factor gene expression in monocytic cells is mediated by binding of c-Rel/p65 heterodimers. *Mol Cell Biol* 1994;14:3772–81.

33. Felts SJ, Stoflet ES, Eggers CT, Getz MJ. Tissue Factor gene transcription in serum-stimulated fibroblasts is mediated by recruitment of c-fos into specific AP-1 DNA-binding complexes. *Biochemistry* 1995;34:12355–62.

34. Cui MZ, Parry GC, Oeth P, Larson H, Smith M, Huang RP, *et al.* Transcriptional regulation of the tissue factor gene in human epithelial cells is mediated by SP1 and EGR-1. *J Biol Chem* 1996;271:2731–9.

35. Mackman N. Regulation of the tissue factor gene. *Thromb Haemost* 1997;78:747–54.

36. Krikun G, Schatz F, Mackman N, Guller S, Lockwood CJ. Transcriptional regulation of the tissue factor gene by progestins in human endometrial stromal cells. *J Clin Endocrinol Metab* 1998;83:926–30.

37. Krikun G, Schatz F, Mackman N, Guller S, Demopoulos R, Lockwood CJ. Regulation of tissue factor gene expression in human endometrium by transcription factors Sp1 and Sp3. *Mol Endocrinol* 2000;14:393–400.

38. Vassalli JD, Sappino AP, Belin D. The plasminogen activator/plasmin system. *J Clin Invest* 1991;88:1067–72.

39. Stassen JM, Arnout J, Deckmyn H. The hemostatic system. Curr Med Chem 2004;11:2245–60.

40. Mignatti P, Rifkin DB. Biology and biochemistry of proteinases in tumor invasion. *Physiol Rev* 1993;73:161–95.

41. Koh SC, Wong PC, Yuen R, Chua SE, Ng BL, Ratnam SS. Concentration of plasminogen activators and inhibitor in the human endometrium at different phases of the menstrual cycle. *J Reprod Fertil* 1992;96:407–13.

42. Schatz F, Aigner S, Papp C, Toth-Pal E, Hausknecht V, Lockwood CJ. Plasminogen activator activity during decidualization of human endometrial stromal cells is regulated by plasminogen activator inhibitor 1. *J Clin Endocrinol Metab* 1995;80:2504–10.

43. Schatz F, Lockwood CJ. Progestin regulation of plasminogen activator inhibitor type 1 in primary cultures of endometrial stromal and decidual cells. *J Clin Endocrinol Metab* 1993;77:621–5.

44. Aplin JD. Cellular biology of the endometrium. In: Wynn RM, Jolie WP, editors. *Biology of the Uterus.*, 2nd ed. New York: Plenum Press; 1988. p. 187–202.

45. Wewer UM, Faber M, Liotta LA, Albrechtsen R. Immunochemical and ultrastructural assessment of the nature of the pericellular basement membrane of human decidual cells. *Lab Invest* 1985;53:624–33.

46. Kislaus LL, Herr JC, Little CD. Immunolocalization of extracellular matrix proteins and collagen synthesis in first trimester human decidua. *Anat Rec* 1987;218:402–15.

47. Church HJ, Vicovac LM, Williams JDL, Hey NA, Aplin JD. Laminins 2 and 4 are expressed by human decidual cells. *Lab Invest* 1996;74:21–32.

48. Ossowski L. Invasion of connective tissue by human carcinoma cell lines: requirement for urokinase, urokinase receptor, and interstitial collagenase. *Cancer Res* 1992;52:6754–60.

49. Liu D, Aguirre Ghiso J, Estrada Y, Ossowski L. EGFR is a transducer of the urokinase receptor initiated signal that is required for in vivo growth of a human carcinoma. *Cancer Cell* 2002;1:445–57.

50. Hollas W, Blasi F, Boyd D. Role of the urokinase receptor in facilitating extracellular matrix invasion by cultured colon cancer. *Cancer Res* 1991;51:3690–5.

51. Liu J, Chakraborty C, Graham CH, Barbin YP, Dixon SJ, Lala PK. Noncatalytic domain of uPA stimulates human extravillous trophoblast migration by using phospholipase C, phosphatidylinositol 3-kinase and mitogen-activated protein kinase. *Exp Cell Res* 2003;286:138–51.

52. Nordengren J, Pilka R, Noskova V, Ehinger A, Domanski H, Andersson C, *et al.* Differential localization and expression of urokinase plasminogen activator (uPA), its receptor (uPAR), and its inhibitor (PAI-1) mRNA and protein in endometrial tissue during the menstrual cycle. Mol Hum Reprod 2004;10:655–63.

53. Floridon C, Nielsen O, Holund B, Sunde L, Westergaard JG, Thomsen SG, *et al.* Localization and significance of urokinase plasminogen activator and its receptor in placental tissue from intrauterine, ectopic and molar pregnancies. *Placenta* 1999;20:711–21.

54. Chen ZL, Strickland S. Neuronal death in the hippocampus is promoted by plasmin-catalyzed degradation of laminin. *Cell* 1997;91:917–25.

55. Bonnefoy A, Legrand C. Proteolysis of subendothelial adhesive glycoproteins (fibronectin, thrombospondin, and von Willebrand factor) by plasmin, leukocyte cathepsin G, and elastase. *Thromb Res* 2000;98:323–32.

56. Nakagami Y, Abe K, Nishiyama N, Matsuki N. Laminin degradation by plasmin regulates long-term potentiation. *J Neurosci* 2000;20:2003–10.

57. Birkedal-Hansen H, Moore WG, Bodden MK, Windsor LJ, Birkedal-Hansen B, DeCarlo A, *et al.* Matrix metalloproteinases: a review. *Crit Rev Oral Biol Med* 1993;4:197–250.

58. Nagase H. Stromelysins 1 and 2. In: Parks WC, Mecham R, editors. *Matrix Metalloproteinases.* San Diego: Academic Press; 1988. p. 43–84.

59. He CS, Wilhelm SM, Pentland AP, Marmer BL, Grant GA, Eisen AZ, *et al.* Tissue cooperation in a proteolytic cascade activating human interstitial collagenase. *Proc Natl Acad Sci U S A* 1989;86:2632–6.

60. Ogata Y, Enghild JJ, Nagase H. Matrix metalloproteinase 3 (stromelysin) activates the precursor for the human matrix metalloproteinase. *J Biol Chem* 1992;267:3581–4.

61. Knauper V, Lopez-Otin C, Smith B, Knight G, Murphy G. Biochemical characterization of human collagenase-3. *J Biol Chem* 1996;271:1544–50.

62. McDonnell S, Wright JH, Gaire M, Matrisian LM. Expression and regulation of stromelysin and matrilysin by growth factors and oncogenes. *Biochem Soc Trans* 1994;22:58–63.

63. Gaire M, Magbanua Z, McDonnell S, McNeil L, Lovett DH, Matrisian LM, *et al.* Structure and expression of the human gene for the matrix metalloproteinase matrilysin. *J Biol Chem* 1994;269:2032–40.

64. Matrisian LM. Matrix metalloproteinase gene expression. *Ann NY Acad Sci* 1994;732:42–50.

65. Lambert E, Dasse E, Haye B, Petitfrere E. TIMPs as multifacial proteins. *Crit Rev Oncol Hematol* 2004;49:187–98.

66. Rodgers WH, Matrisian LM, Giudice LC, Dsupin B, Cannon P, Svitek C, *et al.* Patterns of matrix metalloproteinase expression in cycling endometrium imply differential functions and regulation by steroid hormones. *J Clin Invest* 1994;94:946–53.

67. Casslen B, Urano S, Ny T. Progesterone regulation of plasminogen activator inhibitor 1 (PAI-1) antigen and mRNA levels in human endometrial stromal cells. *Thromb Res* 1992;66:75–87.

68. Casslen B, Urano S, Lecander I, Ny T. Plasminogen activators in the human endometrium, cellular origin and hormonal regulation. *Blood Coagul Fibrinolysis* 1992;3:133–8.

69. Lockwood CJ, Krikun G, Hausknecht VA, Papp C, Schatz F. Matrix metalloproteinase and matrix metalloproteinase inhibitor expression in endometrial stromal cells during progestin-initiated decidualization and menstruation-regulated progestin withdrawal. *Endocrinol* 1998;139:4607–13.

70. Schatz F, Papp C, Aigner S, Krikun G, Hausknecht V, Lockwood CJ. Biological mechanisms underlying the clinical effects of RU 486: modulation of cultured endometrial stromal cell stromelysin-1 and prolactin expression. *J Clin Endocrinol Metab* 1997;82:188–93.

71. Bruner KL, Eisenberg E, Gorstein F, Osteen KG. Progesterone and transforming growth factor-beta coordinately regulate suppression of endometrial matrix metalloproteinases in a model of experimental endometriosis. *Steroids* 1999;64:648–53.

72. Hampton AL, Nie G, Salamonsen LA. Progesterone analogues similarly modulate endometrial matrix metalloproteinase-1 and matrix metalloproteinase-3 and their inhibitor in a model for long-term contraceptive effects. *Mol Hum Reprod* 1999;5:365–7.

73. Salamonsen LA, Butt AR, Hammond FR, Garcia S, Zhang J. Production of endometrial matrix metalloproteinases, but not their tissue inhibitors, is modulated by progesterone withdrawal in an in vitro model for menstruation. *J Clin Endocrinol Metab* 1997;82:1409–15.

74. Christian M, Mak I, White JO, Brosens JJ. Mechanisms of decidualization. *Reprod Biomed Online* 2002;4 Suppl 3:24–30.

75. Dunn CL, Kelly RW, Critchley HOD. Decidualization of the human endometrial stromal cell: an enigmatic transformation. *Reprod Biomed Online* 2003;7:151–61.

76. Moffett-King A. Natural killer cells and pregnancy. *Nat Rev Immunol* 2002;2:656–63.

77. Croy BA, Chantakru S, Esadeg S, Ashkar AA, Wei Q. Decidual natural killer cells: key regulators of placental development (a review). *J Reprod Immunol* 2002;57:151–68.

78. Koopman LA, Kopcow HD, Rybalov B, Boyson JE, Orange JS, Schatz F, *et al.* Human decidual natural killer cells are a unique NK cell subset with immunomodulatory potential. *J Exp Med* 2003;198:1201–12.

79. Dimitriadis E, Robb L, Salamonsen LA. Interleukin 11 advances progesterone-induced decidualization of human endometrial stromal cells. *Mol Hum Reprod* 2002;8:636–43.

80. Brosens JJ, Hayashi N, White JO. Progesterone receptor regulates decidual prolactin expression in differentiating human endometrial stromal cells. *Endocrinology* 1999;140:4809–20.

81. Giangrande PH, McDonnell DP. The A and B isoforms of the human progesterone receptor: two functionally different transcription factors encoded by a single gene. *Recent Prog Horm Res* 1999;54:291–313.

82. Christian M, Pohnke Y, Kempf R, Gellersen B, Brosens JJ. Functional association of PR and CCAAT/enhancer-binding protein beta isoforms: promoter-dependent cooperation between PR-B and liver-enriched inhibitory protein, or liver-enriched activatory protein and PR-A in human endometrial stromal cells. *Mol Endocrinol* 2002;16:141–54.

Chapter 4
Adhesion molecules and implantation

John D Aplin

The timing of implantation

There is evidence that the uterus is receptive to an implanting blastocyst from approximately 7 to 11 days after the luteinising hormone (LH) peak.[1-3] Effective receptivity may well end in the human when corpus luteum rescue is no longer feasible, rather than as a result of a change in uterine properties. Thus the risk of early pregnancy loss increases with later implantation, from 13% on day 9 after ovulation to 82% on day 12 or later.[4] Many conceptuses fail to implant because of genetic or metabolic abnormalities.[5,6] Poor uterine receptivity has been widely proposed as another cause of implantation failure,[7-9] but it remains unclear to what extent this may be because of defective synchronisation between embryo development and maternal differentiation, undetected embryo abnormalities, or a real failure of uterine capability to support implantation of a normal conceptus. For practical reasons, the term 'implantation failure' is often used to include a range of outcomes from blastocyst non-attachment to biochemical (human chorionic gonadotrophin (hCG)-positive) pregnancies that do not give rise to a functioning embryonic heart, that is to say, those that fail in the first 4–5 weeks. Such a definition encompasses implantation and placental organogenesis; this article mostly addresses the former, drawing pertinent comparative information from animal models. Knowledge of early placental development is emerging from mouse genetics[10] and culture models[11-13] but this lies outside the scope of the present discussion.

The embryo–endometrial dialogue

Pre-implantation endocrine patterns of human conception cycles closely resemble those seen in non-conception cycles, although circulating luteal-phase oestrogen and progesterone levels are rather higher in the former.[14] However, there is evidence that an embryo–maternal dialogue can influence the receptive phase, and that such signals pass bidirectionally. Thus, for example, mouse embryos replaced at the pronuclear stage, and simultaneously into the contra-lateral oviduct at the eight-cell stage, will implant, although in the former case this is delayed by at least one day. Developmental synchronisation has occurred by the neural plate stage of development.[15]

Tubal and uterine secretions contribute to the pre-implantation embryonic environment and have a clear impact on pregnancy outcome. Granulocyte-macrophage colony-stimulating factor (GM–CSF) produced by the uterine epithelium and stimulated by oestradiol[16] participates in pre-implantation maternal–embryonic signalling. The embryo expresses a GM–CSF receptor.[17] Mice genetically altered to lack GM–CSF produce blastocysts with fewer cells in the inner cell mass (ICM), and these give rise to small pups. The defect can be rescued by culturing null pre-implantation embryos in medium supplemented with GM–CSF before replacement. Human embryos also contain GM–CSF receptors, indicating the possibility of a similar mechanism.[18,19]

Calcitonin is an endometrial gland cell secretory product expressed in response to progesterone,[20] and is important for pregnancy outcome in rodents, as indicated by a reduction in implantation rates if maternal expression in rats is blocked using antisense oligonucleotide.[21] Calcitonin acts on the pre-implantation embryo by binding a G-protein-coupled receptor, triggering an increase in intracellular calcium, activation of adenyl cyclase and expression of the fibronectin receptor, integrin $\alpha_5\beta_1$.[22] Binding to fibronectin in the maternal stroma is likely to be important in trophoblast invasion in the post-implantation phase. Other data indicate that calcium is likely to be important in signalling at implantation.[23–25]

Systemic maternal and local embryonic signalling occur via distinct molecular pathways. The connexins Cx26 and Cx43, protein components of the gap junctions that laterally couple uterine epithelial cells, are induced by oestrogen, and downregulated by progesterone in the mouse pre-implantation phase. They are then locally induced by the embryo in the implantation chamber via an oestrogen receptor-independent mechanism. Candidate inducers include embryo-derived catecholoestrogen,[26,27] and the proinflammatory mediators interleukin 1β (IL1β) and prostaglandin $F_{2\alpha}$.[28] Implantation and decidualisation have some resemblance to a local inflammatory response. Prostaglandins appear to be involved in the mouse as key modulators of downstream signalling pathways leading to decidualisation; thus the Cox2 null mouse is infertile and its uterine stroma fails to decidualise.[29–31] The epidermal growth factor (EGF) family of ligands and cognate receptors are also involved in the peri-implantation dialogue in mice.[27] Ron, a tyrosine kinase receptor that interacts with signalling pathways involving the EGF receptor, is also required for progression through the implantation phase.[32] The relevance of these pathways in humans remains to be elucidated.

Hatching

Before an embryo can attach to the uterine surface, it must hatch from the zona pellucida. Two mouse serine proteases, ISP1 and ISP2 (implantation serine proteases 1 and 2), have been implicated in hatching. ISP1 is produced by the embryo, while ISP2 is produced by uterine glands. These enzymes may also be required for local proteolysis of maternal tissue as part of the process of invasion.[33]

The maternal barrier

The maternal surface is nonreceptive except during the implantation phase. Like other epithelial surfaces, it contains an apical glycocalyx (thick glycoprotein coat) which allows the diffusion of small molecules but inhibits cell adhesion.[2] In this way it acts as a component of the innate immune system, protecting the upper female tract from infectious agents. The cell surface mucin MUC1 is present in the uterine glycocalyx.[34–37] In mice and rats, MUC1 is downregulated precisely at the time of implantation under the control of maternal steroids.[38] Consistent with this, it emerges as a highly upregulated (6-fold) gene at day 4 in pregnant mice that have been treated at day 3 with a single dose of antiprogestin.[39] There is evidence that another surface mucin, MUC4, is also downregulated in rodents.[40] In contrast, humans express high levels of MUC1 throughout the receptive phase, although its pattern of glycosylation changes. Certain mucin-associated oligosaccharides are useful markers of endometrial differentiation[37] and pathology.[41,42] Experimental studies of human implantation in which embryos hatch and attach to endometrial epithelial cells in monolayer culture have shown that MUC1 disappears from a small area of cells that surrounds the attached embryo.[43,44] Maternal cells further away continue to express the glycoprotein, thus presumably maintaining their barrier property and minimising access of pathogens to the underlying tissue and vasculature. It has been shown that proteolytic cleavage events catalysed by either a disintegrin and metalloprotease 17/tumour necrosis factor α converting enzyme (ADAM17/TACE) or membrane-type 1 matrix metalloproteinase (MT1-MMP) can mediate release of MUC1 from the surface of cultured cells; both these enzymes are expressed in the maternal epithelium.[45,46]

These observations further illustrate the highly localised dialogue that occurs between embryonic and maternal cells. Since blastocysts of high quality are expected to produce the strongest signals, they also lead to a hypothesis that embryo selection occurs at implantation as a result of the need for embryos to overcome an endometrial surface barrier.[2,6]

Embryo attachment

Embryo apposition is followed by attachment of trophectoderm to uterine epithelium. Numerous molecular changes have been reported that correlate with the receptive phase and it is likely that a cascade of adhesion events is required,[2,47–51] but there exists insufficient evidence either in human or other animal species to identify unequivocally the interactions that attach the implanting embryo to the endometrium. Indeed, this is one of the important unsolved problems of contemporary biology.

Several approaches have been taken, giving rise to the panel of molecular markers shown in Table 4.1. The term 'marker' is used advisedly because, while the inclusion criteria include the ability to function as an adhesion molecule, as well as presence at the implantation site, *in vivo* functional evidence is so far mostly lacking (reviewed by Aplin and Kimber[51]). Broadly, the approaches include identification of candidate molecules active in other cell adhesion systems, use of mouse genetics to examine fertility impairment of these candidates, serendipitous infertility in mouse genetic models, identification of candidates using *in vitro* implantation models or *in utero* gene knockdown approaches, and larger-scale screening of relevant mRNA populations in human or animal models.

Candidate adhesion molecules

Integrin $\alpha_v\beta_3$ has been suggested to be important in embryo attachment.[7] The β_3 subunit exhibits regulated expression such that the heterodimer $\alpha_v\beta_3$ is present in human endometrial epithelium only from about day 19. There is evidence for

Table 4.1. Adhesion molecules proposed to play a role in implantation; cell surface and extracellular (secreted, either luminally or in the ECM) components are listed; for brevity, molecular families are specified rather than individual members; decreased expression in the implantation phase has been reported in some components (e.g. some collagens); some genes (e.g. SPARC) have been reported as either down- or upregulated at implantation phase, perhaps reflecting different behaviour in different cell types; primary references can be retrieved via open access from Aplin and Kimber;[51] earlier evidence is given in detail in Aplin (1997)[2]

Adhesion molecule	Location[a]	Maternal/embryonic	Species[c]	Method of identification[d]
Integrins	cs	endo, bl	h, pr, m, rabbit, ruminant, pig	cand, KO (β1), mic
Basigin/EMMPRIN/CD147	cs	endo, bl	m, rat	KO
Cadherins	cs	endo, bl	h, m	cand, mic
Trophinin	cs	endo, bl	h, m, pig	model, KO
CD44	cs	endo, bl	h, m	cand
Selectins and ligands (SLex)	cs, s	endo, bl	h, m	cand
Other glycans: H type I, Ley	cs, s	endo	h, m	cand
Glycam 1	cs, s	endo	sheep, pig	cand
HB-EGF	cs, s	endo, bl	h, m, rat, hamster, rabbit	model
Laminins	s	endo	h, m, rat	cand, mic
Fibulins	s	endo	h, m, pig	cand, mic
Tenascins	s	endo	h, m	cand, mic
Collagens	s	endo	h	cand, mic
SPARC/osteonectin	s	endo	h, m	cand, mic
Thrombospondins	s	endo	h, m	cand, mic
Perlecan	s	endo, bl	m, rat	mic
Mucin (MUC1)	cs, s	endo, bl	h, pr, m, rat, rabbit, ruminant	cand, mic
Mucin (MUC4)	cs, s	endo	rat	cand, mic

[1] cs = cell surface; s = secreted
[b] endo = endometrium; bl = blastocyst
[c] m = mouse; h = human; pr = non-human primate
[d] cand = candidate gene; mic = microarray; KO = mouse genetics; model = *in vitro* implantation model

expression of this integrin at the trophectodermal surface of the embryo in some species, as well as in trophoblast. One of its ligands, osteopontin, a secretory product of endometrial glands, is associated with the apical surface of luminal epithelial cells, and is directly regulated by progesterone, with maximal abundance in the secretory phase.[52,53] A decrease in implantation rates has been reported in rabbits treated *in utero* with reagents that block $\alpha_v\beta_3$ function.[54] An interesting series of investigations has compared the expression of $\alpha_v\beta_3$ with a putative morphological marker of receptivity, the uterodomes that appear at the luminal epithelial surface in the mid-secretory phase.[55-58] Both were effective as markers of cycle progression, and they appeared to be under independent regulation, but variations in the timing of expression of each appeared to be compatible with implantation. Significant cycle-to-cycle variation was noted in the timing of marker appearance in the same women.

Expression of integrin $\alpha_4\beta_1$ is highest in human glandular epithelium between the mid-proliferative and mid-secretory phases. In mice, in addition to its presence on the surface of activated blastocysts, $\alpha_4\beta_1$ appears on the basal luminal epithelial surface and stromal cells in response to oestrogen, and intrauterine injection of monoclonal antibody to α_4 reduced implantation rates.[59] Fibronectin and vascular cell adhesion molecule 1 (VCAM-1) act as ligands for this integrin but it is not yet clear what interaction the intervention is targeting.

Heparin-binding EGF-like growth factor (HB-EGF) appears in epithelial cells immediately adjacent to the implanting embryo just 6–7 hours before it attaches. HB-EGF has been suggested to play two different roles: in addition to accelerating embryo development, it has a membrane-bound variant that can mediate intercellular attachment by binding to ErbB4 and heparan sulphate proteoglycan, both of which are present on the blastocyst.[60]

Mouse genetic models

Numerous genes whose products have been predicted to play a role in implantation have been targeted, and fertility tested in homozygous null offspring. The leukaemia inhibitory factor (LIF)-null mouse[61] is a fascinating and influential paradigm of implantation failure associated with defective maternal paracrine signalling and decidualisation. Many other gene deletions, however, have failed to confirm the direct involvement of the corresponding candidate gene product. Thus, for example, mice lacking integrin α_v or any one of the β subunits with which it associates are fertile, as are osteopontin-null mice. CD44 is an alternative receptor for osteopontin, and again null animals are fertile. Selectin–carbohydrate interactions have been suggested to mediate early attachment, but L-, P- and E-selectin null mice all appear fertile, as do the various double knockouts. More subtle abnormalities may remain to be uncovered. Mice lacking trophinin, a homotypic adhesion molecule, implant but fail slightly later;[62] human fallopian tube epithelium expresses trophinin at ectopic sites in response to hCG,[63] suggesting trophinin's role in the two species may differ. Of course, lack of phenotype does not provide unequivocal proof of non-involvement, but rather just indicates that the gene is non-essential. In fact, it may be that single-gene approaches are limited precisely because there are several adhesion mechanisms available.

Binding to extracellular matrix (ECM) in the maternal stroma is important once the epithelium is breached; trophoblast integrins act as receptors for ECM ligands. Mouse embryos that lack integrin β_1, which dimerises with various α chains to produce a repertoire of ECM receptors, fail to complete implantation, probably because they lack the ability to bind the maternal ECM.[64] ECM remodelling occurs during the secretory phase and decidualisation,[65] with the loss of components such as collagen VI[66,67] and decorin[68] and increases in laminins[69,70] and fibulin 1.[71]

Basigin (EMMPRIN, CD147) is an immunoglobulin superfamily member with putative roles in cell interaction, MMP activation and orientation of ion transporters in the plasma membrane. It is expressed in the endometrial epithelium and also in decidual cells. Transfer of wild-type blastocysts into basigin-null females results in a very low rate of implantation.[72]

Adhesion molecules and the endometrial transcriptome

The search for elusive markers of endometrial receptivity has recently involved the use of microarrays to delineate alterations in the endometrial transcriptome that occur at receptivity. Several studies[73–76] have used a design that compares endometrium in mid-secretory-phase with pre-implantation stages (either early secretory or proliferative). In one study,[76] patient-to-patient variation was eliminated by sampling tissue from the same individual at two different stages of the same cycle. While some known genes have exhibited alterations consistent with previous data – osteopontin upregulation is a notable example – and some interesting genes have emerged that will require functional study, other candidate genes are conspicuous by their absence (trophinin, integrin β_3). It is clear that a significant number of genes are downregulated at this time, with others increasing. Growth factors (such as LIF), tyrosine kinase family receptors or transcription factors (e.g. HOXA10) may directly or indirectly influence the downstream expression of a set of target genes, including those that may directly be involved in cell interactions at implantation. It will be necessary to ask whether expression of 'master genes' with the ability to alter endometrial 'settings' (patterns of gene expression) is altered in infertile women.

In any case, consistent patterns of receptive-state gene expression have not yet emerged from the transcriptomic analysis. A number of reasons can be adduced. There is no ideal control tissue, as proliferative or early secretory phases, although nonreceptive to the embryo, are not true 'neutral' states. The shifting cell populations characteristic of cycling endometrium affect the profile of genes detected in tissue biopsies that contain vascular, stromal and immune elements as well as gland and luminal epithelium. The scale of transcriptional alteration may be quite small (frequently less than 2-fold) and fail to reach statistical significance despite being biologically relevant. It is clear that the receptive endometrium encompasses an envelope of states reflecting a range of histological[42,58,77,78] and, by inference, transcriptomic features. Some of these problems are being addressed by improved experimental design, using purified cell populations (e.g. uterine epithelium[79]) or animal models in which there is scope for improving the resolution of the analysis. Examples include comparing LIF-null with wild-type uterine cells[80,81] and double-screening using the infertile progesterone receptor-null mouse alongside wild-type animals treated with a contraceptive dose of antiprogestin.[39] The latter approach has led to the identification of immune response gene 1 (*Irg1*), encoding a protein predicted to be involved in lipid metabolism, in the implantation-phase luminal epithelium.[82] *In vivo* uterine administration of antisense oligonucleotide to *Irg1* blocks implantation. LIF upregulates *Irg1* expression in mice[80] and is linked to the protein kinase C (PKC) signalling pathway.[83] Other such studies have yielded genes that appear not to be functionally involved in implantation (e.g. cochlin[81]). At the very least, microarrays provide a medium-sensitivity index of the genes that are expressed in the tissue.

Profound alterations in cell surface composition and organisation can occur without any change in transcription. Post-translational modification by phosphorylation, sulphation, glycosylation, lipid conjugation, cross-linking or proteolysis is common. Redistribution of existing gene products into different membrane compartments or supramolecular assemblies may be just as important as *de novo* transcription in the conversion to a receptive state. Critically, the biochemical dialogue between the embryo and the endometrium that determines endometrial receptivity at the attachment site cannot emerge from an analysis of either one alone.

Endometrial receptivity in fertile and infertile women

Infertile endometrium displays molecular alterations that are not always evident histologically. For example, epithelial expression of a mucin-associated glycan at day LH+7, when correlated with histology and endocrine measurements, showed in women with unexplained infertility[41] or recurrent miscarriage[42] that aberrant expression could occur in the context of either normal or temporally retarded histology. Such studies, however, can only be correlative until a clear functional link is made to the molecular apparatus of implantation.

Clinical and treatment implications

Some variation in the differentiation state of the endometrium is compatible with implantation. Similarly, blastocysts with varying characteristics, such as greater or fewer cells,[84] imprinting alterations[85] or chromosomal abnormalities,[6] may implant. The embryo–endometrial dialogue has been hitherto largely inaccessible to experimental or clinical manipulation, but one can anticipate that future advances will be concerned with identifying, and seeking to augment, local signalling pathways at implantation.[86] The development of improved, more accessible *in vitro* models of implantation in the human will be important, and the emergence of human trophoblast stem cell lines[87] should offer opportunities in this respect.

Embryo quality is a central issue. Treatments to improve endometrium or prevent miscarriage are not appropriate if pregnancy loss is occurring as a result of karyotypic or structural abnormalities. Conversely, studies designed to establish efficacy of a given treatment must take account of the fact that many pregnancies will be lost as a result of embryonic abnormality. Future treatments may address the ovarian pathology of abnormal oocyte production, improve the developmental trajectory of the pre-implantation zygote or improve the maternal uterine environment. Enhancing the embryo–endometrial dialogue to maintain normal early pregnancy would be appropriate only after loss of *normal* pregnancies. Similarly, any treatment aimed at improving the rate of normal pregnancy following recurrent aneuploidy should include only couples known recurrently to lose *abnormal* pregnancies.

Conclusion

Is the improvement of implantation rates a suitable goal for medical research? Implantation failure and early pregnancy loss impose a less severe biological burden than the evasion of natural selection by a fraction of abnormal embryos. High rates of early pregnancy failure in humans reflect the high rate of embryo abnormality in our species and the fact that the optimal time period in which to select a healthy conceptus are the pre-implantation and early post-implantation phases.

The quality of the pre-implantation embryo is critical for optimal fetal development and the health of offspring. In mice, blastocysts that have larger numbers of cells go on to produce larger pups.[84] Epidemiological evidence shows that low birthweight is a risk factor for high blood pressure, heart disease and diabetes.[88] Facilitating the implantation of poor-quality embryos would be counterproductive if sustaining good health into old age is an agreed aim. On the other hand, with high-quality embryos, pregnancy is possible in both infertile and postmenopausal women. This is not to argue that the uterus is a passive vehicle; instead it is an active participant in a two-way molecular dialogue with the embryo, and this process itself contributes to embryo selection. Both uterine receptivity and embryo quality are influenced by locally produced growth factors and cytokines, and these in turn depend on the ovary. Improved endometrial receptivity is achievable with improved knowledge of the components of this dialogue, but can only become a reasonable therapeutic objective when defective receptivity can be unequivocally specified as the cause of infertility.

References

1. Bergh PA, Navot D. The impact of embryonic development and endometrial maturity on the timing of implantation. *Fertil Steril* 1992;58:537–42.
2. Aplin JD. Adhesion molecules in implantation. *Rev Reprod* 1997;2:84–93.
3. Aplin JD. Implantation. In: Simpson E, editor. *Encyclopedia of Hormones*. San Diego: Academic Press; 2003. p. 289–97.
4. Wilcox AJ, Baird DD, Weinberg CR. Time of implantation of the conceptus and loss of pregnancy. *N Engl J Med* 1999;340:1796–9.
5. Pellicer A, Rubio C, Vidal F, Minguez Y, Gimenez C, Egozcue J, et al. In vitro fertilization plus preimplantation genetic diagnosis in patients with recurrent miscarriage: an analysis of chromosome abnormalities in human preimplantation embryos. Fertil Steril 1999;71:1033–9.
6. Quenby S, Vince G, Farquharson R, Aplin J. Recurrent miscarriage: a defect in nature's quality control? *Hum Reprod* 2002;17:1959–63.
7. Lessey BA. Uterine factors in implantation. In: *The Endometrium*. Glasser SR, Aplin JD, Giudice L, Tabibzadeh S, editors. London: Taylor and Francis; 2002. p. 208–28.
8. Chang PL, Sauer MV. The oocyte donation model: lessons on endometrial receptivity. In: *The Endometrium*. Glasser SR, Aplin JD, Giudice L, Tabibzadeh S, editors. London: Taylor and Francis; 2002. p. 495–509.
9. Sharkey AM, Smith SK. The endometrium as a cause of implantation failure. *Best Pract Res Clin Obstet Gynaecol* 2003;17:289–307.
10. Rossant J, Cross JC. Placental development: lessons from mouse mutants. *Nat Rev Genet* 2001;2:538–48.
11. Aplin JD, Haigh T, Vicovac L, Church HJ, Jones CJ. Anchorage in the developing placenta: an overlooked determinant of pregnancy outcome? *Hum Fertil* 1998;1:75–9.
12. Aplin JD. Maternal influences on placental development. *Semin Cell Dev Biol* 2000;11:115–25.
13. Aplin JD, Haigh T, Lacey H, Chen CP, Jones CJ. Tissue interactions in the control of trophoblast invasion. *J Reprod Fertil Suppl* 2000;55:57–64.
14. Baird DD, Wilcox AJ, Weinberg CR, Kamel F, McConnaughey DR, Musey PI, et al. Preimplantation hormonal differences between the conception and non-conception menstrual cycles of 32 normal women. *Hum Reprod* 1997;12:2607–13.
15. Ueda O, Yorozu K, Kamada N, Jishage K, Kawase Y, Toyoda Y, et al. Possible expansion of 'Window of Implantation' in pseudopregnant mice: time of implantation of embryos at different stages of development transferred into the same recipient. *Biol Reprod* 2003;69:1085–90.
16. Robertson SA, Mayrhofer G, Seamark RF. Ovarian steroid hormones regulate granulocyte-macrophage colony-stimulating factor synthesis by uterine epithelial cells in the mouse. *Biol Reprod* 1996;54:183–96.

17. Robertson SA, Sjoblom C, Jasper MJ, Norman RJ, Seamark RF. Granulocyte-macrophage colony-stimulating factor promotes glucose transport and blastomere viability in murine preimplantation embryos. *Biol Reprod* 2001;64:1206–15.

18. Sjoblom C, Wikland M, Robertson SA. Granulocyte-macrophage colony-stimulating factor promotes human blastocyst development in vitro. *Hum Reprod* 1999;14:3069–76.

19. Sjoblom C, Wikland M, Robertson SA. Granulocyte-macrophage colony-stimulating factor (GM-CSF) acts independently of the beta common subunit of the GM-CSF receptor to prevent inner cell mass apoptosis in human embryos. *Biol Reprod* 2002;67:1817–23.

20. Kumar S, Zhu LJ, Polihronis M, Cameron ST, Baird DT, Schatz F, *et al*. Progesterone induces calcitonin gene expression in human endometrium within the putative window of implantation. *J Clin Endocrinol Metab* 1998;83:4443–50.

21. Zhu LJ, Bagchi MK, Bagchi IC. Attenuation of calcitonin gene expression in pregnant rat uterus leads to a block in embryonic implantation. *Endocrinology* 1998;139:330–9.

22. Wang J, Rout UK, Bagchi IC, Armant DR. Expression of calcitonin receptors in mouse preimplantation embryos and their function in the regulation of blastocyst differentiation by calcitonin. *Development* 1998;125:4293–302.

23. Luu KC, Nie GY, Salamonsen LA. Endometrial calbindins are critical for embryo implantation: evidence from in vivo use of morpholino antisense oligonucleotides. *Proc Natl Acad Sci U S A* 2004;101:8028–33.

24. Liu Z, Armant DR. Lysophosphatidic acid regulates murine blastocyst development by transactivation of receptors for heparin-binding EGF-like growth factor. *Exp Cell Res* 2004;296:317–26.

25. Passey RJ, Williams E, Lichanska AM, Wells C, Hu S, Geczy CL, *et al*. A null mutation in the inflammation-associated S100 protein S100A8 causes early resorption of the mouse embryo. *J Immunol* 1999;163:2209–16.

26. Paria BC, Lim H, Wang XN, Liehr J, Das SK, Dey SK. Coordination of differential effects of primary estrogen and catecholestrogen on two distinct targets mediates embryo implantation in the mouse. *Endocrinology* 1998;139:5235–46.

27. Paria, BC, Reese, J, Das, SK, Dey, SK. Deciphering the cross-talk of implantation: advances and challenges. *Science* 2002;296:2185–8.

28. Grummer R, Hewitt SW, Traub O, Korach KS, Winterhager E. Different regulatory pathways of endometrial connexin expression: preimplantation hormonal-mediated pathway versus embryo implantation-initiated pathway. *Biol Reprod* 2004;71:273–81.

29. Lim H, Paria BC, Das SK, Dinchuk JE, Langenbach R, Trzaskos JM, *et al*. Multiple female reproductive failures in cyclooxygenase 2-deficient mice. *Cell* 1997;91:197–208.

30. Cheng JG, Stewart CL. Loss of cyclooxygenase-2 retards decidual growth but does not inhibit embryo implantation or development to term. *Biol Reprod* 2003;68:401–4.

31. Wang H, Ma WG, Tejada L, Zhang H, Morrow JD, Das SK, *et al*. Rescue of female infertility from the loss of cyclooxygenase-2 by compensatory upregulation of cyclooxygenase-1 is a function of genetic background. *J Biol Chem* 2004;279:10649–58.

32. Hess KA, Waltz SE, Chan EL, Degen SJ. Receptor tyrosine kinase Ron is expressed in mouse reproductive tissues during embryo implantation and is important in trophoblast cell function. *Biol Reprod* 2003;68:1267–75.

33. O'Sullivan CM, Rancourt SL, Liu SY, Rancourt DE. A novel murine tryptase involved in blastocyst hatching and outgrowth. *Reproduction* 2001;122:61–71.

34. Hey NA, Graham RA, Seif MW, Aplin JD. The polymorphic epithelial mucin MUC1 in human endometrium is regulated with maximal expression in the implantation phase. *J Clin Endocrinol Metab* 1994;78:337–42.

35. Hey NA, Li TC, Devine PL, Graham RA, Saravelos H, Aplin JD. MUC1 in secretory phase endometrium: expression in precisely dated biopsies and flushings from normal and recurrent miscarriage patients. *Hum Reprod* 1995;10:2655–62.

36. Aplin JD, Hey NA. MUC1, endometrium and embryo implantation. *Biochem Soc Trans* 1995;23:826–31.

37. Aplin JD, Hey NA, Graham RA. Human endometrial MUC1 carries keratan sulfate: characteristic glycoforms in the luminal epithelium at receptivity. *Glycobiology* 1998;8:269–76.

38. DeSouza MM, Surveyor GA, Price RE, Julian J, Kardon R, Zhou X, *et al*. MUC1/episialin: a critical barrier in the female reproductive tract. *J Reprod Immunol* 1999;45:127–58.

39. Cheon YP, Li Q, Xu X, DeMayo FJ, Bagchi IC, Bagchi MK. A genomic approach to identify novel progesterone receptor regulated pathways in the uterus during implantation. *Mol Endocrinol* 2002;16:2853–71.

40. McNeer RR, Carraway CA, Fregien NL, Carraway KL. Characterization of the expression and steroid hormone control of sialomucin complex in the rat uterus: implications for uterine receptivity. *J Cell Physiol* 1998;176:110–9.

41. Graham RA, Seif MW, Aplin JD, Li TC, Cooke ID, Rogers AW, et al. An endometrial factor in unexplained infertility. *BMJ* 1990;300:1428–31.

42. Serle E, Aplin JD, Li TC, Warren MA, Graham RA, Seif MW, et al. Endometrial differentiation in the peri-implantation phase of women with recurrent miscarriage: a morphological and immunohistochemical study. *Fertil Steril* 1994;62:989–96.

43. Aplin JD, Meseguer M, Simon C, Ortiz ME, Croxatto H, Jones CJ. MUC1, glycans and the cell-surface barrier to embryo implantation. *Biochem Soc Trans* 2001;29:153–6.

44. Meseguer M, Aplin JD, Caballero-Campo P, O'Connor JE, Martin JC, Remohi J, et al. Human endometrial mucin MUC1 is upregulated by progesterone and down-regulated in vitro by the human blastocyst. *Biol Reprod* 2001;64:590–601.

45. Thathiah A, Blobel CP, Carson DD. Tumor necrosis factor-alpha converting enzyme/ADAM 17 mediates MUC1 shedding. *J Biol Chem* 2003;278:3386–94.

46. Thathiah A, Carson DD. MT1-MMP mediates MUC1 shedding independent of TACE/ADAM17. *Biochem J* 2004;382:363–73.

47. Campbell S, Swann HR, Seif MW, Kimber SJ, Aplin JD. Cell adhesion molecules on the oocyte and preimplantation human embryo. *Hum Reprod* 1995;10:1571–8.

48. Hey NA, Aplin JD. Sialyl-Lewis x and Sialyl-Lewis a are associated with MUC1 in human endometrium. *Glycoconj J* 1996;13:769–79.

49. Kimber SJ, Spanswick C. The adhesion cascade. In: *The Endometrium*. Glasser SR, Aplin JD, Giudice L, Tabibzadeh S, editors. London: Taylor and Francis; 2002. p. 229–48.

50. Bloor DJ, Metcalfe AD, Rutherford A, Brison DR, Kimber SJ. Expression of cell adhesion molecules during human preimplantation embryo development. *Mol Hum Reprod* 2002;8:237–45.

51. Aplin JD, Kimber SJ. Trophoblast-uterine interactions at implantation. *Reprod Biol Endocrinol* 2004;2:48.

52. Apparao KB, Murray MJ, Fritz MA, Meyer WR, Chambers AF, Truong PR, et al. Osteopontin and its receptor alphavbeta(3) integrin are coexpressed in the human endometrium during the menstrual cycle but regulated differentially. *J Clin Endocrinol Metab* 2001;86:4991–5000.

53. Johnson GA, Burghardt RC, Bazer FW, Spencer TE. Osteopontin: roles in implantation and placentation. *Biol Reprod* 2003;69:1458–71.

54. Illera MJ, Lorenzo PL, Gui YT, Beyler SA, Apparao KB, Lessey BA. A role for alphavbeta3 integrin during implantation in the rabbit model. *Biol Reprod* 2003;68:766–71.

55. Creus M, Ordi J, Fabregues F, Casamitjana R, Ferrer B, Coll E, et al. alphavbeta3 integrin expression and pinopod formation in normal and out-of-phase endometria of fertile and infertile women. Hum Reprod 2002;17:2279–86.

56. Creus M, Ordi J, Fabregues F, Casamitjana R, Carmona F, Cardesa A, et al. The effect of different hormone therapies on integrin expression and pinopode formation in the human endometrium: a controlled study. *Hum Reprod* 2003;18:683–93.

57. Ordi J, Creus M, Ferrer B, Fabregues F, Carmona F, Casamitjana R, et al. Midluteal endometrial biopsy and alphavbeta3 integrin expression in the evaluation of the endometrium in infertility: implications for fecundity. Int *J Gynecol Pathol* 2002;21:231–8.

58. Ordi J, Creus M, Quinto L, Casamitjana R, Cardesa A, Balasch J. Within-subject between-cycle variability of histological dating, alpha v beta 3 integrin expression, and pinopod formation in the human endometrium. *J Clin Endocrinol Metab* 2003;88:2119–25.

59. Basak S, Dhar R, Das C. Steroids modulate the expression of alpha4 integrin in mouse blastocysts and uterus during implantation. *Biol Reprod* 2002;66:1784–9.

60. Paria BC, Elenius K, Klagsbrun M, Dey SK. Heparin-binding EGF-like growth factor interacts with mouse blastocysts independently of ErbB1: a possible role for heparan sulfate proteoglycans and ErbB4 in blastocyst implantation. *Development* 1999;126:1997–2005.

61. Chen JR, Cheng JG, Shatzer T, Sewell L, Hernandez L, Stewart CL. Leukemia inhibitory factor can substitute for nidatory E and is essential to inducing a receptive uterus for implantation but is not essential for subsequent embryogenesis. *Endocrinology* 2000;141:4365–72.

62. Nadano D, Sugihara K, Paria BC, Saburi S, Copeland NG, Gilbert DJ, et al. Significant differences between mouse and human trophinins are revealed by their expression patterns and targeted disruption of mouse trophinin gene. *Biol Reprod* 2002;66:313–21.

63. Nakayama J, Aoki D, Suga T, Akama TO, Ishizone S, Yamaguchi H, et al. Implantation-dependent expression of trophinin by maternal fallopian tube epithelia during tubal pregnancies: possible role of human chorionic gonadotrophin on ectopic pregnancy. *Am J Pathol* 2003;163:2211–9.

64. Stephens LE, Sutherland AE, Klimanskaya IV, Andrieux A, Meneses J, Pedersen RA, *et al.* Deletion of beta 1 integrins in mice results in inner cell mass failure and peri-implantation lethality. *Genes Dev* 1995;9:1883–95.

65. Aplin JD. Endometrial extracellular matrix. In: *The Endometrium.* Glasser SR, Aplin JD, Giudice L, Tabibzadeh S, editors. London: Taylor and Francis; 2002. p. 294–307.

66. Mulholland J, Aplin JD, Ayad S, Hong L, Glasser SR. Loss of collagen type VI from rat endometrial stroma during decidualization. *Biol Reprod* 1992;46:1136–43.

67. Mylona P, Kielty CM, Hoyland JA, Aplin JD. Expression of type VI collagen mRNAs in human endometrium during the menstrual cycle and first trimester of pregnancy. *J Reprod Fertil* 1995;103:159–67.

68. San Martin S, Soto-Suazo M, De Oliveira SF, Aplin JD, Abrahamsohn P, Zorn TM. Small leucine-rich proteoglycans (SLRPs) in uterine tissues during pregnancy in mice. *Reproduction* 2003;125:585–95.

69. Aplin JD, Charlton AK, Ayad S. An immunohistochemical study of human endometrial extracellular matrix during the menstrual cycle and first trimester of pregnancy. *Cell Tissue Res* 1988;253:231–40.

70. Church HJ, Vicovac LM, Williams JD, Hey NA, Aplin JD. Laminins 2 and 4 are expressed by human decidual cells. *Lab Invest* 1996;74:21–32.

71. Haendler B, Yamanouchi H, Lessey BA, Chwalisz K, Hess-Stumpp H. Cycle-dependent endometrial expression and hormonal regulation of the fibulin-1 gene. *Mol Reprod Dev* 2004;68:279–87.

72. Igakura T, Kadomatsu K, Kaname T, Muramatsu H, Fan QW, Miyauchi T, *et al.* A null mutation in basigin, an immunoglobulin superfamily member, indicates its important roles in peri-implantation development and spermatogenesis. *Dev Biol* 1998;194:152–65.

73. Kao LC, Tulac S, Lobo S, Imani B, Yang JP, Germeyer A, *et al.* Global gene profiling in human endometrium during the window of implantation. *Endocrinology* 2002;143:2119–38.

74. Carson DD, Lagow E, Thathiah A, Al-Shami R, Farach-Carson MC, Vernon M, *et al.* Changes in gene expression during the early to mid-luteal (receptive phase) transition in human endometrium detected by high-density microarray screening. *Mol Hum Reprod* 2002;8:871–9.

75. Borthwick JM, Charnock-Jones DS, Tom BD, Hull ML, Teirney R, Phillips SC, *et al.* Determination of the transcript profile of human endometrium. *Mol Hum Reprod* 2003;9:19–33.

76. Riesewijk A, Martin J, van Os R, Horcajadas JA, Polman J, Pellicer A, *et al.* Gene expression profiling of human endometrial receptivity on days LH+2 versus LH+7 by microarray technology. *Mol Hum Reprod* 2003;9:253–64.

77. Meyer WR, Novotny DB, Fritz MA, Beyler SA, Wolf LJ, Lessey BA. Effect of exogenous gonadotropins on endometrial maturation in oocyte donors. *Fertil Steril* 1999;71:109–14.

78. Murray MJ, Meyer WR, Zaino RJ, Lessey BA, Novotny DB, Ireland K, *et al.* A critical analysis of the accuracy, reproducibility, and clinical utility of histologic endometrial dating in fertile women. *Fertil* 2004;81:1333–43.

79. Ho Hong S, Young Nah H, Yoon Lee J, Chan Gye M, Hoon Kim C, Kyoo Kim M. Analysis of estrogen-regulated genes in mouse uterus using cDNA microarray and laser capture microdissection. *J Endocrinol* 2004;181:157–67.

80. Sherwin JR, Freeman TC, Stephens RJ, Kimber S, Smith AG, Chambers I, *et al.* Identification of genes regulated by leukemia-inhibitory factor in the mouse uterus at the time of implantation. *Mol Endocrinol* 2004;18:2185–95.

81. Rodriguez CI, Cheng G Jr, Liu L, Stewart CL. Cochlin, a secreted VWA domain containing factor, is regulated by LIF in the uterus at the time of implantation. *Endocrinology* 2004;145:1410–18.

82. Cheon YP, Xu X, Bagchi MK, Bagchi IC. Immune-responsive gene 1 is a novel target of progesterone receptor and plays a critical role during implantation in the mouse. Endocrinology 2003;144:5623–30.

83. Chen B, Zhang D, Pollard JW. Progesterone regulation of the mammalian ortholog of methylcitrate dehydratase (immune response gene 1) in the uterine epithelium during implantation through the protein kinase C pathway. *Mol Endocrinol* 2003;17:2340–54.

84. Kwong WY, Wild AE, Roberts P, Willis AC, Fleming TP. Maternal undernutrition during the preimplantation period of rat development causes blastocyst abnormalities and programming of postnatal hypertension. *Development* 2000;127:4195–202.

85. Mann MR, Lee SS, Doherty AS, Verona RI, Nolen LD, Schultz RM, *et al.* Selective loss of imprinting in the placenta following preimplantation development in culture. *Development* 2004;131:3727–35.

86. Paria BC, Ma W, Tan J, Raja S, Das SK, Dey SK, *et al.* Cellular and molecular responses of the

uterus to embryo implantation can be elicited by locally applied growth factors. *Proc Natl Acad Sci U S A* 2001;98:1047–52.

87. Gerami-Naini B, Dovzhenko OV, Durning M, Wegner FH, Thomson JA, Golos TG. Trophoblast differentiation in embryoid bodies derived from human embryonic stem cells. *Endocrinology* 2004;145:1517–24.

88. Barker DJ, Eriksson JG, Forsen T, Osmond C. Fetal origins of adult disease: strength of effects and biological basis. *Int J Epidemiol* 2002;31:1235–9.

Chapter 5
Vascular growth and modelling in the endometrium

D Stephen Charnock-Jones

The formation of an appropriate circulatory system is a critical step in the development of a multicellular organism. This is self-evident given the numerous critical functions performed by the circulatory system, including oxygen and waste transport, nutritional support, homeostasis and immune defence. This is borne out by the fact that many knockout mice die *in utero* because of defects in the various components of the circulatory system, such as blood cells, endothelial cells, other cells making up the vascular structures, and cardiovascular defects.

While embryonic development clearly depends on the appropriate vascular structures it is also true that tissue function in adult life depends critically on the appropriate function on endothelial cells. This is particular apparent in tissues that grow rapidly, both normal and pathological. For example, following ovulation the corpus luteum develops rapidly and concurrent with luteal growth is a remarkable degree of angiogenesis. By simply blocking the actions of a single growth factor that is critical to the growth of the luteal endothelial cells, i.e. vascular endothelial growth factor A (VEGF A), luteal growth and function (such as progesterone production) can be abolished.[1] In a pathological setting, the growth of hormone-dependent prostate tumours is dependent on the endothelial cells since upon hormone re-administration it is in fact the endothelial cells that respond before the tumour epithelial cells.[2]

In most organs in the adult the tissue and consequently the vasculature change only gradually. However, the endometrium undergoes profound change on a regular basis and the coordination of growth and function of the numerous cell types involved is critical for successful reproduction.

The generation of an appropriate environment for embryonic development requires the development of a receptive endometrium, which is, in turn, dependent upon both epithelial and stromal differentiation. Should implantation not occur, menstruation ensues, followed by the complete regrowth of the upper two-thirds of the endometrium. These changes are orchestrated by the ovarian sex hormones oestradiol and progesterone, although many of their effects are mediated indirectly by locally acting factors.[3] Nonetheless, the endometrium, including the endothelial cells within it, are exposed to cyclic fluctuations in a large range of stimuli that govern angiogenesis, regression, homeostasis, blood flow, nutrient supply, tissue fluid balance, oxygenation and waste-product removal. The appropriate response of the vascular cells to these multiple stimuli is the coordinated growth of a mature vascular tree that is able to generate and support a receptive endometrium and, should fertilisation occur, support embryonic development.

Examination of routinely fixed sections of endometrial tissue reveals a striking feature of the endometrial vasculature, namely the presence of the so-called spiral arterioles. As will be discussed below, these become extremely tortuous during the secretory phase of the cycle and numerous profiles of the same vessel appear in a single section owing to the tightly coiled nature of the arteriole. These spiral arterioles branch from the smaller basal arteries that supply the lower layer of the endometrium (basalis). The basal arteries in turn branch from radial arteries within the myometrium.[4] While the spiral arterioles are a prominent histological feature of the endometrium, the majority of capillaries are not visible. This is because the vessels collapse following biopsy or hysterectomy and without specific immunohistochemical staining the vessels are easily overlooked. Nonetheless, staining with appropriate endothelial-specific markers reveals a dense subepithelial capillary plexus, with capillaries forming a less dense network elsewhere in the endometrium.[5]

The capillaries in the upper (functional) layer of the endometrium are lined by a single continuous layer of endothelial cells that may be surrounded by pericytes. However, the extent of pericyte coverage differs in various regions of the endometrium, with more complete coverage being observed in the basal layer.[6] The larger vessels are surrounded by one or many layers of smooth-muscle cells. The presence of such vascular smooth muscles enables these vessels to regulate blood flow within the endometrium.

Changes in vascular structure during the menstrual cycle

Given the profound changes that occur in the endometrial thickness and structure during the menstrual cycle, one would expect that endothelial growth might show similar changes over the menstrual cycle. However, both the microvascular density and the endothelial proliferation rate remain relatively constant throughout the entire menstrual cycle.[7,8] These results, particularly relating to endothelial proliferation rate, seem surprising given that vascular repair occurs early in the proliferative phase and the endometrial thickness increases rapidly at this time. Furthermore, during the secretory phase of the cycle there is little increase in tissue thickness and yet apparently the endothelial proliferation rate is similar to that observed during the earlier phases.

So, while there do seem to be relatively few changes in proliferation rate and vascular density, the vasculature within the endometrium clearly does alter throughout the menstrual cycle. Immediately following menstruation tissue and blood vessel repair takes place. Although there are observations concerning the repair of the denuded endometrial surface, very little is known about the process of vascular repair immediately following menstruation. During the remaining period of the proliferative phase, the endometrium undergoes rapid growth under the influence of oestradiol. The spiral arterials elongate and a functional capillary network is established during this phase.

Following ovulation and the start of the secretory phase, endometrium proliferation in the functional layer ceases and differentiation begins to take place. This process is driven by the rising concentrations of progesterone produced by the corpus luteum. In the latter half of the luteal phase the endometrial stromal cells, particularly those close to the spiral arterioles, begin to decidualise (differentiate). During this phase of the cycle the spiral arterioles continue to grow and they become extremely tortuous and highly coiled. Measurement of vascular smooth-muscle proliferation rates indicates that this does rise during the mid and late secretory phases.[9]

The spiral arterioles with their unusual structure play an important role in menstruation should fertilisation and implantation not occur. While a detailed description of the regulation of this process is beyond the scope of this chapter, suffice it to say that there is profound contraction of the muscle cells within the spiral arterioles, leading to tissue ischaemia and breakdown. This is triggered by the fall in luteal progesterone and is accompanied by changes in local protease, prostaglandin, cytokine and haemostatic factor production.[10] The acute constriction leads to local ischaemia and an increase in apoptosis, tissue breakdown and, subsequently, shedding of the upper two-thirds of the endometrium (functional layer) into the uterine cavity.

Development of functional receptive endometrium

Endothelial cells from different tissues differ in a variety of ways and, as previously described, the vasculature within the endometrium shows considerable variation at different anatomical sites and it also varies during the menstrual cycle.[5,11–13] In light of this, one might wonder whether this regional specialisation has important functional consequences. Previously it had been presumed that the vasculature is merely 'plumbing' to supply nutrients and remove waste products from a tissue. However, this notion is increasingly recognised as being somewhat inaccurate. There is increasing evidence showing that there is dialogue between endothelial cells found at different sites within the body. These differences can be found at the transcriptional, antigenic and morphological levels. More intriguing still are the data which suggest that the endothelial cells actually play an active part in defining tissue structure, architecture and function.[14]

While there is a paucity of data relating to signals emanating from endothelial cells within the endometrium, there is at least one report in the literature that perturbing endothelial function can alter endometrial epithelial behaviour.[15] However, numerous cell types found within the endometrium produce factors known to regulate endothelial behaviour. Several of these, such as members of the VEGF and angiopoietin families, are known to have their principal actions on endothelial cells and several have been shown to be regulated by ovarian steroids.[16–25] However, studies in knockout mice have revealed that the regulation of endothelial function is far more complex and involves additional factors and more subtle regulatory mechanisms.

Angiogenesis, which is defined as the growth of new vessels from pre-existing vessels, clearly occurs in the endometrium since the microvascular density remains relatively stable even as the tissue mass increases.

Sprouting angiogenesis is the most common form of angiogenesis and occurs during vessel growth in the developing brain, the corpus luteum and in many solid tumours. The steps required for this process have become considerably clearer in recent years and many of the key factors involved in these various steps, i.e. the control points of the process, have been elucidated.[14,26,27] The principal steps have been identified as follows:

1. vasodilation and an increase in vascular permeability
2. activation of proteases leading to degradation of the capillary basement membrane

3.   increase and proliferation of endothelial cells
4.   migration of endothelial cells, usually towards a chemotactic stimulus
5.   assembly of endothelial cells to form a tube
6.   recruitment of pericytes to the outside of the capillary to stabilise the newly formed vessel.

In addition to this form of angiogenesis, other processes such as elongation,[28] intus-susception[29] and intercalation of circulating endothelial progenitors may play a role.[30] However, it seems unlikely that sprouting angiogenesis occurs in the endometrium and more recent evidence has revealed that elongation of endothelial cells in the walls of existing capillaries would seem to play a major role.[31]

Key factors regulating endometrial endothelial cell function

The sequence of VEGF A was described in 1989 and its pivotal role in endothelial biology has now been well established by numerous genetic and other functional studies in a wide variety of models.[32] This factor is essential for endothelial cell differentiation and the fact that deletion of even a single allele leads to embryonic fatality suggests that during development the precise level of VEGF A plays an important role.[33,34] This factor has now been implicated in regulating the vessels associated with growth of various tissues, for example lung, bone, peripheral motor neurones, kidney and developing pancreas.[35-40] Ablation of this factor either genetically or by using antibodies or receptor antagonists has revealed its pivotal role. However, while VEGF A is necessary for endothelial function, simply adding excess does not lead to the growth of mature, well-organised functional vessels. This is particularly apparent in many tumours which frequently overexpress VEGF A (and many other factors). In more-refined experiments where VEGF A production is directed by a tissue-specific promoter, additional, but malformed, vessels are formed.[41]

The regulation of biologically active VEGF A is achieved at many different levels. The rate of transcription is directly regulated by hypoxia[42] but it is also regulated by steroid hormones.[16,17,24,43] There is also post-transcriptional regulation of message stability, which is mediated by elements in the $3'$ untranslated regions of the transcript.[44] VEGF A exists in at least five different splice variants and these have differing properties.[24,45,46] However, the balance of these splice variants is regulated transiently by progesterone in human endometrium.[47] The various isoforms of VEGF A differ in their affinity for heparin sulphate obtained within the extracellular matrix. The shorter form ($VEGF_{121}$) is freely diffusible whereas the long form ($VEGF_{189}$) is bound tightly to proteoglycans.[45] There is thus the possibility of a freely diffusible form and a reservoir form of the growth factor. Importantly, the long forms of VEGF A can be released by proteolytic cleavage of the immobilised factor.[48,49] The biological activity of the VEGF protein is then modulated by binding to the competitive antagonist soluble FLT1. This is a soluble form of the extracellular domain of the high-affinity VEGF receptor that is produced by alternative splicing.[50] While it is produced in large amounts by the placenta, it is also produced by endothelial cells and is regulated in the endometrium.[51-53]

Thus while the pivotal role of VEGF A has been established in many systems, the numerous subtle ways in which the local activity of this factor is regulated suggests significant complexity and it is the local level that is important.[54]

Another family of growth factors that act on endothelial cells through tyrosine kinase receptors is the angiopoietins. Angiopoietin 1 and 2 (ANG1 and ANG2) both act by binding to the TIE2 receptor. These factors are produced by cells in the vessel wall and they are essential for the stabilisation of endothelial cells. ANG1 is an endothelial cell survival factor and reduces vascular permeability.[55–57] ANG2 is generally believed to be an antagonist of ANG1 and is regulated differentially.[58,59]

The VEGF system interacts with several other signalling families to cooperatively regulate vessel growth and adaptation. These studies necessitate *in vivo* work as it not currently possible to grow or even maintain functional vessels in long-term culture. The most informative of these have been performed using genetically modified mice in which specific growth factors are overexpressed in selected tissues – for example in the skin under the control of the keratin 14 promoter. These studies have shown that overexpression of any of VEGF A, ANG1 or placenta growth factor (PlGF) leads to an increase in vessel number and, in the case of VEGF A and PlGF, an increase in vascular permeability.[41,60] However, overexpression of the closely related growth factors VEGF C and VEGF D does not lead to an increase in vessel number but to an increase in the number of lymphatics.[61] Use of such models clearly indicates the importance of the factor in question in vessel growth and behaviour (at least in skin). However, it is intriguing that when VEGF A and ANG1 are both expressed in the skin there is an increase in vessel number but normal vascular permeability is restored.[62] This suggests combinations of factors are important for the regulation of vessel growth and function.

Similar studies have employed the 5′ promoter regions and the 3′ intron of the alpha myosin heavy chain gene to specifically express VEGF-A, ANG1 or ANG2 in cardiac muscle. These data show that ANG2 can collaborate with VEGF A to induce capillary angiogenesis *in vivo* and also that ANG1 can act as a negative regulator of VEGF A-induced angiogenesis in the specific tissue investigated, in this case the heart.[63]

In the endometrium, factors from both the VEGF and the angiopoietin family are present and several vary during the menstrual cycle. (For examples, see Li *et al.*[25] and Hirchenhain *et al.*[64]) An additional feature, which is not always recognised, is that sometimes the cells that produce these factors are transient or are localised at specific sites within the endometrium. For example, the endometrial natural killer (NK) cells, as well as increasingly markedly in the late secretory phase, also tend to cluster in a subepithelial location. They also contain mRNAs encoding ANG2 and PlGF.[25]

However, it is clear that, while the factors known to play a role in sprouting angiogenesis are present in the endometrium, the capillaries and the tissue actually grow by a different mechanism. This reveals our fundamental lack of knowledge in the subtle regulation of endothelial cell function. There are preliminary reports in the literature and we have obtained some initial data which reveal that interfering with VEGF function in nonpregnant endometrium can have direct effects on the processes surrounding implantation. However, it would be naive to think that VEGF alone is the key factor determining every aspect of endothelial function. While it is a pivotal factor, it is clearly regulated by many stimuli, for example steroids, hypoxia, glucose and other locally acting growth factors such as sonic hedgehog.[65] So, while VEGF itself is regulated by many factors, some of which may alter the splicing of the VEGF transcript, the resulting peptide also interacts with other factors.

Although the cooperative effects of VEGF and angiopoietins have been demonstrated in several model systems, it is becoming clear that many other families of growth factors play a role in modulating endothelial cell behaviour. For example, the neuropilin and semaphorin family, which were originally described as axonal guidance molecules (receptor and ligand, respectively), has been shown to affect angiogenesis and cardiac development.[66] Neuropilin itself has been identified as a self surface molecule that is able to bind directly to VEGF A and together with receptor VEGF R2 interacts to regulate endothelial growth.[67]

Other molecules originally described in the nervous system or known to be important during early development have similarly been shown to affect capillary growth. For example the Notch/jagged family,[68] the hedgehog family[65] and members of the WNT family.[69] It is likely that the list of molecules involved in determining the structure of vascular networks will lengthen. It is becoming recognised that the vascular network in a tissue is more than the simple supply route for nutrients: rather, the endothelial cells are able to influence cell and tissue function. However, the complexity suggests that it is an understanding of these multifactorial interactions that will yield the most benefit. Techniques that begin to make this task tractable (genomics and proteomics), are now becoming widely available. Gene array technology in particular allows the identification of all the transcripts present in a tissue at any point in time.[70] While this technique yields little spatial information, laser capture and micro dissection should address this need.

These new methods, if combined with studies in functionally relevant models and with subsequent confirmation in a clinical setting, offer the prospect of new targets for diagnostic and therapeutic interventions.

References

1. Ferrara N, Chen H, Davis-Smith T, Gerber HP, Nguyen TN, Peers D, et al. Vascular endothelial growth factor is essential for corpus luteum angiogenesis. Nat Med 1998;4:336–40.
2. Franck-Lissbrant I, Haggstrom S, Damber JE, Bergh, A. Testosterone stimulates angiogenesis and vascular regrowth in the ventral prostate in castrated adult rats. Endocrinology 1998;139:451–6.
3. Cooke PS, Buchanan DL, Young P, Setiawan T, Brody J, Korach KS, et al. Stromal estrogen receptors mediate mitogenic effects of estradiol on uterine epithelium. Proc Natl Acad Sci U S A 1997;94:6535–40.
4. Ramsey EM. Vascular anatomy. In: Wynn RM, editor. Biology of the Uterus. New York: Plenum Press; 1982. p. 59–76.
5. Zhang EG, Smith SK, Charnock-Jones DS. Expression of CD105 (endoglin) in arteriolar endothelial cells of human endometrium throughout the menstrual cycle. Reproduction 2002;124:703–11.
6. Hull ML, Charnock-Jones DS, Chan CL, Bruner-Tran KL, Osteen KG, Tom BD, et al. Antiangiogenic agents are effective inhibitors of endometriosis. J Clin Endocrinol Metab 2003;88:2889–99.
7. Rogers PAW, Au SL, Affandi B. Endometrial microvascular density during the normal menstrual cycle and following exposure to long-term levonorgestrel. Hum Reprod 1993;8:1396–404.
8. Goodger AM, Rogers PAW. Endometrial endothelial cell proliferation during the menstrual cycle. Hum Reprod 1994;9:399–405.
9. Abberton KM, Taylor NH, Healy DL, Rogers PAW. Vascular smooth muscle alpha-actin distribution around endometrial arterioles during the menstrual cycle: Increased expression during the perimenopause and lack of correlation with menorrhagia. Hum Reprod 1996;11:204–11.
10. Kelly RW, King AE, Critchley HOD. Inflammatory mediators and endometrial function – focus on the perivascular cell. J Reprod Immunol 2002;57:81–93.
11. Garlanda C, Dejana, E. Heterogeneity of endothelial cells. Specific markers. Arterioscler Thromb Vasc Biol 1997;17:1193–202.
12. Pettersson A, Nagy JA, Brown LF, Sundberg C, Morgan E, Jungles S, et al. Heterogeneity of the angiogenic response induced in different normal adult tissues by vascular permeability factor/vascular endothelial growth factor. Lab Invest 2000;80:99–115.
13. Girard JP, Baekkevold ES, Yamanaka T, Haraldsen G, Brandtzaeg P, Amalric F. Heterogeneity of endothelial cells: the specialized phenotype of human high endothelial venules characterized by suppression subtractive hybridization. Am J Pathol 1999;155:2043–55.
14. Cleaver O, Melton DA. Endothelial signaling during development. Nat Med 2003;9:661–8.

15. Hastings JM, Licence DR, Burton GJ, Charnock-Jones DS, Smith SK. Soluble vascular endothelial growth factor receptor 1 inhibits edema and epithelial proliferation induced by 17 beta-estradiol in the mouse uterus. *Endocrinology* 2003;144:326–34.

16. Cullinan-Bove K, Koos RD. Vascular endothelial growth factor/vascular permeability factor expression in the rat uterus: Rapid stimulation by estrogen correlates with estrogen-induced increases in uterine capillary permeability and growth. *Endocrinology* 1993;133:829–37.

17. Hyder SM, Stancel GM, Chiappetta C, Murthy L, Boettger-Tong HL, Makela, S. Uterine expression of vascular endothelial growth factor is increased by estradiol and tamoxifen. *Cancer Res* 1996;56:3954–60.

18. Iruela-Arispe ML, Porter P, Bornstein P, Sage EH. Thrombospondin-1, an inhibitor of angiogenesis, is regulated by progesterone in the human endometrium. *J Clin Invest* 1996;97:403–12.

19. Sangha RK, Xiao Feng L, Shams M, Ahmed A. Fibroblast growth factor receptor-1 is a critical component for endometrial remodeling: Localization and expression of basic fibroblast growth factor and FGF-R1 in human endometrium during the menstrual cycle and decreased FGF-R1 expression in menorrhagia. *Lab Invest* 1997;77:389–402.

20. Shweiki D, Itin A, Neufeld G, Gitay-Goren H, Keshet E. Patterns of expression of vascular endothelial growth factor (VEGF) and VEGF receptors in mice suggest a role in hormonally regulated angiogenesis. *J Clin Invest* 1993;91:2235–43.

21. Hirchenhain J, Huse I, Hess A, Bielfeld P, De Bruyne F, Krussel JS. Differential expression of angiopoietins 1 and 2 and their receptor Tie-2 in human endometrium. *Mol Hum Reprod* 2003;9:663–9.

22. Rowe AJ, Wulff C, Fraser HM. Localization of mRNA for vascular endothelial growth factor (VEGF), angiopoietins and their receptors during the peri-implantation period and early pregnancy in marmosets (Callithrix jacchus). *Reproduction* 2003;126:227–38.

23. Krikun G, Critchley H, Schatz F, Wan L, Caze R, Baergen RN, et al. Abnormal uterine bleeding during progestin-only contraception may result from free radical-induced alterations in angiopoietin expression. *Am J Pathol* 2002;161:979–86.

24. Charnock-Jones DS, Sharkey AM, Rajput-Williams J, Burch D, Schofield JP, Fountain SA, et al. Identification and localization of alternately spliced mRNAs for vascular endothelial growth factor in human uterus and estrogen regulation in endometrial carcinoma cell lines. *Biol Reprod* 1993;48:1120–8.

25. Li XF, Charnock-Jones DS, Zhang E, Hiby S, Malik S, Day K, et al. Angiogenic growth factor messenger ribonucleic acids in uterine natural killer cells. *J Clin Endocrinol Metab* 2001;86:1823–34.

26. Jain RK. Molecular regulation of vessel maturation. *Nat Med* 2003;9:685–93.

27. Carmeliet P. Angiogenesis in health and disease. *Nat Med* 2003;9:653–60.

28. Ausprunk DH, Knighton DR, Folkman J. Differentiation of vascular endothelium in the chick chorioallantois: a structural and autoradiographic study. *Dev Biol* 1974;38:237–48.

29. Djonov V, Schmid M, Tschanz SA, Burri PH. Intussusceptive angiogenesis: its role in embryonic vascular network formation. *Circ Res* 2000;86:286–92.

30. Asahara T, Masuda H, Takahashi T, Kalka C, Pastore C, Silver M, et al. Bone marrow origin of endothelial progenitor cells responsible for postnatal vasculogenesis in physiological and pathological neovascularization. *Circ Res* 1999;85:221–8.

31. Gambino LS, Wreford NG, Bertram JF, Dockery P, Lederman F, Rogers PAW. Angiogenesis occurs by vessel elongation in proliferative phase human endometrium. *Hum Reprod* 2002;17:1199–206.

32. Ferrara N. Vascular endothelial growth factor: basic science and clinical progress. *Endocr Rev* 2004;25:581–611.

33. Carmeliet P, Ferreira V, Breier G, Pollefeyt S, Kieckens L, Gertenstein M, et al. Abnormal blood vessel development and lethality in embryos lacking a single VEGF allele. *Nature* 1996;380:435–9.

34. Ferrara N, Carver-Moore K, Chen H, Dowd M, Lu L, O'Shea HS, et al. Heterozygous embryonic lethality induced by targeted inactivation of the VEGF gene. Nature 1996;380:439–42.

35. Compernolle V, Brusselmans K, Acker T, Hoet P, Tjwa M, Beck H, et al. Loss of HIF-2alpha and inhibition of VEGF impair fetal lung maturation, whereas treatment with VEGF prevents fatal respiratory distress in premature mice. *Nat Med* 2002;8:702–10.

36. Gerber HP, Vu TH, Ryan AM, Kowalski J, Werb Z, Ferrara N. VEGF couples hypertrophic cartilage remodeling, ossification and angiogenesis during endochondral bone formation. *Nat Med* 1999;5:623–8.

37. Lammert E, Gu G, McLaughlin M, Brown D, Brekken R, Murtaugh LC, et al. Role of VEGF-A in vascularization of pancreatic islets. *Curr Biol* 2003;13:1070–4.

38. Lammert E, Cleaver O, Melton D. Induction of pancreatic differentiation by signals from blood

vessels. *Science* 2001;294:564–7.

39. Lambrechts D, Storkebaum E, Morimoto M, Del-Favero J, Desmet F, Marklund SL, Wyns S, *et al*. VEGF is a modifier of amyotrophic lateral sclerosis in mice and humans and protects motoneurons against ischemic death. *Nat Genet* 2003;34:383–94.

40. Oosthuyse B, Moons L, Storkebaum E, Beck H, Nuyens D, Brusselmans K, *et al*. Deletion of the hypoxia-response element in the vascular endothelial growth factor promoter causes motor neuron degeneration. *Nat Genet* 2001;28:131–8.

41. Detmar M, Brown LF, Schon MP, Elicker BM, Velasco P, Richard L, *et al*. Increased microvascular density and enhanced leukocyte rolling and adhesion in the skin of VEGF transgenic mice. *J Invest Dermatol* 1998;111:1–6.

42. Levy AP, Levy NS, Wegner S, Goldberg MA. Transcriptional regulation of the rat vascular endothelial growth factor gene by hypoxia. *J Biol Chem* 1995;270:13333–40.

43. Mueller MD, Vigne JL, Minchenko A, Lebovic DI, Leitman DC, Taylor RN. Regulation of vascular endothelial growth factor (VEGF) gene transcription by estrogen receptors alpha and beta. *Proc Natl Acad Sci U S A* 2000;97:10972–7.

44. Levy NS, Chung S, Furneaux H, Levy AP. Hypoxic stabilization of vascular endothelial growth factor mRNA by the RNA-binding protein HuR. *J Biol Chem* 1998;273:6417–23.

45. Houck KA, Ferrara N, Winer J, Cachianes G, Li B, Leung DW. The vascular endothelial growth factor family: Identification of a fourth molecular species and characterization of alternative splicing of RNA. *Mol Endocrinol* 1991;5:1806–14.

46. Poltorak Z, Cohen T, Sivan R, Kandelis Y, Spira G, Vlodavsky I, *et al*. VEGF145, a secreted vascular endothelial growth factor isoform that binds to extracellular matrix. *J Biol Chem* 1997;272:7151–8.

47. Ancelin M, Buteau-Lozano H, Meduri G, Osborne-Pellegrin M, Sordello S, Plouet J, *et al*. A dynamic shift of VEGF isoforms with a transient and selective progesterone-induced expression of VEGF(189) regulates angiogenesis and vascular permeability in human uterus. *Proc Natl Acad Sci U S A* 2002;99:6023–8.

48. Plouet J, Moro F, Bertagnolli S, Coldeboeuf N, Mazarguil H, Clamens S, *et al*. Extracellular cleavage of the vascular endothelial growth factor 189-amino acid form by urokinase is required for its mitogenic effect. *J Biol Chem* 1997;272:13390–6.

49. Houck KA, Leung DW, Rowland AM, Winer J, Ferrara N. Dual regulation of vascular endothelial growth factor bioavailability by genetic and proteolytic mechanisms. *J Biol Chem* 1992;267:26031–7.

50. Kendall RL, Thomas KA. Inhibition of vascular endothelial cell growth factor activity by an endogenously encoded soluble receptor. *Proc Natl Acad Sci U S A* 1993;90:10705–9.

51. Graubert MD, Ortega MA, Kessel B, Mortola JF, Iruela-Arispe ML. Vascular repair after menstruation involves regulation of vascular endothelial growth factor-receptor phosphorylation by sFLT-1. *Am J Pathol* 2001;158:1399–410.

52. He Y, Smith SK, Day KA, Clark DE, Licence DR, Charnock-Jones DS. Alternative splicing of vascular endothelial growth factor (VEGF)-R1 (FLT-1) pre-mRNA is important for the regulation of VEGF activity. *Mol Endocrinol* 1999;13:537–45.

53. Clark DE, Smith SK, He Y, Day KA, Licence DR, Corps AC, *et al*. A vascular endothelial growth factor antagonist is produced by the human placenta and released into the maternal circulation. *Biol Reprod* 1998;59:1540–8.

54. Ozawa CR, Banfi A, Glazer NL, Thurston G, Springer ML, Kraft PE, *et al*. Microenvironmental VEGF concentration, not total dose, determines a threshold between normal and aberrant angiogenesis. *J Clin Invest* 2004;113:516–27.

55. Fujikawa K, de Aos Scherpenseel I, Jain SK, Presman E, Christensen RA, Varticovski L. Role of PI 3-kinase in angiopoietin-1-mediated migration and attachment-dependent survival of endothelial cells. *Exp Cell Res* 1999;253:663–72. Erratum in: *Exp Cell Res* 2000;255:133.

56. Kim I, Kim HG, So JN, Kim JH, Kwak HJ, Koh GY. Angiopoietin-1 regulates endothelial cell survival through the phosphatidylinositol 3′-Kinase/Akt signal transduction pathway. *Circ Res* 2000;86:24–9.

57. Thurston G, Rudge JS, Ioffe E, Zhou H, Ross L, Croll SD, *et al*. Angiopoietin-1 protects the adult vasculature against plasma leakage. *Nat Med* 2000;6:460–3.

58. Zhang EG, Smith SK, Baker PN, Charnock-Jones DS. The regulation and localization of angiopoietin-1, -2, and their receptor Tie2 in normal and pathologic human placentae. *Mol Med* 2001;7:624–35.

59. Hanahan D. Signaling vascular morphogenesis and maintenance. *Science* 1997;277:48–50.

60. Suri C, McClain J, Thurston G, McDonald DM, Zhou H, Oldmixon EH, *et al*. Increased

vascularization in mice overexpressing angiopoietin-1. *Science* 1998;282:468–71.

61. Veikkola T, Jussila L, Makinen T, Karpanen T, Jeltsch M, Petrova TV, *et al*. Signalling via vascular endothelial growth factor receptor-3 is sufficient for lymphangiogenesis in transgenic mice. *EMBO J* 2001;20:1223–31.

62. Thurston G, Suri C, Smith K, McClain J, Sato TN, Yancopoulos GD, *et al*. Leakage-resistant blood vessels in mice transgenically overexpressing angiopoietin-1. *Science* 1999;286:2511–4.

63. Visconti RP, Richardson CD, Sato TN. Orchestration of angiogenesis and arteriovenous contribution by angiopoietins and vascular endothelial growth factor (VEGF). *Proc Natl Acad Sci U S A* 2002;99:8219–24.

64. Hirchenhain J, Huse I, Hess A, Bielfeld P, De Bruyne F, Krussel JS. Differential expression of angiopoietins 1 and 2 and their receptor Tie-2 in human endometrium. *Mol Hum Reprod* 2003;9:663–9.

65. Pola R, Ling LE, Silver M, Corbley MJ, Kearney M, Blake *et al*. The morphogen Sonic hedgehog is an indirect angiogenic agent upregulating two families of angiogenic growth factors. *Nat Med* 2001;7:706–11.

66. Gitler AD, Lu MM, Epstein JA. PlexinD1 and semaphorin signaling are required in endothelial cells for cardiovascular development. *Dev Cell* 2004;7:107–16.

67. Klagsbrun M, Takashima S, Mamluk R. The role of neuropilin in vascular and tumor biology. *Adv Exp Med Biol* 2002;515:33–48.

68. Alva JA, Iruela-Arispe ML. Notch signaling in vascular morphogenesis. *Curr Opin Hematol* 2004;11:278–83.

69. Goodwin AM, D'Amore PA. Wnt signaling in the vasculature. *Angiogenesis* 2002;5:1–9.

70. Borthwick JM, Charnock-Jones DS, Tom BD, Hull ML, Teirney R, Phillips SC, *et al*. Determination of the transcript profile of human endometrium. *Mol Hum Reprod* 2003;9:19–33.

Chapter 6
Tissue remodelling at the fetal–maternal interface: the regulation of matrix metalloproteinase 9 transcription

Marie Cohen and Paul Bischof

Introduction

As life moved out of the oceans, new reproductive strategies developed to account for the loss of nutrients and oxygen normally provided by the water environment. Despite the fact that many examples of viviparity exist in invertebrates, fish, amphibians and reptiles, placentation is a relatively new acquisition in evolution. The establishment of an intimate trophic connection between mother and embryo is a characteristic of mammals. Implantation and the ensuing placentation are thus new strategies in reproduction, which allow the development of a small number of fetuses in the protective maternal organism. As the mammals evolved from small rodent-like creatures with short gestational periods to larger animals with prolonged gestations, the placenta had to adapt to the increasing needs of the growing fetus.

Orchestrating the blastocyst–endometrial summit requires perfect synchronisation between embryonic development and endometrial maturation. This synchronisation does not only involve the embryo and the endometrium but also the maternal pituitary and the ovary. As a result of ovarian oestradiol and progesterone secretions, the endometrium proliferates and differentiates. During the mid-luteal phase (days 22–24 of a 28-day cycle) decidualisation starts around the endometrial spiral arteries and extends to the whole endometrium within a few days. The endometrial extracellular matrix (ECM) becomes distended because water is attracted, possibly owing to the decidual secretion of hygroscopic molecules such as heparan sulphate proteoglycans.[1,2] This is the milieu in which the blastocyst is going to implant. Thus when a blastocyst implants into a decidualised endometrium, the tissue has already changed the composition of its ECM, cells are distended by oedema, and proteoglycans are abundant in the tissue. Although the 'soil' has been prepared, the embryo still has to overcome several barriers such as the endometrial basement membrane and the various collagens of the ECM before it can implant.

Mammalian embryos will initiate implantation-type reactions in many different non-uterine sites, such as the eye,[3] kidney,[4] spleen and testis.[5,6] The embryo expresses thus an intrinsic invasive potential, which is neither related to the cellular and biochemical nature of the invaded host tissue nor to its hormonal status. Most of this is not true for the endometrium because it protects itself from implantation except during a limited period known as the receptive phase or the implantation window. This particular receptivity seems to be the property of the endometrial epithelial lining since experimental removal of the uterine epithelium allows the blastocyst to 'implant' completely.[7] The hormonal requirements of the implantation window have been well defined in rats[8] but not in humans.

Human blastocysts are particularly more invasive than other mammalian embryos and this property is due to an abundant secretion of proteases by the trophectodermal cells of the blastocyst and the cytotrophoblastic cells (CTB) of the early placenta. Human extravillous CTB, these motile and highly invasive trophoblastic cells (used as an *in vitro* model of trophectodermal cells) are invasive because they secrete proteases.[9–12] Serine protease, cathepsin and metalloproteinase have been implicated in the invasive process.[13]

Matrix metalloproteinases

Matrix metalloproteinases (MMPs), also called matrixins, are a family of at least 20 human zinc-dependent endopeptidases collectively capable of degrading essentially all components of the ECM. According to their substrate specificity and structure, members of the MMP gene family can be classified into four subgroups:

- Gelatinases (MMP2 and 9) digest collagen type IV (the major constituent of basement membranes) and denatured collagen (gelatine).
- Collagenases (MMP1, 8 and 13) digest collagen type I, II, III, VII and X, and they are thus appropriately designed for digesting the collagen of the ECM of the interstitium.
- Stromelysins (MMP3, 7, 10, 11 and 12) have a relatively, broad substrate specificity and digest collagen type IV, V, VII as well as laminin, fibronectin, elastin, proteoglycans and gelatine.
- The substrate of the membrane metalloproteinases (MMP14, 15 and 16) is essentially proMMP2 and these enzymes allow activation of MMP2 at the cell surface on the invasive front. The substrate for MMP17 has not been clearly determined so far.

In general, MMPs contain a signal peptide (which indicates that they are secreted proteins), a propeptide, a catalytic domain with the highly conserved zinc-binding site, and a haemopexin-like domain linked to the catalytic domain by a hinge region.[13] In addition, MMP2 and MMP9 contain a fibronectin type II insert within the catalytic domain whereas the membrane-type MMPs (MT-MMPs) MMP14 to 17 have a transmembrane domain in the C-terminal end of the haemopexin-like domain. Most MMPs are secreted as inactive proenzymes (zymogens), which become activated in the extracellular compartments with the exception of MMP11 and MT-MMPs. Activation occurs by dissociation of a Zn^{2+}–Cys interaction that leads to the loss of the propeptide. Several enzymes are capable of activating the pro-matrixins, the most prominent of them being plasmin.[14] The activity of MMPs in the extracellular space is specifically inhibited by tissue inhibitor of metalloproteinases (TIMP), which binds to the highly conserved zinc-binding site of active MMPs at molar equivalence. The TIMP gene family consists of four structurally related members, TIMP1, 2, 3 and 4, that besides inhibiting MMPs also exert other biologically important functions.[15] TIMP3 is produced by CTB and plays an important role in regulating CTB invasion.[16]

In vitro, CTB invade a reconstituted basement membrane (Matrigel™),[17–19] and they thus behave like metastatic cells. This invasive behaviour is due to the ability of CTB to secrete MMPs since TIMP inhibits their invasiveness.[20] Several studies have localised MMP proteins[21–23] and mRNA[22,23] in human trophoblast. Furthermore, cultured CTB secrete MMPs[9–11,24] but CTB from early pregnancy are more invasive and secrete more MMPs than CTB isolated from term placenta.[25] Not all MMPs are equally important for trophoblast invasion. Gelatinase B (MMP9) is considered to be instrumental in trophoblast invasion since *in vitro* it mediates CTB invasion into a Matrigel.[11,20]

Regulation of the *MMP9* gene by transcription factors

Although CTB behave like metastatic cells, *in vivo* they are only transiently invasive (first trimester) and their invasion is normally limited only to the endometrium and to the proximal third of the myometrium.[26] This temporal and spatial regulation of trophoblast invasion is believed to be mediated in an autocrine way by trophoblastic factors and in a paracrine way by uterine factors. Several types of regulators have been investigated: hormones, cytokines, growth factors and ECM glycoproteins. (For a review, see Bischof and Campana.[27]) Cytokines influence the secretion and/or activity of MMPs and, although there is a certain degree of cell specificity, proinflammatory cytokines tend to exert a stimulating effect whereas anti-inflammatory cytokines are generally inhibitors of MMPs.

The *MMP9* gene contains 13 exons and 12 introns for a total size of 7.7 kbp. The regulatory region (5′ flanking) of this gene has been described in two studies[28,29] showing multiple cis-regulatory elements (Figure 6.1). These cis-regulatory elements are specific DNA sequences that bind trans-activators or trans-repressors (transcription factors), which are thus proteins encoded by other genes.

Activator protein 1

It was observed that all genes inducible by the tumour promoter TPA (phorbol myristate acetate) have a consensus sequence (TGAG/CTCA) known as the TRE site (TPA responsive element) that binds activator protein 1 (AP1). AP1 transcription factors are dimeric leucine zipper proteins usually formed by members of the Jun and Fos family. Jun and Fos are oncogene products and their genes belong to the family of early response genes. There are several reports showing that AP1 is involved in MMP9 expression in tumour cell lines such as HT1080 fibrosarcoma cells,[29] OVCAR cells[30] and UM-SCC-1 cells.[31] We have observed that the phorbol ester TPA not only increases MMP9 activity in CTB but also increases MMP9 (but not MMP2) mRNA.[32] The maximum mRNA response appears only after 24 h of incubation and cycloheximide significantly inhibits the stimulatory effect of TPA on MMP9 message. Thus TPA must stimulate the synthesis of MMP9 by inducing early response genes. A band-shift assay with ^{32}P-labelled sense and antisense oligonucleotides corresponding to the *MMP9* TRE sequence showed that TPA induces an increase in the binding of CTB nuclear proteins to this TRE sequence. In the presence of a mixture of monoclonal antibodies to Jun and Fos, we observed a reduction of the amount of CTB nuclear proteins bound to the TRE sequence. Thus TPA induces the transcription of *c-Jun* and *c-Fos* oncogenes in CTB. These proteins bind to a TRE sequence, possibly the ones in the promoter region of the *MMP9* gene. Transient

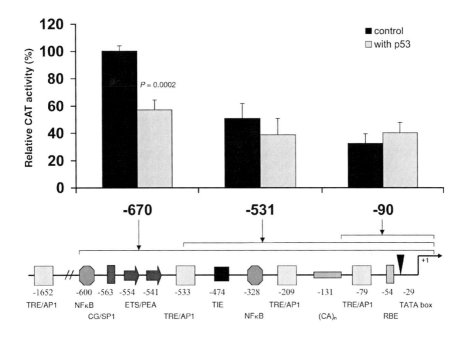

Figure 6.1. Influence of p53 on various deletions of *hMMP9* promoter. CTB were co-transfected with 3 μg of −90hMMP9CAT or −531hMMP9CAT or −670hMMP9CAT-reporter plasmid together with 0.5 μg of wild-type p53 expression or control vector. After incubation (48 h), the cells were harvested and CAT activity assayed and normalised to the total amount of cell proteins in the cellular lysate. Three different CTB preparations were transfected in triplicate and the results expressed as mean ± SEM. Promoter activities were calculated relative to the control (−670hMMP9CAT in the absence of wild-type p53) set at 100%. A paired Student's *t* test was used to compare cells co-transfected with wild-type p53 or not. The lower part of the figure presents a schematic view of the regulatory region of the hMMP9 gene. Binding sites are listed in order of appearance. RBE = retinoblastoma control element; TRE/AP1 = TPA response element/activator protein 1; $(CA)_n$ = cytosine adenine repeats; NFκB = nuclear factor kappa B; TIE = transforming growth factor beta inhibitory element; ETS/PEA = erythroblastosis twenty-six specific/polyoma enhancing element; CG/SP1 = cytosine guanine/specificity protein 1.

transfection of CTB with antisense and sense probes (as controls) to *c-Jun* and *c-Fos* demonstrates that expression of *c-Jun* and *c-Fos* oncogenes is a prerequisite for trophoblastic MMP9 expression.[32]

Other transcription factors

Although AP1 plays an important role in transcriptional activation of *MMP9*, basal transcription as well as cytokine-induced trans-activation require specific interactions with other cis-acting elements. As shown in Figure 6.1, transfection of CTB with various deletions of the *MMP9* promoter driving a reporter gene (chloramphenicol acetyl transferase, CAT) indicates that the first TRE (−79) but not the second (−209) is essential but not sufficient for *MMP9* transcription. Indeed, the region of the *MMP9* promoter spanning the nucleotides −531 to −670 significantly increases the CAT activity compared with the regions spanning nucleotides 1 to −531. Specificity protein-1 (SP1) and nuclear factor kappa B (NFκB) are present in this region and are known to cooperate with TRE for a complete activation of the *MMP9* gene.[33] It is not yet known whether this is also true for CTB.

NFκB is a heterodimeric protein complex formed by REL DNA binding proteins (the products of the *c-Rel* oncogene family), usually p50 and p65 (RELA). This protein complex is maintained in an inactive state in the cytoplasm through binding to members of the IκB family of inhibitors. This binding prevents the nuclear translocation of NFκB and transcriptional activation. When NFκB is activated by various inducers such as cytokines, phosphorylation of IκB-NFκB complexes occurs, IκB is degraded and NFκB translocates to the nucleus, where it binds to a DNA consensus sequence (GGAATTCCCC) located in the regulatory region of certain genes including *MMP9* (−328, −600). Several reports have shown that some of the cytokines that regulate trophoblast invasion activate or repress NFκB. Interleukin 1 (IL1), a stimulator of *MMP9* in CTB[34] induces NFκB activation in A549 epithelial cells[35] and in rat pancreatic beta cells.[36] Tumour necrosis factor (TNF), another potent stimulator of trophoblastic *MMP9*,[34] also activates NFκB in A549 epithelial cells,[35] in myocytes,[36] in neurons[37] and in B16 melanoma cells.[38]

The *ETS* gene family encodes transcription factors that bind to a consensus sequence (C/A)GGA(A/T) named PEA3 (polyoma enhancer A binding protein 3) which can be found in the regulatory region of the *MMP9* gene (−554, −541). ETS proteins do not usually dimerise to bind DNA but prefer to form complexes with other transcription factors such as AP1 for which they function as co-activators.[39] In the case of the *MMP9* gene, AP1 seems also to be involved since PEA3 is coupled to the third TRE (−533). However, this changes with the cell type: in OVCAR cells *MMP9* transcription depends on ETS–AP1 complexes[30] but not in UM-SCC-1 cells.[31] The situation in CTB is unknown. That the ETS proteins might be involved in the regulation of trophoblast invasion comes from the following observations: knockout mice for *Ets2* have deficient MMP9 expression, decreased trophoblast proliferation and persistence of ECM.[40] Furthermore, noninvasive MCF-7 cells transfected with an *Ets* oncogene product become invasive and massively increase their MMP9 secretion.[41]

Regulation of *MMP9* gene by p53

As is the case with many other genes, *MMP9* can be regulated by co-repressors or co-activators. These are proteins that bind to transcription factors (and are sometimes transcription factors themselves), thereby inhibiting or stimulating the transcriptional potential. A good example of this is the p53 phosphoprotein that displays direct and indirect transcriptional regulatory activity. Transcriptional activation by p53 occurs through binding to a DNA consensus sequence consisting of two copies of a 10 bp motif 5′-PuPuPuC(A/T)(T/A)GpyPyPy-3′ separated by 0–13 base pairs.[42] In contrast, p53 downregulates genes that lack p53 binding sites by interfering with other DNA binding proteins such as Fos,[43] SP1[44] or TATA binding proteins.[45] Binding sites for these proteins are present in the MMP9 promoter. It has been shown that p53 trans-activates *MMP2* in an osteogenic sarcoma cell line, U2-OS, and in a fibrosarcoma cell line, HT1080,[46] but trans-represses *MMP1* in human fibroblasts[47] and *MMP13* in squamous cell carcinoma.[48]

The 53 kDa nuclear protein p53 is 393 residues long and consists of a trans-activation domain at the N-terminus, a specific DNA-binding domain, and an oligomerisation domain at the C-terminus. Mutations have been identified in the DNA-binding domain in about 50% of human cancers. As stated by Levine in a review,[49] p53 is the 'gatekeeper' of the genome. Indeed, this protein is responsible, besides its growth-promoting effects, for inducing cell cycle arrest or apoptosis in the case of DNA damage. This avoids the damage in DNA being carried over in daughter cells. p53 is thus a tumour suppressor gene. When p53 is mutated (as in cancer) or otherwise altered, it loses its tumour suppressive activity and becomes oncogenic. The status of p53 in a cell is thus directly related to the acquisition of an invasive phenotype.

In a normal cell, p53 protein is kept at a very low level because of its short half-life (about 20 min). This turnover seems to be a result of the proteolytic degradation of p53 in the proteasome through binding to MDM2 and ubiquitination.[50] Stresses such as ionising radiation induce DNA damage to cells and a rapid increase in cellular p53 (essentially as a result of dissociation from MDM2) and concomitant activation of specific p53-dependent genes. Increased wild-type p53 levels inevitably lead to cell cycle arrest or apoptosis. These important responses are due to the recruitment by p53 of binding proteins such as BRCA1 (breast cancer antigen 1) or BARD1 (BRCA1-associated ring domain). If p53 is the gatekeeper, these proteins are its weapons.

We have performed co-transfection assays with a CAT reporter gene driven by various deletions of *MMP9* promoter and expression vector of p53 in HT1080 cells and CTB. In both cells, p53 downregulated *MMP9* promoter activity in a dose-dependent manner (results not shown). Since there is no p53 consensus sequence in the regulatory region of the *MMP9* promoter, downregulation of *MMP9* must occur by interaction with a cis-acting element. As downregulation was significantly more pronounced with the −670 promoter compared with −531 or −90 (Figure 6.1), one must conclude that p53 interaction must occur within the region spanning −670 to −531 bp of the *MMP9* 5′ flanking region. Although this result represents a novel mechanism regulating *hMMP9* expression, under more physiological conditions, *MMP9* activity as measured by zymography was not increased in human CTB exposed to pifithrin alpha (PFT, an inhibitor of endogenous p53) despite the fact that PFT stimulated MMP9 activity in MCF-7 cells (Figure 6.2). This result shows that placental wild-type p53, although present (immunoprecipitated and identified on Western blots), is unable to exert one of its functions. In contrast to the case with tumours, placental p53 is probably not mutated (under investigation) but, similarly to tumours, placental p53 has lost its onco-suppressive functions by a mechanism that remains to be elucidated. It can thus be concluded that placental p53 has become oncogenic. This observation *per se* can partly explain the invasive properties of human cytotrophoblastic cells.

Trophoblast invasion is compared with tumour invasion because both processes share the same molecular and biochemical parameters to invade neighbouring tissues. However, trophoblast is a 'well-behaved tumour' since its invasive potential is limited under physiological conditions. Understanding the molecular mechanisms that govern these limitations will undoubtedly increase our knowledge of embryo implantation but might also lead to new therapeutic strategies to fight cancer.

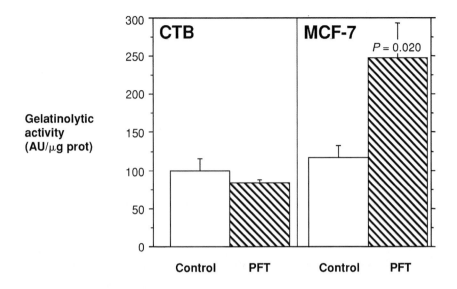

Figure 6.2.   Gelatinolytic activity of CTB and MCF-7 cells treated with pifithrin alpha (PFT). CTB and MCF-7 cells were incubated for 24 h in the presence or absence of PFT (20 μM). After incubation, the cells were harvested and the gelatinolytic activity of *MMP9* was measured by gelatine zymography. Digestion bands on the zymogram were scanned and the digestion areas quantitated by comparison with an activity standard run in parallel. Activities in arbitrary units (AU) were normalised to the total amount of cell proteins and the results expressed in percent of controls (cells without PFT). Three experiments in triplicate were performed with different cell preparations. The results represent the mean ± SEM. A paired Student's *t* test was used to compare treated and untreated cells.

Acknowledgements

The authors wish to express their gratitude to the Swiss National Science Foundation for their financial support.

References

1.   Tellbach M, Salamonsen LA, Van Damme MP. The influence of ovarian steroids on ovine endometrial glycosaminoglycans. *Glycoconj J* 2002;19:385–94.
2.   Greca CP, Abrahamsohn PA, Zorn TM. Ultrastructural cytochemical study of proteoglycans in the endometrium of pregnant mice using cationic dyes. *Tissue Cell* 1998;30:304–11.
3.   Runner MN. Development of mouse eggs in the anterior chamber of the eye. *Anat Rec* 1947;98:1–17.
4.   Fawcett DW. The development of mouse ova under the capsule of the kidney. *Anat Rec* 1950;108:71–91.
5.   Kirby DRS. The development of mouse blastocyst transplanted to the scrotal and cryptorchid testis. *J Anat* 1963;97:119–30.
6.   Kirby DRS. Development of the mouse blastocyst transplanted to the spleen. *J Reprod Fert* 1963;5:1–12.

7. Cowell TP. Implantation and development of mouse eggs transferred to the uteri of non progestational mice. *J Reprod Fertil* 1969;19:239–45.

8. Psychoyos A. Endocrine control of egg implantation. In: Greep RO, Astwood EG, Geiger SR, editors. *Handbook of Physiology*. Washington: American Physiological Society; 1973. Section 7, vol. 2, part 2, p. 187–215.

9. Fisher SJ, Cui T, Zhang L, Hartmann L, Grahl K, Guo-Yang Z, *et al.* Adhesive and degradative properties of human placental cytotrophoblast cells in vitro. *J Cell Biol* 1989;109:891–902.

10. Fisher SJ, Leitch MS, Kantor MS, Basbaum CB, Kramer RH. Degradation of extra-cellular matrix by the trophoblastic cells of first trimester placentas. *J Cell Biochem* 1985;27:31–41.

11. Bischof P, Martelli M, Campana A, Itoh Y, Ogata Y, Nagase H. Importance of metalloproteinases (MMP) in human trophoblast invasion. *Early Pregnancy* 1995;1:263–9.

12. Bischof P, Martelli M. Proteolysis in the penetration phase of the implantation process. *Placenta* 1992;13:17–24.

13. Westermarck J, Kähäri VM. Regulation of matrix metalloproteinase expression in tumour invasion. *FASEB J* 1999;13:781–92.

14. Nagase H. Activation mechanisms of matrix metalloproteinases. *J Biol Chem* 1997;378:151–60.

15. Gomez DE, Alonso DF, Yoshiji H, Thorgeirsson UP. Tissue inhibitor of metalloproteinases: structure, regulation and biological functions. *Eur J Cell Biol* 1997;74:111–22.

16. Bass KE, Li H, Hawkes SP, Howard E, Bullen E, Vu TK, *et al.* Tissue inhibitor of metalloprotreinase-3 is upregulated during human cytotrophoblast invasion in vitro. *Dev Genet* 1999;21:61–7.

17. Kliman HJ, Feinberg RF. Human trophoblast–extracellular matrix (ECM) interactions in vitro: ECM thickness modulates morphology and proteolytic activity. *Proc Natl Acad Sci U S A* 1990;87:3057–61.

18. Graham CH, Connelly I, MacDougall JR, Kerbel RS, Stetler-Stevenson WG, Lala PK. Resistance of malignant trophoblast cells to both the anti-proliferative and anti-invasive effects of transforming growth factor beta. *Exp Cell Res* 1994;214:93–9.

19. Graham CH, Lala PK. Mechanism of control of trophoblast invasion in situ. *J Cell Physiol* 1991;148:228–34.

20. Librach CL, Werb Z, Fitzgerald ML, Chiu K, Corwin NM, Esteves RA, *et al.* 92 kDa type IV collagenase mediates invasion of human cytotrophoblasts. *J Cell Biol* 1991;113:437–49.

21. Fernandez PL, Merino MJ, Nogales FF, Charonis AS, Stettler-Stevenson W, Liotta L. Immunohistochemical profile of basement membrane proteins and 72 kilodalton type IV collagenase in the implantation placental site. *Lab Invest* 1992;66:572–9.

22. Autio-Harmainen, H, Hurskainen, T, Niskasaari, K, Hoyhtya, M, Tryggvason K. Simultaneous expression of 70 kilodaltons type IV collagenase and type IV collagen alpha 1 (IV) chain genes by cells of early human placenta and gestational endometrium. *Lab Invest* 1992;66:191–200.

23. Polette M, Nawrocki B, Pintiaux A, Massenat C, Maquoi E, Volders L, *et al.* Expression of gelatinases A and B and their tissue inhibitors by cells of early and term human placenta and gestational endometrium. *Lab Invest* 1994;71:838–46.

24. Bischof P, Friedli E, Martelli M, Campana A. Expression of extra-cellular matrix-degrading metalloproteases by cultured human cytotrophoblast cells: Effect of cell adhesion and immunopurification. *Am J Obstet Gynecol* 1991;65:1791–801.

25. Shimonovitz S, Hurwitz A, Dushnik M, Anteby E, Geva-Eldar T, Yagel S. Developmental regulation of the expression of 72 and 92 kd type IV collagenases in human trophoblasts: a possible mechanism for control of trophoblast invasion. *Am J Obstet Gynecol* 1994;171:832–8.

26. Pijnenborg R, Dixon G, Robertson WB, Brosens I. Trophoblastic invasion of human decidua from 8 to 18 weeks of pregnancy. *Placenta* 1980;1:3–19.

27. Bischof P, Campana A. Molecular mediators of implantation. *Baillieres Best Pract Res Clin Obstet Gynaecol* 2000;14:801–14.

28. Huhtala P, Tuuttila A, Chow LT, Lohi J, Keski-Oja, J, Tryggvason K. Complete structure of the human gene 92-kDa type IV collagenase. *J Biol Chem* 1991;266:16485–90.

29. Sato H, Seiki M. Regulatory mechanism of 92 kDa type IV collagenase gene expression which is associated with invasiveness of tumour cells. *Oncogene* 1993;8:395–405.

30. Gum R, Lengyel E, Juarez J, Chen JH, Sato H, Seiki M, *et al.* Stimulation of 92-kDa gelatinase B promoter activity by ras is mitogen-activated protein kinase kinase 1-independent and requires multiple transcription factor binding sites including closely spaced PEA3/ets and AP-1 sequences. *J Biol Chem* 1996;271:10672–80.

31. Gum R, Wang H, Lengyel E, Juarez J, Boyd D. Regulation of 92 kDa type IV collagenase expression by the jun aminoterminal kinase- and the extra-cellular signal-regulated kinase-dependent signaling cascades. *Oncogene* 1997;14:1481–93.

32. Bischof P, Truong K, Campana A. Regulation of trophoblastic gelatinases by proto-oncogenes. *Placenta* 2003;24:155–63.

33. Curran T, Franza BR. Fos and Jun: the AP-1 connection. *Cell* 1988;55:395–7.

34. Meisser A, Chardonnens D, Campana A. Bischof P. Effects of tumour necrosis factor alpha, interleukin-1 alpha, macrophage colony stimulating factor and transforming growth factor beta on trophoblastic matrix metalloproteinases. *Mol Hum Reprod* 1999;5:252–60.

35. Newton R, Adcock IM, Barnes PJ. Superinduction of NF-kappa B by actinomycin D and cycloheximide in epithelial cells. *Biochem Biophys Res Commun* 1996;218:518–23.

36. Kwon G, Corbett JA, Rodi CP, Sullivan P, McDaniel ML. Interleukin-1 beta-induced nitric oxide synthase expression by rat pancreatic beta-cells: evidence for the involvement of nuclear factor kappa B in the signalling mechanism. *Endocrinology* 1995;136:4790–5.

37. Tamatani M, Che YH, Matsuzaki H, Ogawa S, Okado H, Miyake S, *et al.* Tumor necrosis factor induces Bcl-2 and Bcl-x expression through NFkappaB activation in primary hippocampal neurons. *J Biol Chem* 1999;274:8531–8.

38. Englaro W, Bahadoran P, Bertolotto C, Busca R, Derijard B, Livolsi A, *et al.* Tumor necrosis factor alpha-mediated inhibition of melanogenesis is dependent on nuclear factor kappa B activation. *Oncogene* 1999;18:1553–9.

39. Sharrocks AD, Brown AL, Ling Y, Yates PR. The ETS-domain transcription factor family. *Int J Biochem Cell Biol* 1997;12:1371–87.

40. Yamamoto H, Flannery ML, Kupriyanov S, Pearce J, McKercher SR, Henkel GW, *et al.* Defective trophoblast function in mice with a targeted mutation of Ets2. *Genes Dev* 1998;12:1315–26.

41. Kaya M, Yoshida K, Higashino F, Mitaka T, Ishii S, Fujinaga K. A single ets-related transcription factor, E1AF, confers invasive phenotype on human cancer cells. Oncogene 1996;12:221–7.

42. El-Deiry WS, Kern SE, Pietenpol JA, Kinzler KW, Vogelstein B. Definition of a consensus binding site for p53. *Nat Genet* 1992;1:45–9.

43. Donehower LA, Bradley A. The tumor suppressor p53. *Biochim Biophys Acta* 1993;1155:181–205.

44. Borellini F, Glazer RI. Induction of Sp1-p53 DNA-binding heterocomplexes during granulocyte/macrophage colony-stimulating factor-dependent proliferation in human erythroleukemia cell line TF-1. *J Biol Chem* 1993;268:7923–8.

45. Werner H, Karnieli E, Rauscher FJ, LeRoith D. Wild-type and mutant p53 differentially regulate transcription of the insulin-like growth factor I receptor gene. *Proc Natl Acad Sci U S A* 1996;93:8318–23.

46. Bian J, Sun Y. Transcriptional activation by p53 of the human type IV collagenase (gelatinase A or matrix metalloproteinase 2) promoter. *Mol Cell Biol* 1997;17:6330–8.

47. Sun Y, Sun Y, Wenger L, Rutter JL, Brinckerhoff CE, Cheung HS. p53 down-regulates human matrix metalloproteinase-1 (Collagenase-1) gene expression. *J Biol Chem* 1999;274:11535–40.

48. Ala-aho R, Grenman R, Seth P, Kahari VM. Adenoviral delivery of p53 gene suppresses expression of collagenase-3 (MMP13) in squamous carcinoma cells lines. *Oncogene* 2002;21:1187–95.

49. Levine AJ. P53, the cellular gatekeeper for growth and division. *Cell* 1997;88:323–31.

50. Ogawara Y, Kishishita S, Obata T, Isazawa Y, Suzuki T, Tanaka K, *et al.* Akt enhances Mdm2-mediated ubiquitination and degradation of p53. *J Biol Chem* 2002;277:21843–50.

Chapter 7
Embryo interactions in human implantation

Francisco Domínguez, Jose A Horcajadas, Ana Cervero,
Antonio Pellicer and Carlos Simón

Introduction

Embryonic implantation, the process by which the human embryo orientates towards, attaches to and finally invades the underlying maternal endometrial tissue, requires a receptive endometrium, a functionally normal blastocyst and adequate cross-communication between endometrium and blastocyst. During apposition, human blastocysts find a location in which to implant, while they are guided to a specific area in the maternal endometrium. In the adhesion phase, which occurs six to seven days after ovulation, within the 'implantation window', direct contact occurs between the endometrial epithelium and the trophectoderm. Finally, in the invasion phase, the embryonic trophoblast traverses the basement membrane and passes the endometrial stroma to reach the uterine vessels.

Many molecules (hormones, cytokines, integrins, enzymes, etc.) take part in the dialogue between the human blastocyst and the maternal endometrium to achieve implantation. We present here our published data on the embryonic regulation of endometrial epithelial molecules such as chemokine receptors, the leptin system and the relaxin receptor LGR7. A final section on gene profiling is also included.

Chemokine receptors at the maternal–embryonic interface

Chemokines, a family of small polypeptides with molecular weights in the range 8–12 kDa, attract specific leucocyte subsets by binding to cell-surface receptors. In reproductive biology, these molecules have been implicated in crucial processes such as ovulation, menstruation and parturition, and in pathological processes such as preterm delivery, HIV infection, endometriosis and ovarian hyperstimulation syndrome, as well as in embryo implantation.[1,2] More and more evidence suggests that chemokines produced and incorporated by the endometrial epithelium and the human blastocyst are implicated in this molecular network (Table 7.1). During implantation, leucocytes are recruited into the endometrium. The regulation of the uterine tissue during this process is thought to be orchestrated by uterine epithelial cells, which release an array of chemokines in a precise temporal pattern driven by ovarian steroids.[3,4] Chemokines act on a range of leucocyte subsets, which in turn release a number of proteases and other mediators that facilitate embryo invasion.[5]

Table 7.1. Summary of chemokine receptors expressed at the maternal–fetal interface; chemokine ligands are shown in brackets

Chemokine receptor	Reference
Expressed in human endometrium	
CCR2B (MCP 1, 3 and 5)	Dominguez *et al.*[16]
CCR5 (RANTES, MIP1α and β)	Dominguez *et al.*,[16] Mulayim *et al.*[54]
CXCR1 (IL8)	Dominguez *et al.*,[16] Mulayim *et al.*[54]
CXCR2 (IL8)	Mulayim et al.,[54]
CXCR4 (SDF1)	Dominguez *et al.*,[16] Kitaya *et al.*[55]
CXCR3 (MIG, IP10)	Kitaya *et al.*[55]
CCR3 (Eotaxin)	Zhang *et al.*[56]
Expressed in human blastocyst	
CCR2B (MCP 1, 3 and 5)	Dominguez *et al.*[16]
CCR5 (RANTES, MIP1α and β)	Dominguez *et al.*[16]
CCR1 (MIP1, 1α and 3)	Sato *et al.*[57]

Chemokines and their receptors are divided into two families based on structural and genetic considerations. All chemokines are structurally similar, having at least three β-pleated sheets and a C-terminal α-helix. In addition, most chemokines have at least four cysteines in conserved positions. In the CXC chemokine family (α–chemokines), the two cysteines nearest the N-termini of family members are separated by a single (and variable) amino acid. Dimerisation of chemokines is favoured when chemokines bind to cell-surface or connective-tissue components such as glycosaminoglycans.[6] These interactions strongly suggest that chemokine dimerisation is a critical *in vivo* process.

Chemokine receptors belong to the superfamily of G-protein-coupled receptors (GPCRs). These receptors display seven sequences of 20–25 hydrophobic residues that form an α-helix and span the plasma membrane, an extracellular N-terminus, three extracellular loops, three intracellular domains, and an intracellular C-terminal tail. These receptors transmit information to the cell about the presence of chemokine gradients in the extracellular environment. They are named depending on the structure of their ligand (CXC or CC). CXCR4 is expressed in neutrophils, mono-cytes, B and T lymphocytes, and its primary ligand is the stromal cell-derived factor 1 (SDF1).[7] CCR5, a receptor of regulated on activation, normal T-cell-expressed and secreted (RANTES) and macrophage inflammatory protein 1 (MIP1) α and β, is expressed in monocytes, dendritic cells, activated T lymphocytes and natural killer (NK) cells.[8] CCR2B, expressed in monocytes, basophils, dendritic cells, NK cells and activated T lymphocytes, is the main receptor for monocyte chemotactic proteins (MCP) 1, 2, 3 and 4.[9] CXCR1, a receptor of interleukin 8 (IL8) and granulocyte chemotactic protein 2 (GCP2), is expressed mainly in neutrophils and dendritic cells.[10]

A specific molecular cross-talk between embryo and endometrium has been reported to take place during the human implantation process.[11,12] The endometrial epithelium is a key site where molecular interactions between the embryo and endometrium seem to be initiated,[13,14] and from which chemokines are produced and secreted.[15]

The mRNA expression of the four chemokine receptors was analysed throughout the natural cycle using quantitative fluorescent polymerase chain reaction (QF-PCR). CXCR1 and CCR5 receptors showed a progesterone-dependent pattern in the early secretory phase (40- and 47-fold increases, respectively) that continued into the mid-secretory phase (157- and 176-fold increases, respectively) and was maximum in the late secretory phase (628- and 560-fold increases, respectively). Unlike the other receptors studied, CXCR4 presented a more pronounced upregulation in the mid-luteal phase rather than in the early and late luteal phases (an eighteen-fold increase in mid-luteal versus early luteal phase, and a two-fold increase when we compared mid-luteal with late luteal phase). This receptor, which is located in the endometrial epithelium, is therefore specifically upregulated during the implantation window.[16]

To study the '*in vivo*' hormonal regulation of chemokine receptors CXCR1, CCR2, CCR5 and CXCR4, endometrial biopsies were obtained on different days of hormone replacement therapy (HRT) cycles. Immunohistochemistry was carried out for protein localisation.

On day 13 ($n = 3$), when women were treated solely with oestradiol, a very weak staining for CCR2B, CCR5 and CXCR4 was localised in the luminal and glandular epithelium and endothelial cells. During the pre-receptive and receptive periods (days 18 and 21, respectively), an increase of staining intensity for CXCR1 receptor was noted in the glandular compartment. A slight signal was observed in stromal cells. CCR5 receptor was also immunolocalised, mainly at the luminal epithelium but also in the stromal and perivascular cells, showing a slight increase compared with the nonreceptive phase. CCR2B receptor showed a moderate increase in staining on days 18 and 21 in the luminal epithelium while no staining was observed in endothelial cells or stroma. CXCR4 receptor showed the same staining as CCR5, and was mainly expressed in the epithelium on days 18 and 21. Endothelial and stromal cells were also positive.[16]

The embryonic impact on immunolocalisation and polarisation of chemokine receptors CXCR1, CXCR4, CCR5 and CCR2B in cultured endometrial epithelial cells (EEC) was investigated using our apposition model for human implantation. When the blastocyst was absent, CXCR1, CXCR4 and CCR5 produced barely detectable staining in only a few cells at the EEC monolayer. However, when a human blastocyst was present, there was an increase in the number of stained cells for CXCR1, CXCR4 and CCR5, and polarisation of these receptors in one of the cell poles of the endometrial epithelium became evident. Immunolocalisation and polarisation changes in CCR2B receptor were not present in the EEC monolayer and this receptor was not upregulated by the presence of the human blastocyst.

Finally, we detected immunoreactive CCR2B and CCR5 receptors in the human blastocyst. CCR2B staining was localised mainly at the inner cell mass, whereas CCR5 staining could be visualised across the trophectoderm. In all cases ($n = 3$), CCR5 staining was more intense than that of CCR2B receptor, while the pellucide zone was not stained in any case. Immunoreactive CXCR4 and CXCR1 were not detected in human blastocysts when the same technique was used.

Relevance of leptin and leptin receptor in human endometrium

Obesity is a condition that is reaching epidemic proportions in the USA. The prevalence of obesity has doubled in the past decade[17] and one of the pathological consequences is infertility, indicating a link between adipose tissue and the reproductive system.[18] High body mass index (BMI) has been associated with low *in vitro* fertilisation (IVF) pregnancy rates,[19] suggesting the involvement of endometrial receptivity and implantation in these conditions.

Leptin is a 16 kDa non-glycosylated polypeptide of 146 amino acids discovered in 1994 by Zhang *et al.*[20] It is the *OB* gene product, a small pleiotrophic peptide initially thought to be secreted by adipose tissue. Leptin secretion is tightly linked to food consumption, energy balance and body weight.[21] Leptin has also been implicated in the regulation of reproductive function.[18]

Leptin receptor is the product of the *LEPR* or *OBR* gene and belongs to the class I superfamily of cytokine receptors. The full-length receptor has the signalling capabilities of an IL6-type receptor and also has its helical structure.[22] In humans and rodents, two major forms of leptin receptors (OB-R) are expressed. The short form (OB-RS) is detected in many organs and is considered to lack signalling capability[23] as it has a truncated intracellular domain.[24] The long form (OB-RL), with a complete intracellular domain, predominates in the hypothalamus and anterior pituitary, and is also expressed in low amounts in peripheral tissues.[25]

OB-RL activation involves the signal transduction cascade of Janus kinases (JAKs) and signal transducers and activators of transcription (STATs). Leptin binding leads to receptor oligomerisation and activation of the JAK/STAT pathway.[21]

An early observation indicated that *ob/ob* female mice (which lack functional leptin) and *db/db* mice (which lack functional leptin receptor) are characterised by obesity and sterility.[21,26] Fertility in the *ob/ob* animals can be restored by exogenous administration of leptin but not by food restriction, indicating that leptin *per se* is required for normal reproductive functioning.[27] Moreover, impaired reproductive function of *ob/ob* male mice is corrected only with leptin treatment.[28]

Similar findings in congenital leptin deficiency[29] and leptin mutation[30] have also been reported in humans. However, there are discrepancies in reports concerning normal reproduction in leptin-deficient women with lipoatropic diabetes.[31] In keeping with its predominant role as a signal for starvation,[32] leptin also seems to be important in mediating undernutrition-induced deficits in reproductive function. In starved mice, the lack of reproductive function coincides with the fall of plasma leptin level and several neuroendocrine changes. An exogenous leptin injection restores fertility in these mice.[33] In addition, leptin infusions restore ovulatory function in an animal model of starvation.

Human obesity is not characterised by leptin deficiency. It is interesting to consider that obesity is a state of leptin resistance and, therefore, this idea will focus on the status of the leptin receptor (OB-RL). However, evidence for this hypothesis is limited,[34] with only a few cases of splice-site mutation in the leptin receptor (which leads to a truncated form of the receptor with no signalling function)[35] having been reported.

Although the leptin system clearly influences reproduction, whether leptin exerts its effect as an endocrine or paracrine mediator is yet to be resolved. A large body of data supports the notion that the reproductive actions of leptin involve a direct effect on the brain, specifically the hypothalamus. Leptin receptor and actions of leptin have been described in the pituitary in both rodents and humans.[36] Expression of functional leptin receptors has also been detected in rodents[37] and humans,[38] and follicular and serum leptin production seems to be influenced by the ovarian functional state.[39] The mechanism linking leptin, luteinising hormone (LH) and oestradiol levels has not been clearly established. Endocrine data from IVF patients suggest that leptin production may be influenced by the ovarian functional state.[39]

In recent years, three different groups[40–42] have reported the expression of the leptin system in the human endometrium. All three groups affirm that the long form of leptin receptor (OB-RL) mRNA is detectable by Northern blot analysis[41] and reverse transcription polymerase chain reaction (RT-PCR) in the human endometrium. Furthermore, OB-RL protein has been detected by Western blot analyses,[40,41] and immunohistochemically OB-RL has been located in glandular and luminal epithelium.[40,42] In addition, OB-RL has been detected by RT-PCR and Western blot in cultured human EEC.[40] Interestingly, the Japanese group reported that OB-R mRNA expression peaked in the early secretory phase when semi-quantitative RT-PCR was employed[41] and the German group obtained similar findings at the protein level using semi-quantitative immunohistochemistry.[42]

Our group has described, for the first time, the expression of leptin and leptin receptor (long form) in the secretory endometrium and how leptin secretion is regulated in EEC by the human embryo during the apposition phase.[40]

Using our co-culture model, leptin and leptin receptor mRNA and protein were identified in secretory endometrium and in EEC co-cultured with human embryos, by RT-PCR and immunoblot, respectively. We also reported that individual human blastocysts and EEC secrete leptin. We found that the concentration of immunoactive leptin secreted by competent blastocysts was significantly higher than that secreted by arrested blastocysts cultured alone.[40] In contrast, leptin secreted from co-cultures of arrested blastocysts with EEC was significantly higher than that secreted from co-cultures of competent blastocysts with EEC. These findings suggest that the endometrium is a target tissue for circulating leptin and, in addition, is a site of local production. Expression of components of the leptin signalling system in the endometrium and EEC and regulation of leptin secretion by EEC due to the presence of the human embryo implicate the leptin system in the human implantation process.

In the embryonic context, leptin and STAT3 proteins have been immunolocalised in a polarised manner in mouse and human oocytes and in pre-implantation embryos.[43] Both molecules were found in pre-implantation embryos, with differences in the allocation of blastomeres occurring after the first cell division (2–4 cell stage). A cell-borne concentration gradient of these proteins extended along the surface of the embryo at the morula stage. A potential role of these proteins in early development has been suggested because of the fact that at the morula stage inner blastomeres contain little leptin/STAT3, while outer cells contain both leptin/STAT3-rich and -poor cells. In humans, this pattern has also been observed at the blastocyst stage.[43] The data presented by our group suggest a role for leptin during the pre-implantation phase in humans.[40] Higher levels of leptin were present in conditioned media from single human blastocysts, suggesting that this molecule may be a marker of embryonic vitality. However, when competent blastocysts were co-cultured with EEC, leptin concentrations in conditioned media did not differ from those of EEC cultured alone. This finding suggests various possibilities: leptin secreted by a competent blastocyst may bind to EEC or the secretion of leptin is regulated in EEC and/or in the human blastocyst. In any case, all these findings strongly suggest that this molecule takes part in the embryonic–endometrial dialogue during the adhesion phase of human embryonic implantation (Figure 7.1).

Relaxin and relaxin receptor LGR7

Relaxin is a peptide hormone produced by the corpus luteum during the luteal phase of the menstrual cycle and during the first trimester of pregnancy. It is composed of two peptide chains, A and B, of 24 and 29 amino acids, respectively, linked by disulphide bridges. Relaxin belongs structurally to a family of closely related protein hormones that includes, besides insulin and relaxin, insulin-like growth factor 1 (IGF1), IGF2, the relaxin-like factor (RLF/INSL3) and other novel relaxin/insulin-like factors 2 (INSL4) and 1 (INSL6).[44]

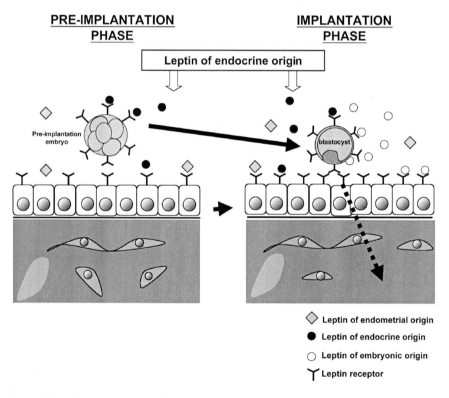

Figure 7.1.   General hypothesis of the human leptin system interactions at the maternal–embryonic interface during the pre-implantation and implantation phases; reproduced with permission from Cervero *et al.*[58] (*The Journal of Clinical Endocrinology & Metabolism,* © 2004 The Endocrine Society)

Relaxin has been associated with a wide range of functions related to pregnancy, such as parturition and lactation.[45] In nonpregnant women, the peak of circulating relaxin coincides with the window of endometrial receptivity and both *in vivo* and *in vitro* experiments have shown that it plays a role in the decidualisation process. Although relaxin is a well-studied hormone, very little was known about its receptor. Hsu and co-workers[46] have shown that LGR7 and LGR8, two leucine-rich, repeat-containing G-protein-coupled receptors, *in vitro* bind relaxin as a high-affinity ligand, resulting in cyclic adenosine monophosphate (cAMP) signalling. LGR7 has higher affinity for relaxin and the potency of LGR8 is somewhat lower.

LGR7 expression in human endometrial samples throughout the natural menstrual cycle was initially analysed by semi-quantitative RT-PCR. Maximal LGR7 RNA expression was observed during the proliferative phase. In general, LGR7 expression decreased during the early secretory phase and remained low for the rest of the secretory phase, with the exception of one woman in the late secretory phase group.[47]

To investigate LGR7 expression at the protein level, immunohistochemical analyses were performed with the 7BP antibody. Specific LGR7 expression was observed in all phases of the menstrual cycle. As observed in the QF-PCR experiments, the highest expression levels were obtained during the proliferative phase and the lowest levels during the secretory phase. In the early- to mid-proliferative phase, when the endometrium is under the influence of oestradiol, LGR7 staining was present in both the stromal and the epithelial compartment. This immunoreactive pattern was maintained in the late proliferative and early secretory phase. However, during the mid-secretory phase, LGR7 immunoreactive protein disappeared from the stromal compartment and staining was only observed in the glandular and the luminal epithelial. During late secretory phase, staining appeared again in both stromal and epithelial compartments.[47]

Our study established the presence of immunoreactive LGR7 protein in the human endometrium during all phases of the menstrual cycle, and also during the window of implantation. However, it could be hypothesised that regulation of LGR7 would not be necessary to suggest a specific role for it in the implantation process.

Gene profiling

Advances in gene expression profiling facilitated by the development of DNA micro-arrays[48] represent major progress in global gene expression analysis. The availability of this technology makes it possible to investigate the endometrial receptivity process from a global genomic perspective.[49–51] Our group has used human endometrial samples and oligonucleotide microarray technology (Human Genome U95A Array, Affymetrix GeneChip® Array) to determine global changes in gene expression at the moment of acquiring endometrial receptivity. To gain new insights into this complex process, we took a different approach from previously published related studies: we investigated endometrial biopsies obtained from the same woman in one menstrual cycle in pre-receptive (LH + 2) versus receptive (LH + 7) endometrium.[52] This study design allowed us to avoid masking effects occurring with the use of sample clustering, both by pooling endometria from different women and by grouping sampling days. Our approach revealed a consistent pattern of differentially expressed genes, even taking into account the human individual biological divergence. For identifying trends of gene expression across samples, a method known as principal component analysis (PCA) was performed.[53] Only those genes that appeared regulated in at least four out of five women were selected. Secondly, for these genes, the average expression and fold-change levels were calculated based on all five women.

Using the predefined criterion of a fold-change regulation higher than 3 in at least four out of five women, we identified 211 regulated genes among which were 12 expressed sequence tags (ESTs).[52] In total, 153 of these genes were specifically upregulated in the LH + 7 samples. Likewise, 58 downregulated genes were identified.

In validation studies we quantified the expression pattern of four differentially expressed genes by QF-PCR in LH + 2 versus LH + 7 endometria in three different women. Using QF-PCR, we investigated the expression of the three selected upregulated genes, glutathione peroxidase 3 (GPX3), claudin 4 and solute carrier family 1 member 1 (SLC1A1), during the entire menstrual cycle. All results obtained in this study matched with the chip data.

The results obtained corroborated the regulation profiles observed with DNA chip hybridisation experiments. In QF-PCR experiments, GPX3 was, on average, 113-fold upregulated in three independent LH + 7 versus LH + 2 samples, which is in agreement with the mean 66-fold upregulation obtained in the five woman studied by microarray. Human claudin 4 analysis showed that this gene was, on average, 2.9-fold upregulated in LH + 7 versus LH + 2 samples whereas, in the microarrays, a mean of 17-fold upregulation was registered.

Validation for downregulated genes was accomplished with the acyl-coenzyme A: acyltransferase (ACAT) gene (a cadherin-associated protein). Again, QF-PCR results demonstrated a decrease (38-fold) for *ACAT* in independent LH + 7 versus LH + 2 samples, confirming the microarray data (on average, 8-fold downregulation).

The gene expression localisation of two upregulated genes was detected by *in situ* hybridisation. The genes selected were GPX3 and SLC1A1. The experiments were performed on three sets of endometrial biopsies. For GPX3, a clear gene expression pattern was observed, showing low or no staining in the proliferative phase. The increasing amounts of glandular and luminal epithelial expression during the secretory phase were consistent with the pattern observed by QF-PCR.[52] For SLC1A1, we found increased staining in glandular epithelium during the secretory phase compared with the mid-luteal glandular expression pattern,[52] which again is consistent with the observed expression pattern by QF-PCR analysis.

Recently, and in a short period of time, four papers focusing on endometrial gene expression profiling have been published.[49–52] Although all used the same technology, some differences in the experimental design and in the analysis of the data were observed. The menstrual day for sample collection and pooling or not of the isolated RNA are two very important differences in these papers. Furthermore, in data analysis, three of them required a minimum fold increase of 2.0 in order to consider there to be evident gene regulation. However, Riesewijk and co-workers[52] used a 3.0-fold increase and performed the microarray analysis using samples from the same woman at two different stages of a single menstrual cycle.

We compared the results considering only those genes up- or downregulated in the receptive phase with a fold change of > 3.0. Only three upregulated genes, osteopontin, apolipoprotein D and Dickkopf, and one downregulated gene, olfactomedin, are present in the four studies. Another eight upregulated genes were present in the study by Riesewijk *et al.* and also in two out of the other three studies.

The data published in these studies offer the opportunity to develop an endo-metrial database of genes expressed during the window of implantation. We consider that all the published data are complementary, not only owing to different study designs but also to differences in the software and statistics used for analysis of the hybridisation data. Taken together, these results contribute to gaining an insight into the complexity of endometrial receptivity and the large number of known and new factors involved in achieving a successful embryo implantation.

References

1. Cocchi F, DeVico AL, Garzino-Demo A, Arya SK, Gallo RC, Lusso P. Identification of RANTES, MIP-1 alpha, and MIP-1 beta as the major HIV-suppressive factors produced by CD8+ T cells. *Science* 1995;270:1811–5.
2. Simón C, Caballero-Campo P, García-Velasco JA, Pellicer A. Potential implications of chemokines in reproductive function: an attractive idea. *J Reprod Immunol* 1998;38:169–93.
3. Robertson SA, Mayrhofer G, Seamark RF. Ovarian steroid hormones regulate granulocyte-macrophage colony-stimulating factor synthesis by uterine epithelial cells in the mouse. *Biol Reprod* 1996;54:265–77.
4. Wood GW, Hausmann X, Choudhuri R. Relative role of CSF-1, MCP-1/JE, and RANTES in macrophage recruitment during successful pregnancy. *Mol Reprod Dev* 1997;46:62–70.
5. Dudley DJ, Trantman MS, Mitchel MD. Inflammatory mediators regulate interleukin-8 production by cultured gestational tissues: evidence for a cytokine network at the chorio–decidual interface. *J Clin Endocrinol Metab* 1993;76:404–10.
6. Witt DP, Lander AD. Differential binding of chemokines to glycosaminoglycan subpopulations. *Curr Biol* 1994;4:394–400.
7. Nagasawa T, Nakajima T, Tachibana K, Iizasa H, Bleul CC, Yoshie O, *et al*. Molecular cloning and characterization of a murine pre-B-cell growth-stimulating factor/stromal cell-derived factor 1 receptor, a murine homolog of the human immunodeficiency virus 1 entry coreceptor fusin. *Proc Natl Acad Sci U S A* 1996;93:14726–9.
8. Chantakru S, Kuziel WA, Maeda N, Croy BA. A study on the density and distribution of uterine Natural Killer cells at mid pregnancy in mice genetically-ablated for CCR2B, CCR5 and the CCR5 receptor ligand, MIP-1 alpha. *J Reprod Immunol* 2001;49:33–47.
9. Polentarutti N, Allavena P, Bianchi G, Giardina G, Basile A, Sozzani S, *et al*. IL-2-regulated expression of the monocyte chemotactic protein-1 receptor (CCR2B) in human NK cells: characterization of a predominant 3.4-kilobase transcript containing CCR2B and CCR2A sequences. *J Immunol* 1997;158:2689–94.
10. Differential usage of the CXC chemokine receptors 1 and 2 by interleukin-8, granulocyte chemotactic protein-2 and epithelial-cell-derived neutrophil attractant-78. *Eur J Biochem* 1998;255:67–73.
11. Glasser SR, Mulholland J, Mani SK. Blastocyst endometrial relationships: reciprocal interactions between uterine epithelial and stromal cells and blastocysts. *Trophoblast Res* 1991;5:225–80.
12. De los Santos MJ, Mercader A, Frances A, Portoles E, Remohi J, Pellicer A, *et al*. Immunoreactive human embryonic interleukin-1 system and endometrial factors regulating their secretion during embryonic development. *Biol Reprod* 1996;54:563–74.
13. Simon C, Gimeno MJ, Mercader A, O'Connor JE, Remohi J, Polan ML, *et al*. Embryonic regulation of integrins beta 3, alpha 4, and alpha 1 in human endometrial epithelial cells in vitro. *J Clin Endocrinol Metab* 1997;82:2607–16.
14. Galan A, O'Connor JE, Valbuena D, Herrer R, Remohi J, Pampfer S, *et al*. The human blastocyst regulates endometrial epithelial apoptosis in embryonic adhesion. *Biol Reprod* 2000;63:430–9.
15. Caballero-Campo P, Dominguez F, Coloma J, Meseguer M, Remohi J, Pellicer A, *et al*. Hormonal and embryonic regulation of chemokines IL-8, MCP-1 and RANTES in human endometrium during the window of implantation. *Mol Hum Reprod* 2002;8:375–84.
16. Dominguez F, Galan A, Martin JJ, Remohi J, Pellicer A, Simon C. Hormonal and embryonic regulation of chemokine receptors CXCR1, CXCR4, CCR5 and CCR2B in the human endometrium and the human blastocyst. *Mol Hum Reprod* 2003;9:189–98.
17. Houseknecht KL, Baile CA, Matteri RL, Spurlock ME. The biology of leptin: a review. *J Anim Sci* 1998;76:1405–20.
18. Frisch RE. The right weight: body fat, menarche and ovulation. *Baillieres Clin Obstet Gynaecol* 1990;4:419–39.
19. Wang JX, Davies M, Norman RJ. Body mass and probability of pregnancy during assisted reproduction treatment: retrospective study. *BMJ* 2000;321:1320–1.

20. Zhang Y, Proenca R, Maffei M, Barone M, Leopold L, Friedman JM. Positional cloning of the mouse obese gene and its human homologue. *Nature* 1994;372:425–32.
21. Friedman JM, Halaas JL. Leptin and the regulation of body weight in mammals. *Nature* 1988;395:763–70.
22. Baumann H, Morella KK, White DW. The full-length leptin receptor has signaling capabilities of interleukin 6-type cytokine receptors. *Proc Natl Acad Sci U S A* 1996;93:8374–8.
23. Wang Y, Kuropatwinski KK, White DW. Leptin receptor action in hepatic cells. *J Biol Chem* 1997;272:16216–23.
24. Campfield LA, Smith FJ, Burn P. The OB protein (leptin) pathway – a link between adipose tissue mass and central neural networks. *Horm Metab Res* 1996;28:619–32.
25. Finn PD, Cunningham MJ, Pau KY, Spies HG, Clifton DK, Steiner RA. The stimulatory effect of leptin on the neuroendocrine reproductive axis in the monkey. *Endocrinology* 1998;139:4652–62.
26. Ingalls AM, Dickie MM, Snell GD. Obese, a new mutation in the house mouse. *J Hered* 1950;41:317–18.
27. Barash IA, Cheung CC, Weigle DS. Leptin is a metabolic signal to the reproductive system. *Endocrinology* 1996;137:3144–7.
28. Mounzih K, Lu R, Chehab FF. Leptin treatment rescues the sterility of genetically obese ob/ob males. *Endocrinology* 1997;138:1190–3.
29. Montague CT, Farooqi IS, Whitehead JP. Congenital leptin deficiency is associated with severe early-onset obesity in humans. *Nature* 1997;387:903–8.
30. Strobel A, Issad T, Camoin L, Ozata M, Strosberg AD. A leptin missense mutation associated with hypogonadism and morbid obesity. *Nat Med* 1998;18:213–15.
31. Andreelli F, Hanaire-Broutin H, Laville M, Tauber JP, Riou JP, Thivolet C. Normal reproductive function in leptin-deficient patients with lipoatropic diabetes. *J Clin Endocrinol Metab* 2000;85:715–19.
32. Schneider JE, Goldman MD, Tang S, Bean B, Ji H, Friedman MI. Leptin indirectly affects estrous cycles by increasing metabolic fuel oxidation. *Horm Behav* 1998;33:217–28.
33. Ahima RS, Prabakaran D, Mantzoros C. Role of leptin in the neuroendocrine response to fasting. *Nature* 1996;382:250–2.
34. Conway GS, Jacobs HS. Leptin: a hormone of reproduction. *Hum Reprod* 1997;12:633–5.
35. Clement K, Vaisse C, Lahlou N. A mutation in the human leptin receptor gene causes obesity and pituitary dysfunction. *Nature* 1998;392:398–401.
36. Shimon I, Yan X, Magoffin DA, Friedman TC, Melmed S. Intact leptin receptor is selectively expressed in human fetal pituitary and pituitary adenomas and signals human fetal pituitary growth hormone secretion. *J Clin Endocrinol Metab* 1998;83:4059–64.
37. Zachow RJ, Magoffin DA. Direct intraovarian effects of leptin: impairment of the synergistic action of the insulin-like growth factor I on follicle-stimulating hormone-dependent estradiol-17 beta production by rat ovarian granulosa cells. *Endocrinology* 1997;138:847–50.
38. Karlsson C, Lindell K, Svensson E, Bergh C, Lind P, Billig H, *et al.* Expression of functional leptin receptors in human ovary. *J Clin Endocrinol Metab* 1997;82:4144–8.
39. Bützow TL, Moilanen JM, Lehtovirta M. Serum and follicular fluid leptin during in vitro fertilization: Relationship among leptin increase, body fat mass, and reduced ovarian response. *J Clin Endocrinol Metab* 1999;84:3135–9.
40. González RR, Caballero-Campo P, Jasper M, Mercader A, Devoto L, Pellicer A, *et al.* Leptin and leptin receptor are expressed in the human endometrium and endometrial leptin secretion is regulated by the human blastocyst. *J Clin Endocrinol Metab* 2000;85:4883–8.
41. Kitawaki J, Koshiba H, Ishihara H. Expression of leptin receptor in human endometrium and fluctuation during the menstrual cycle. *J Clin Endocrinol Metab* 2000;85:1946–50.
42. Alfer J, Müller-Schöttle F, Classen-Linke I. The endometrium as a novel target for leptin: differences in fertility and subfertility. *Mol Hum Reprod* 2000;6:595–601.
43. Antczak M, Van Blerkom JV. Oocyte influences on early development: the regulatory proteins leptin and STAT3 are polarized in mouse and human oocytes and differentially distributed within the cells of the preimplantatation stage embryo. *Mol Hum Reprod* 1997;2:1067–86.
44. Ivell R, Bathgate RA. Reproductive biology of the relaxin-like factor (RLF/INSL3). *Biol Reprod* 2002;67:699–705.
45. Telgmann R, Gellersen B. Marker genes of decidualization activation of the decidual prolactin gene. *Hum Reprod Update* 1998;4:472–9.
46. Hsu SY, Kudo M, Chen T, Nakabayashi K, Bhalla A, van der Spek PJ, *et al.* The three subfamilies of leucine rich repeat-containing G protein coupled receptors (LGR): Identification of LGR6 and LGR7 and the signalling mechanism for LGR7. *Mol Endocrinol* 2000;14:8,1257–71.

47. Luna JJ, Riesewijk A, Horcajadas JA, Van Os R, Dominguez F, Mosselman S, *et al.* Gene expression pattern and immunoreactive protein localization of LGR7 receptor in human endometrium throughout the menstrual cycle. *Mol Hum Reprod* 2004;10:85–90.

48. Schena M, Shalon D, Davis RW, Brown PO. Quantitative monitoring of gene expression patterns with a complementary DNA microarray. *Science* 1995;270:467–70.

49. Kao LC, Tulac S, Lobo S, Imani B, Yang JP, Germeyer A, *et al.* Global gene profiling in human endometrium during the window of implantation. *Endocrinology* 2002;143:2119–38.

50. Carson, DD, Lagow E, Thathiah A, Al-Shami R, Farach-Carson MC, Vernon M, *et al.* Changes in gene expression during the early to mid-luteal (receptive phase) transition in human endometrium detected by high-density microarray screening. *Mol Hum Reprod* 2002;8:971–9.

51. Borthwick JM, Charnock-Jones DS, Tom BD, Hull ML, Teirney R, Phillips SC, *et al.* Determination of the transcript profile of human endometrium. *Mol Hum Reprod* 2003;9:19–33.

52. Riesewijk A, Martín J, van Os R, Horcajadas JA, Polman J, Pellicer A, *et al.* Gene expresion plofiling of human endometrial receptivity on days LH+2 versus LH+7 by microarray technology. *Mol Hum Reprod* 2003;9:253–64.

53. Joliffe I. Principal *Component Analysis.* Springer Series in Statistics. New York: Springer-Verlag; 1986.

54. Mulayim N, Palter SF, Kayisli UA, Senturk L, Arici A. Chemokine receptor expression in human endometrium. *Biol Reprod* 2003;68:1491–5.

55. Kitaya K, Nakayama T, Daikoku N, Fushiki S, Honjo H. Spatial and temporal expression of ligands for CXCR3 and CXCR4 in human endometrium. *J Clin Endocrinol Metab* 2004;89:2470–6.

56. Zhang J, Lathbury LJ, Salamonsen LA. Expression of the chemokine eotaxin and its receptor, CCR3, in human endometrium. *Biol Reprod* 2000;62:404–11.

57. Sato Y, Higuchi T, Yoshioka S, Tatsumi K, Fujiwara H, Fujii S. Trophoblasts acquire a chemokine receptor, CCR1, as they differentiate towards invasive phenotype. *Development* 2003;130:5519–32.

58. Cervero A, Horcajadas JA, MartIn J, Pellicer A, Simon C. The leptin system during human endometrial receptivity and preimplantation development. *J Clin Endocrinol Metab* 2004;89:2442–51.

Chapter 8

Experimental models of implantation of the human embryo: reconstructing the endometrial–embryo dialogue *in vitro*

Helen Mardon

Implantation failure: a major challenge in *in vitro* fertilisation

Failure of the embryo to implant successfully into the endometrium is one of the major causes of infertility. Many causes of infertility, such as sperm dysfunction and certain disorders of the fallopian tube or ovary, can now be identified and either treated or bypassed by *in vitro* fertilisation (IVF). However, up to 20% of cases of infertility have no apparent cause and are labelled 'unexplained', and for which there is no treatment other than IVF.[1] Approximately one-third of normal human pregnancies end in miscarriage and 22% of these occur before pregnancy is detected clinically, probably as a result of failure of the embryo to implant properly. The frequent failure of IVF treatment, despite the repeated replacement of apparently high-quality embryos, demonstrates that a woman's fertility ultimately depends on the ability of the embryos to implant successfully into the endometrium.

The successful establishment of a pregnancy is also influenced by other factors in addition to endometrial receptivity and morphological quality of the embryo, and the failure of the embryo to implant may also result from impairment of the genetic potential of the embryo, which remains an intractable problem. The pregnancy rates from donated oocytes in older women (> 40 years) are similar to those of younger women in egg-donation IVF cycles, and in both groups the majority of embryos fail to implant and establish a pregnancy.[2] The ability of the endometrium to facilitate implantation is therefore likely to be a key factor underlying fertility where the embryonic genetic potential is thought to be optimal, as in egg donation.

Stages of human embryo implantation

The function of the endometrium is to receive the implanting blastocyst and support pregnancy. This is achieved by its unique capacity to undergo remarkable cyclical regeneration and remodelling in preparation for implantation and in response to steroid hormones and the local signalling pathways elicited as a result of their action. Early embryo implantation involves three main events. In the first stage, the pre-implantation blastocyst and the endometrium are primed for implantation. This involves successful hatching of the blastocyst and expression of molecules on the trophectoderm that are permissive for uterine–embryo interaction. At the same time, the endometrium must be receptive for embryo attachment, which occurs during a window of implantation from about day 20 to day 24 of the endometrial cycle.[3] Coordination of these events in the two tissues is thus critical. Development to the blastocyst stage appears to be to some extent autonomously driven, as blastocyst formation from fertilised eggs can be obtained in defined complex serum-free medium. However, there is growing evidence to suggest that there is considerable cross-signalling by soluble factors that facilitates the priming of the blastocyst and endometrium immediately prior to implantation.[4] During the second stage of implantation, the hatched blastocyst attaches to and penetrates the luminal epithelium of the endometrium. It is likely that signals from both soluble factors and immobilised extracellular matrix (ECM) ligands are involved in these processes. The third stage involves invasion of the trophoblast through the epithelial basement membrane and the underlying stromal ECM. Subsequent proliferation and differentiation of the trophoblast results in the colonisation of the maternal blood supply and establishment of a functional placenta.

Blastocyst implantation is mediated via soluble and ECM-bound signalling molecules, although the precise molecular mechanisms that are involved in the human are not understood. Functional studies using animal models, particularly murine, have revealed a number of molecules that have a role in implantation. Genetic studies using gene knockout methodology have identified a number of growth factors and receptors, including the epidermal growth factor (EGF) and its receptor (EGFR),[5] leukaemia inhibitory factor (LIF)[6] and the interleukin 11 (IL11) receptor α,[7,8] that have a function in embryo implantation. Many other molecules, including IL11,[8] heparin-binding EGF-like growth factor (HB-EGF),[9,10] matrix metalloproteinases (MMPs) and their inhibitors (TIMPs),[11,12] have been implicated in implantation in animals by virtue of their appearance *in vivo* in the endometrium at sites of implantation and from evidence from *in vitro* experiments.

Although murine models are powerful and provide clues about molecules that may be involved in embryo implantation in the human, differences in the reproductive physiology between the two species means that knowledge gained from the mouse does not necessarily translate directly to the human. Primates provide a more physiologically relevant model. Valuable information about early implantation events is emerging from *in vivo* and *in vitro* studies in baboons[13,14] and the rhesus monkey.[15] Important insights into implantation have also been gleaned from some striking analyses of marmoset early implantation sites.[16] Thus there are compelling data from animal studies concerning mechanisms of implantation, but the cellular and molecular mechanisms involved in implantation of the human embryo remain poorly understood.

Implantation in the human

Previous studies in the human have largely been confined to description of the expression profiles of various molecules in the endometrium obtained at various stages of the menstrual cycle. The levels of a number of molecules have been shown to peak during the window of implantation, particularly the ECM receptor integrin $\alpha_v\beta_3$,[17] LIF[18] and HB-EGF.[19–21] The expression of molecules in human peri-implantation blastocysts is less well studied. Integrin subunits α_3, α_v, β_1, β_4 and β_5[22] and EGFR[23] are expressed on early, pre-implantation human embryos, indicating that these molecules may have a function in the implantation in the human.

More recently, gene profiling studies of human endometrium during the window of implantation using oligonucleotide microarrays have revealed additional genes that are significantly upregulated during the window of implantation.[3,24,25] These include genes encoding proteins with functions that predictably might be relevant to implantation, such as the adhesion molecule osteopontin, proteinases and immune modulators, together with more surprising candidates such as apolipoprotein E. Other genes are downregulated, including those coding for the breakdown of the ECM, such as MMP7.[24] The data emerging from gene profiling by DNA array technology are undoubtedly proving to be informative even if the technology as applied in these studies has some limitations, as discussed in detail in Chapter 16.

In contrast to the early stages of implantation (the first two weeks of pregnancy), tissues and cells from the maternal–fetal interface during the later stages of first-trimester pregnancy, when the placenta is being established, have been widely studied.[26] Although there are likely to be significant differences in the processes occurring in early and late first-trimester trophoblast invasion, a study has suggested that one cell–cell adhesion mechanism, involving L-selectin, may be common to both.[27] Genbacev and co-workers showed that the trophectoderm of peri-implantation human blastocysts expresses L-selectin and the luminal epithelium of human endometrium expresses L-selectin ligands in the receptive phase of the cycle, suggesting a role for the interaction of these molecules in blastocyst attachment. They also demonstrated that cytotrophoblast isolated from first-trimester placenta bind, via cell-surface L-selectin, to the luminal epithelium in sections of luteal-phase endometrium. Together, these observations suggest a mechanism for initial blastocyst attachment to the luminal epithelium that is similar to that of L-selectin-mediated leucocyte recruitment to sites of vascular damage. This is achieved via the making and breaking of L-selectin–ligand interactions, which impedes the passage of the leucocyte, causing it to roll along the vessel wall.[28] Various ligand–receptor interactions are then induced which mediate extravasion of the leucocyte. It is intriguing to speculate that similar processes occur in implantation of the human embryo.

Analyses of early implantation sites in tubal pregnancies such as those reported recently[29] may be particularly useful for investigating the mechanisms underlying the initial stages of embryo attachment and invasion since there are similarities (as well as differences) between tubal and endometrial implantation. However the analysis of the early stages of normal human implantation remains an intractable problem, largely because early implantation sites in the human are inaccessible to experimental manipulation *in vivo* and much of the literature on human blastocyst implantation is essentially descriptive.

Functional models for implantation in the human

There are few models of human embryo implantation that have been exploited to dissect the implantation process and from which information about the function of specific molecules involved has been obtained. Many studies have investigated either endometrial tissue (or cells) or human embryos. These studies are undoubtedly informative, but the function of specific molecules in implantation must also be investigated in the context of endometrial–blastocyst interactions. Three experimental models of human implantation that have been designed to address this problem will be discussed below. These are solid-phase embryo cultures, endometrial cell–embryo co-cultures and three-dimensional cultures, the application of each investigating a different process in implantation.

Solid-phase assays for blastocyst attachment and trophoblast outgrowth

Solid-phase assays have been used previously to determine the function and signalling properties of ECM components in the adhesion and trophoblast outgrowth of mouse blastocysts. Using these assays it has been shown that fibronectin supports blastocyst attachment and trophoblast outgrowth.[30–33] Similar assays have been applied to test the function of HB-EGF, in isolation, for mediating the attachment of human peri-implantation blastocysts.

HB-EGF has a function in diverse biological processes such as wound healing, tumour growth, smooth muscle cell hyperplasia, angiogenesis and reproduction.[34] It is synthesised as a 208 amino acid transmembrane precursor (tm–HB-EGF) containing EGF, heparin-binding, transmembrane and cytoplasmic domains. The ectodomain can be secreted as a 12–22 kDa soluble form of HB-EGF (sol-HB-EGF) by proteolytic cleavage.[35,36] Thus tm–HB-EGF and sol-HB-EGF can act as juxtacrine and paracrine growth factors in the human endometrium,[37] as well as adhesion molecules. Their biological functions are mediated by the EGF receptor EGFR (ErbB1) and ErbB4 that in turn can exist as surface cleaved ectodomains and soluble intracellular domains that localise to the nucleus.[38,39] Thus tm–HB-EGF is a good candidate for mediating human blastocyst attachment because:

1. it has been shown to attach to mouse blastocysts[9]
2. tm–HB-EGF is expressed on the luminal surface of receptive-stage endometrium[40]
3. its specific receptor, ErbB4, is expressed on the polar trophectoderm of peri-implantation human blastocysts.[40]

We designed a solid-phase assay to test this function in human blastocyst attachment.[40] In this assay, recombinant HB-EGF was expressed as a fusion protein with the Fc region of immunoglobulin G (IgG) and the fusion protein adsorbed onto glass coverslips coated with protein A so that the anchored HB-EGF ectodomain was in the correct orientation to allow it to interact with the blastocyst (Figure 8.1A). Hatched, expanded, good-quality day 6 human blastocysts, assessed according to morphology, were cultured from day 2 embryos donated for research by couples undergoing IVF. The blastocysts were placed on the coated coverslips and cultured for 48 hours in the presence or absence of sol-HB-EGF as a competitor. Using this assay we were able to demonstrate that tm–HB-EGF supports blastocyst attachment but not trophoblast outgrowth (Figure 8.1B and C), and that it promotes blastocyst survival and development as assessed by the increased levels of human chorionic gonadotrophin (hCG) in the culture supernatants of blastocysts cultured on tm–HB-EGF-coated coverslips.[40] Such relatively simple solid-phase models thus have the significant advantage that they allow the function of specific molecules to be determined in isolation. However, the absence of endometrial cells and their products means that these assays encapsulate a particular process in implantation and do not necessarily permit analyses of dynamic processes.

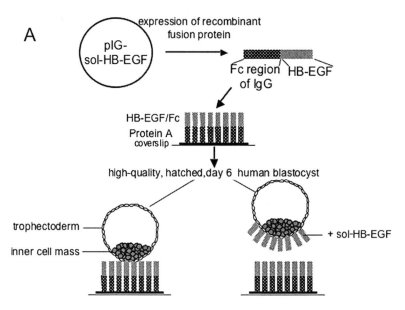

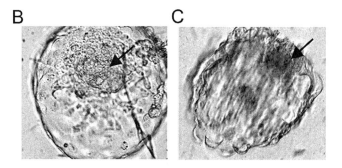

Figure 8.1. Solid-phase assay to test function of purified molecules in implantation; the design of the assays of recombinant HB-EGF using the expression vector pIG is illustrated in A; human blastocysts cultured on HB-EGF-coated coverslip in the absence (B) or presence (C) of a soluble inhibitor of HB-EGF; the blastocyst in A is attached to the coverslip via the HB-EGF receptor expressed on the trophectoderm, whereas in B it remains in suspension

Endometrial cell–blastocyst co-cultures

The interaction of the blastocyst with various cellular components of the endo-metrium can be investigated in co-cultures of isolated cells and peri-implantation blastocysts. Lindenberg and co-workers[41] obtained striking images of human blastocysts adhering to a monolayer of endometrial epithelium *in vitro* via the polar trophectoderm. More recently, Meseguer *et al.*[42] have described an elegant, well-characterised *in vitro* model system for investigating embryo-driven induction of endometrial epithelium receptivity and the converse priming of the embryo for implantation by the endometrial epithelium. These experimental systems in which human embryos are co-cultured with monolayer human endometrial epithelial cells have revealed the modulation of expression of a number of molecules by the blastocyst and are described in detail in Chapter 7.[43]

The molecular mechanisms underpinning regulated trophoblast invasion of the endometrial stroma can also be investigated by the use of such endometrial cell–blastocyst co-cultures (Figure 8.2A).[44] High-resolution image analysis of blastocysts invading monolayers of endometrial stromal cell systems has been used to investigate the nature and extent of trophoblast invasion. The model is highly reproducible and we have demonstrated that the blastocysts remain expanded but unattached to the stromal cell layer for approximately 10–15 hours. They then attach to the dorsal surface of the stromal cells and remain attached for a further 5–10 hours (Figure 8.2B). The blastocysts then contract and become less expanded before entering the invasive stage (Figure 8.2C). The trophoblast invades the stromal cells along the same axis as the elongated cells, and the blastocyst as a whole acquires a bipolar axis (Figure 8.2D). This suggests that the endometrial stroma may provide specific directional cues for invading trophoblast during implantation but the nature of such cues remains to be determined.

Analyses of Z-images of stained wholemounts of these 'implantation sites' reveal that the invasive trophoblast completely penetrates the stromal cell layer and establishes contact with the underlying stromal ECM (Figure 8.2E).[44] A prominent adhesive structure anchors the trophoblast to the stromal ECM. These structures are adjacent to the basal membrane of the trophoblast cells and contain actin and cytokeratin filaments (Figure 8.2F). In fact they resemble podosomes, which are phagocytic foci found in scavenger cells such as macrophages and osteoclasts as well as in outgrowing trophoblast in mouse embryos.[45] These observations suggest that, prior to colonisation of the maternal vasculature, trophoblast may perform a nutritional function by scavenging endometrial ECM breakdown products. Indeed further analyses of ECM receptors and associated molecules in trophoblast podosomes will shed light on their precise nature and function.

Blastocysts implanting into stromal cells secrete high levels of hCG, a secreted product of trophoblast, compared with blastocysts maintained on plastic or on Matrigel™,[44,46] suggesting that the stromal cells provide factors that promote blastocyst development and invasion. The implantation model described here is robust in that it is reproducible, supports invasion and appears to support prolonged development and wellbeing of the blastocysts exposed to endometrial stromal cells. The model will allow the functional dissection of molecules or groups of molecules specifically in the stromal invasion stage of implantation by the addition of specific antagonists or function blocking agents. In particular, soluble growth factors and cytokines and ECM-associated factors that mediate the invasion process can be identified, and their function determined.

The cell–embryo co-culture model also has the potential to be used as an indicator of embryo quality. Currently, the benefits of new treatments or culture conditions for IVF can only be assessed on the basis of embryo morphology or whether the embryos form pregnancies when transferred back to the woman. The availability of *in vitro*

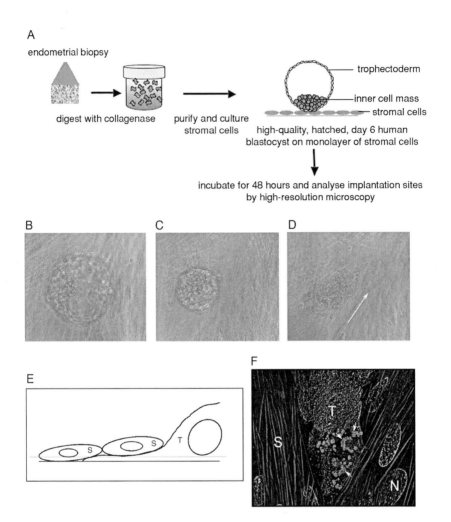

Figure 8.2. Endometrial stromal cell–embryo co-culture model of implantation; the design of the model is illustrated in A; real-time imaging of a human blastocyst attaching to and invading the confluent stromal layer is shown at 10 (B), 15 (C) and 40 hours (D) after placing the blastocyst onto the cells; the expanded blastocyst is attached to the cells in B, undergoes contraction in C, and the trophoblast invades the stromal layer along a bipolar axis (white arrow in D); Z-images, obtained by deconvolution, adjacent to the coverslip, indicated by the line in E and as shown in F, reveal that the trophoblast (T) penetrate the stromal cells (S) and migrate along the ECM underneath them; trophoblast surrounded by stromal cells with distinct elongated actin filaments are shown in F, where distinct podosome-like structures (arrows) in the trophoblast comprising an actin core surrounded by a cytokeratin ring can be seen; the nuclei are indicated by N; parts B to F reproduced by permission of Oxford University Press/*Human Reproduction* from Carver J, Martin K, Spyropoulou I, Barlow D, Sargent I, Mardon H. An in-vitro model for stromal invasion during implantation of the human blastocyst. *Hum Reprod* 2003;18:283–90, © European Society of Human Reproduction and Embryology

models such as the one we present here will enable embryos to be assessed in terms of their ability to implant, thereby providing a useful measure of embryo quality in response to a particular treatment.

Three-dimensional co-cultures of endometrial cells and blastocysts

The cell–blastocyst co-culture models allow us to investigate the interaction of trophoblast with specific endometrial cell types. More complex, three-dimensional models are required to dissect further all the stages of early implantation in a physiological context. Such a model for implantation in the human has been established, in which human blastocysts are cultured on a three-dimensional structure comprising a reconstituted endometrial stroma and epithelium separated by a basement membrane.[47] Such a three-dimensional reconstituted endometrial structure, illustrated in Figure 8.3, was generated by mixing isolated endometrial stromal cells with collagen type I on a filter in a tissue culture well insert. The basement membrane preparation Matrigel is then layered on the surface of the gel, and isolated endometrial epithelial cells seeded onto this. An important aspect of this model is that the epithelial monolayer that forms on the basement membrane is polarised, as it is *in vivo*. Analyses of three-dimensional models such as this are as yet limited to the microscopic analysis of the initial attachment of the blastocyst to, and its penetration of, the endometrial epithelial layer. A significant advantage of this model is that it facilitates implantation of the human blastocyst through the two cell layers and has the potential to allow all three stages of implantation (attachment, epithelial penetration and stromal invasion) to be visualised.[48] Further refinement and improvement of the three-dimensional culture system towards a superior relevant system physiologically could be achieved by inclusion of additional endometrial cell types such as endothelial cells and glandular epithelium.

Establishing models for human implantation

Each of the experimental systems described above critically relies upon high-quality human blastocysts. In addition, accurate clinical diagnosis and the application of strict histopathological criteria to endometrial tissue samples from which the cells are derived for the co-culture and three-dimensional models is essential. Ideally, cells and cell lines should be established from endometrial tissue biopsies obtained from healthy, fertile women (who are undergoing sterilisation) of reproductive age, and who have not received recent hormonal medication. Further characterisation of the cell lines with time in culture is also critical to ensure that the cells are homogeneous and phenotypically similar to their *in vivo* equivalent such that the integrity of the endometrial cell type is sustained as far as possible.[40]

Conclusions

Model systems for the study of complex processes such as implantation of the human embryo can involve varying degrees of complexity. It is likely that each stage of the implantation process involves multiple molecular mechanisms and, the more complex the model, the more of these putative mechanisms may be operating within the model. Each of the *in vitro* models described above thus has advantages as well as limitations. However, the application of a combination of these experimental systems

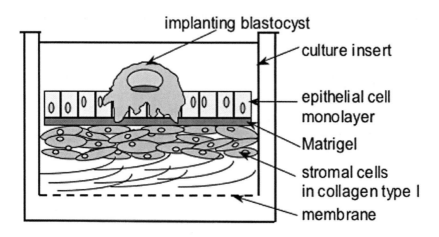

Figure 8.3. Three-dimensional model of implantation; endometrial stromal cells are mixed with ECM such as collagen type I and placed on a tissue culture well insert, overlaid with Matrigel and purified endometrial epithelial cells; the progression of events in implantation from attachment through to invasion of the stromal ECM may be observed by the use of this model

together with the use of specific inhibitors or antagonists provides a potentially powerful tool with which to dissect the molecular, cellular and physiological mechanisms of embryo implantation in the human.

Acknowledgements

The author is extremely grateful to Janet Carver, Natasha Karpovich, Petra Klemmt and Tracey Ward for help with the diagrams and preparation of the manuscript.

References

1. Isaksson R, Tiitinen A. Present concept of unexplained infertility. *Gynecol Endocrinol* 2004;18:278–90.
2. Toner JP, Grainger DA, Frazier LM. Clinical outcomes among recipients of donated eggs: an analysis of the U. S. national experience, 1996–1998. *Fertil Steril* 2002;78:1038–45.
3. Kao LC, Tulac S, Lobo S, Imani B, Yang JP, Germeyer A, *et al.* Global gene profiling in human endometrium during the window of implantation. *Endocrinology* 2002;143:2119–38.
4. Dominguez F, Pellicer A, Simon C. Paracrine dialogue in implantation. *Mol Cell Endocrinol* 2002;186:175–81.
5. Threadgill DW, Dlugosz AA, Hansen LA, Tennenbaum T, Lichti U, Yee D, *et al.* Targeted disruption of mouse EGF receptor: effect of genetic background on mutant phenotype. *Science* 1995;269:230–4.
6. Stewart CL, Kaspar P, Brunet LJ, Bhatt H, Gadi I, Kontgen F, *et al.* Blastocyst implantation depends on maternal expression of leukaemia inhibitory factor. *Nature* 1992;359:76–9.

7. Robb L, Li R, Hartley L, Nandurkar HH, Koentgen F, Begley CG. Infertility in female mice lacking the receptor for interleukin 11 is due to a defective uterine response to implantation. *Nat Med* 1998;4:303–8.
8. Bilinski P, Roopenian D, Gossler A. Maternal IL-11Ralpha function is required for normal decidua and fetoplacental development in mice. *Genes Dev* 1998;12:2234–43.
9. Raab G, Kover K, Paria BC, Dey SK, Ezzell RM, Klagsbrun M. Mouse preimplantation blastocysts adhere to cells expressing the transmembrane form of heparin-binding EGF-like growth factor. *Development* 1996;122:637–45.
10. Das SK, Wang XN, Paria BC, Damm D, Abraham JA, Klagsbrun M, et al. Heparin-binding EGF-like growth factor gene is induced in the mouse uterus temporally by the blastocyst solely at the site of its apposition: a possible ligand for interaction with blastocyst EGF-receptor in implantation. *Development* 1994;120:1071–83.
11. Das SK, Yano S, Wang J, Edwards DR, Nagase H, Dey SK. Expression of matrix metalloproteinases and tissue inhibitors of metalloproteinases in the mouse uterus during the peri-implantation period. *Dev Genet* 1997;21:44–54.
12. Bany BM, Schultz GA. Tissue inhibitor of matrix metalloproteinase-3 expression in the mouse uterus during implantation and artificially induced decidualization. *Mol Reprod Dev* 2001;59:159–67.
13. Leach RE, Khalifa R, Armant DR, Brudney A, Das SK, Dey SK, et al. Heparin-binding EGF-like growth factor modulation by antiprogestin and CG in the baboon (Papio anubis). *J Clin Endocrinol Metab* 2001;86:4520–8.
14. Fazleabas AT, Donnelly KM, Srinivasan S, Fortman JD, Miller JB. Modulation of the baboon (Papio anubis) uterine endometrium by chorionic gonadotrophin during the period of uterine receptivity. *Proc Natl Acad Sci U S A* 1999;96:2543–8.
15. Sun XY, Li FX, Li J, Tan YF, Piao YS, Tang S, et al. Determination of genes involved in the early process of embryonic implantation in rhesus monkey (Macaca mulatta) by suppression subtractive hybridization. *Biol Reprod* 2004;70:1365–73.
16. Enders AC, Lopata A. Implantation in the marmoset monkey: expansion of the early implantation site. *Anat Rec* 1999;256:279–99.
17. Lessey BA, Damjanovich L, Coutifaris C, Castelbaum A, Albelda SM, Buck CA. Integrin adhesion molecules in the human endometrium. Correlation with the normal and abnormal menstrual cycle. *J Clin Invest* 1992;90:188–95.
18. Cullinan EB, Abbondanzo SJ, Anderson PS, Pollard JW, Lessey BA, Stewart CL. Leukemia inhibitory factor (LIF) and LIF receptor expression in human endometrium suggests a potential autocrine/paracrine function in regulating embryo implantation. *Proc Natl Acad Sci U S A* 1996;93:3115–20.
19. Yoo HJ, Barlow DH, Mardon HJ. Temporal and spatial regulation of expression of heparin-binding epidermal growth factor-like growth factor in the human endometrium: a possible role in blastocyst implantation. *Dev Genet* 1997;21:102–8.
20. Leach RE, Khalifa R, Ramirez ND, Das SK, Wang J, Dey SK, et al. Multiple roles for heparin-binding epidermal growth factor-like growth factor are suggested by its cell-specific expression during the human endometrial cycle and early placentation. *J Clin Endocrinol Metab* 1999;84:3355–63.
21. Lessey BA, Gui Y, Apparao KB, Young SL, Mulholland J. Regulated expression of heparin-binding EGF-like growth factor (HB-EGF) in the human endometrium: a potential paracrine role during implantation. *Mol Reprod Dev* 2002;62:446–55.
22. Campbell S, Swann HR, Seif MW, Kimber SJ, Aplin JD. Cell adhesion molecules on the oocyte and preimplantation human embryo. *Hum Reprod* 1995;10:1571–8.
23. Chia CM, Winston RM, Handyside AH. EGF, TGF-alpha and EGFR expression in human preimplantation embryos. *Development* 1995;121:299–307.
24. Carson DD, Lagow E, Thathiah A, Al-Shami R, Farach-Carson MC, Vernon M, et al. Changes in gene expression during the early to mid-luteal (receptive phase) transition in human endometrium detected by high-density microarray screening. *Mol Hum Reprod* 2002;8:871–9.
25. Borthwick JM, Charnock-Jones DS, Tom BD, Hull ML, Teirney R, Phillips SC, et al. Determination of the transcript profile of human endometrium. *Mol Hum Reprod* 2003;9:19–33.
26. Zhou Y, Genbacev O, Fisher SJ. The human placenta remodels the uterus by using a combination of molecules that govern vasculogenesis or leukocyte extravasation. *Ann N Y Acad Sci* 2003;995:73–83.
27. Genbacev OD, Prakobphol A, Foulk RA, Krtolica AR, Ilic D, Singer MS, et al. Trophoblast L-selectin-mediated adhesion at the maternal–fetal interface. *Science* 2003;299:405–8.
28. Vestweber D, Blanks JE. Mechanisms that regulate the function of the selectins and their ligands. *Physiol Rev* 1999;79:181–213.

29. Bai SX, Wang YL, Qin L, Xiao ZJ, Herva R, Piao YS. Dynamic expression of matrix metalloproteinases (MMP-2, -9 and -14) and the tissue inhibitors of MMPs (TIMP-1, -2 and -3) at the implantation site during tubal pregnancy. *Reproduction* 2005;129:103–13.

30. Schultz JF, Mayernik L, Rout UK, Armant DR. Integrin trafficking regulates adhesion to fibronectin during differentiation of mouse peri-implantation blastocysts. *Dev Genet* 1997;21:31–43.

31. Yelian FD, Yang Y, Hirata JD, Schultz JF, Armant DR. Molecular interactions between fibronectin and integrins during mouse blastocyst outgrowth. *Mol Reprod Dev* 1995;41:435–48.

32. Wang J, Mayernik L, Armant DR. Integrin signaling regulates blastocyst adhesion to fibronectin at implantation: intracellular calcium transients and vesicle trafficking in primary trophoblast cells. *Dev Biol* 2002;245:270–9.

33. Rout UK, Wang J, Paria BC, Armant DR. Alpha5beta1, alphaVbeta3 and the platelet-associated integrin alphaIIbbeta3 coordinately regulate adhesion and migration of differentiating mouse trophoblast cells. *Dev Biol* 2004;268:135–51.

34. Raab G, Klagsbrun M. Heparin-binding EGF-like growth factor. *Biochim Biophys Acta* 1997;1333:F179–99.

35. Goishi K, Higashiyama S, Klagsbrun M, Nakano N, Umata T, Ishikawa M, et al. Phorbol ester induces the rapid processing of cell surface heparin-binding EGF-like growth factor: conversion from juxtacrine to paracrine growth factor activity. *Mol Biol Cell* 1995;6:967–80.

36. Suzuki M, Raab G, Moses MA, Fernandez CA, Klagsbrun M. Matrix metalloproteinase-3 releases active heparin-binding EGF-like growth factor by cleavage at a specific juxtamembrane site. *J Biol Chem* 1997;272:31730–7.

37. Chobotova K, Muchmore ME, Carver J, Yoo HJ, Manek S, Gullick WJ, et al. The mitogenic potential of heparin-binding epidermal growth factor in the human endometrium is mediated by the epidermal growth factor receptor and is modulated by tumor necrosis factor-alpha. *J Clin Endocrinol Metab* 2002;87:5769–77.

38. Elenius K, Corfas G, Paul S, Choi CJ, Rio C, Plowman GD, et al. A novel juxtamembrane domain isoform of HER4/ErbB4. Isoform-specific tissue distribution and differential processing in response to phorbol ester. *J Biol Chem* 1997;272:26761–8.

39. Lee JC, Wang ST, Chow NH, Yang HB. Investigation of the prognostic value of coexpressed erbB family members for the survival of colorectal cancer patients after curative surgery. *Eur J Cancer* 2002;38:1065–71.

40. Chobotova K, Spyropoulou I, Carver J, Manek S, Heath JK, Gullick WJ, et al. Heparin-binding epidermal growth factor and its receptor ErbB4 mediate implantation of the human blastocyst. *Mech Dev* 2002;119:137–44.

41. Lindenberg S, Hyttel P, Sjogren A, Greve T. A comparative study of attachment of human, bovine and mouse blastocysts to uterine epithelial monolayer. *Hum Reprod* 1989;4:446–56.

42. Meseguer M, Aplin JD, Caballero-Campo P, O'Connor JE, Martin JC, Remohi J, et al. Human endometrial mucin MUC1 is up-regulated by progesterone and down-regulated *in vitro* by the human blastocyst. *Biol Reprod* 2001;64:590–601.

43. Simon C, Dominguez F, Remohi J, Pellicer A. Embryo effects in human implantation: embryonic regulation of endometrial molecules in human implantation. *Ann N Y Acad Sci* 2001;943:1–16.

44. Carver J, Martin K, Spyropoulou I, Barlow D, Sargent I, Mardon H. An in-vitro model for stromal invasion during implantation of the human blastocyst. *Hum Reprod* 2003;18:283–90.

45. Parast MM, Aeder S, Sutherland AE. Trophoblast giant-cell differentiation involves changes in cytoskeleton and cell motility. *Dev Biol* 2001;230:43–60.

46. Martin KL, Barlow DH, Sargent IL. Heparin-binding epidermal growth factor significantly improves human blastocyst development and hatching in serum-free medium. *Hum Reprod* 1998;13:1645–52.

47. Bentin-Ley U, Pedersen B, Lindenberg S, Larsen JF, Hamberger L, Horn T. Isolation and culture of human endometrial cells in a three-dimensional culture system. *J Reprod Fertil* 1994;101:327–32.

48. Bentin-Ley U, Lopata A. In vitro models of human blastocyst implantation. *Baillieres Best Pract Res Clin Obstet Gynaecol* 2000;14:765–74.

SECTION 2
THE EMBRYO

Chapter 9
What makes a good egg?

Alison A Murray and Norah Spears

Introduction

More than 25 years have passed since the birth of the first child born after *in vitro* fertilisation (IVF).[1] While early attempts to carry out IVF were initiated to overcome fallopian tube malfunction, many advances have been made in assisted reproductive technology (ART) and it is now possible to treat a wide range of fertility problems such as male infertility, women with Turner syndrome, and hypogonadotrophic conditions. New techniques have been developed, such as oocyte donation and intracytoplasmic sperm transfer, which have increased the number of patients that can be treated for infertility, currently estimated at one couple in six. Despite these many advances in technology, success rates for all treatment cycles are generally less than 25%.[2]

In vivo, only a species-specific number of ovarian follicles are selected to release their oocytes for fertilisation during each reproductive cycle.[3] While many factors play a role in selecting the follicles (and hence oocytes) for ovulation, the overriding factor is availability and follicular response to the circulating gonadotrophins, follicle-stimulating hormone (FSH) and luteinising hormone (LH). Exogenous administration of these gonadotrophins bypasses the normal selection processes and allows a high number of follicles to reach the ovulatory stage, a technique that the majority of ART protocols use as a means of harvesting a large number of oocytes for fertilisation.[4]

While these superovulatory techniques have been used for many years, it is only more recently that basic research has been conducted to determine the effects of these techniques on oocyte quality. Therefore, while the low success rates in ART may be a consequence of many factors, such as endometrial response to implantation or poor luteal support, the effects of superovulatory levels of gonadotrophins may lead to the production of oocytes with impaired fertilisation ability or compromised developmental competence. As the possibilities within ART increase, it is imperative that we gain a fuller understanding of what makes a good egg, so that we can avoid manipulations that might compromise oocyte developmental competence and hence the quality of life of the resulting offspring.

Follicular growth and development

Oocytes are maintained within follicles that form the basic units that sustain oocytes before their release at ovulation. In the human, 1–2 million follicles are present at birth,[5] of which approximately 400 will sequentially mature and ovulate.[6] The remaining 99.9% begin development but never complete it, instead defaulting to atresia.

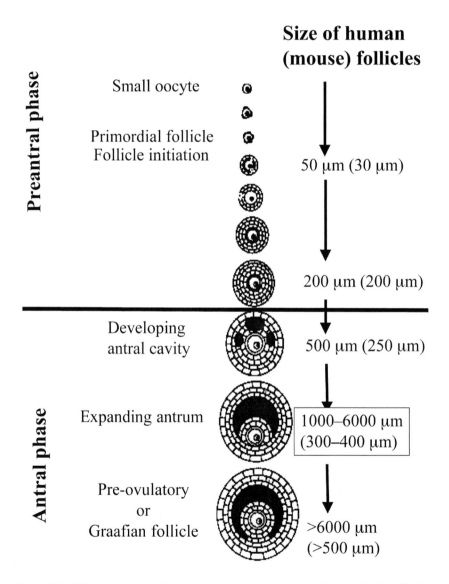

Figure 9.1. Follicle development in the human and mouse; adapted with permission from Gosden *et al.*[131] (*Reproductive Medicine Review*, © 1994 Cambridge University Press)

By birth or shortly afterwards, primary oocytes, arrested at the diplotene stage of the first prophase of meiotic division, associate with a few flattened granulosa cells to form primordial follicles. Follicles are maintained in a quiescent primordial pool, with a continual small proportion leaving that pool and beginning their growth phase (Figure 9.1).[7] The first signs of growth are an increase in oocyte volume and proliferation of the surrounding granulosa cells.[8] Once follicles have started to grow, follicular development can be considered as a two-phase process: a slow-growing (preantral) phase with no absolute requirement for gonadotrophin stimulation and a faster-growing (antral) phase where responsiveness to gonadotrophins is obligatory if the follicle is to proceed to the ovulatory stage. The transition between these two phases is characterised by the formation of a fluid-filled antral cavity and the production of steroid hormones.

By the early preantral stage the follicle has a distinct avascular multi-laminar granulosa cell layer surrounding the oocyte and has also acquired vascularised and distinct thecal cell layers outside the follicle basement membrane. Of the cohort of follicles that leaves the primordial pool at the same time, most will reach the late preantral stage of development, with few lost to atresia.[9] Only a proportion of these follicles, which are advanced enough in development to respond to circulating endocrine signals, will make the transition to the antral stage of follicular growth and progress further.

Irrespective of species, antral formation occurs when 2000–3000 granulosa cells are present within the follicle.[10] Fluid begins to accumulate within the small spaces between the granulosa cells which coalesce to form a large antral cavity. The granulosa cells proliferate rapidly and differentiate into two populations, the mural cells adjacent to the basement membrane and the cumulus cells which surround the oocytes.[11] The antral cavity rapidly enlarges, separating the two cell types, and eventually the oocyte, surrounded by the cumulus cells, becomes embedded in follicular fluid connected to the mural cell layer by a thin stalk of cells.

Ovulation occurs in response to circulating endocrine signals that initiate a number of changes within the follicle. Granulosa cells cease to proliferate and the cumulus cells undergo mucification. Concurrent with cumulus cell expansion, gap junction communication between the oocyte and its surrounding cells is broken, resulting in the oocyte resuming meiosis and reaching the second meiotic block. Follicle rupture occurs at the apex to the stalk attachment, resulting in the release of the mature oocyte to await fertilisation.

Oocyte growth and maturation

Initially, oocyte growth is commensurate with follicle growth. In most species, oocytes are generally thought to have completed their growth phase by the early antral stage of follicular development. In the mouse, the oocyte grows from 15 to 80 μm over a few weeks while in the human the oocyte grows from 35 to 120 μm in a few months. This represents an approximately 100-fold increase in volume.[3,12] There are marked changes in the ultrastructure of the oocyte. From the outset of growth, the oocyte secretes the components that form the zona pellucida and there is the appearance of novel organelles such as the cortical granules: both these features are important in promoting monospermic fertilisation.[13] Other cell structures become far more abundant and disperse throughout the cytoplasm, such as mitochondria and Golgi apparatus.[12,14] The mechanisms that are required for oocyte activation at the time of fertilisation are also acquired throughout oocyte growth.[15]

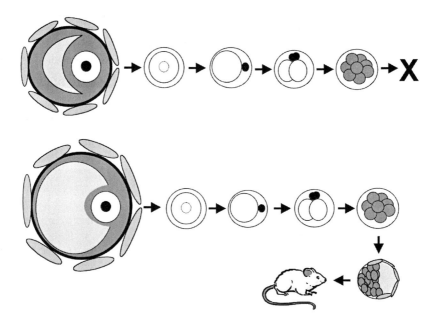

Figure 9.2. Oocyte developmental competence is acquired in a step-wise manner during follicular growth

Throughout the growth phase there is a rapid increase in the rate of transcription and translation. Fully grown mouse oocytes contain around 80 pg of mRNA and 25 ng protein by the time they are fully mature.[16,17] While RNA and protein are normally subject to rapid turnover, oocytes have the capacity to package and store these molecules until they are required at a further point along the developmental pathway.[18,19] Unlike lower species, few maternal-effect genes necessary for development after fertilisation have yet to be identified in mammalian oocytes. Two such genes, *Mater* and *Zar1*, have been found to be necessary in promoting the oocyte-to-embryo transition.[20,21]

By the time of release from the follicle, the oocyte will have achieved both nuclear maturation (resumption of meiosis until the first meiotic division (MI) and production of the first polar body) and cytoplasmic maturation (acquiring the mechanisms that promote monospermic fertilisation and sustain the earliest stages of embryogenesis).[22] Oocytes acquire the ability to resume meiosis and support embryogenesis in a step-wise manner that is highly correlated with follicular development (Figure 9.2). By the time oocytes have completed growth, at the early antral stage of follicular development, they are competent to resume meiosis and undergo germinal vesicle breakdown. They are unable, however, to progress to the second meiotic division (MII), instead arresting for a second time at MI.[23] During the antral stage of follicular development, the oocyte acquires the necessary molecules that permit further meiotic progression.[24] Similarly, aspects of cytoplasmic maturation are acquired sequentially, with oocytes gradually gaining the ability to firstly cleave to two cells (where they arrest if they are not fully mature), subsequently gaining the ability to complete pre-implantation development until, finally, at the pre-ovulatory stage they can support the development of live young.[25]

Until recently, it was assumed that the oocyte played a passive role in follicular development. From recent research it has now become increasingly clear that it plays a major role in controlling follicular development and hence contributes to its own development. There has been much research into oocyte-specific factors that control granulosa cell function. Growth differentiation factor 9 (GDF9) is perhaps the best characterised of these and has been implicated in controlling somatic cell function and differentiation at progressing stages of follicular development.[26] GDF9 is first expressed in the oocytes of growing follicles but not primordial follicles[27] and it has been shown to be an absolute requirement for preantral follicle development.[28] This factor may also be responsible for the acquisition of differentiated thecal layers around the follicle[29] and it has been implicated in controlling the steroidogenic function of the somatic cells, increasing androstenedione output,[30] suppressing FSH-induced oestrogen production and controlling factors that regulate pituitary FSH secretion.[31] GDF9 has also been implicated in influencing the phenotype of granulosa cells[26] and stimulation of cumulus cell expansion prior to ovulation.[32] A second member of the GDF family, bone morphogenetic protein 15 (BMP15) or GDF9B, is also an oocyte-specific factor implicated in controlling follicular function. Mice null for BMP15 are subfertile.[33] In sheep, homozygote carriers of mutations in the gene are infertile while heterozygote carriers have an increased ovulation rate.[34,35] Bmp15 gene defects have also been associated with hypergonadotrophic ovarian failure in humans.[36]

Far less is understood about the role of somatic cells in promoting oocyte maturation. That these cells are necessary to the oocyte has been demonstrated in knockout mice where gap junction communication is disrupted. In this model, oocyte development arrests before they acquire meiotic competence.[37] Some granulosa cell factors, such as kit ligand, have been shown to play a role in oocyte growth.[38] GDF9 has been shown to stimulate expression of kit ligand in the granulosa cells[39] which in turn acts through the c-kit receptor on the oocyte, allowing the oocyte to indirectly control its own growth.

Some other granulosa cell factors such as leptin have been implicated in oocyte transcriptional activity and establishment of cell polarity and lineage during pre-implantation development.[40] In addition, the mechanisms that maintain meiotic arrest within the oocyte are also known to be controlled by the somatic cells.[41]

Although it has been shown that the developmental programmes within oocytes can proceed independently of one another, under normal circumstances these two aspects of maturation are highly coordinated. While the oocyte has achieved some aspects of maturation during the early stages of follicular growth, it is not until the gonadotrophin-dependent stage that many aspects of maturation are acquired. Therefore, it would seem logical that the gonadotrophins and hence also steroids could influence the developmental competence of the oocyte.

Gonadotrophin and steroid action within the ovary

Until fairly recently, most preparations of gonadotrophins used for ovulation induction contained both FSH and LH and little was known about the individual roles that these play in the development of the follicle and maturation of the oocyte. With the availability of recombinant forms of both FSH and LH, it is now possible to determine more precisely what effects each of these has on both the follicle and oocyte. From the growing number of studies using these recombinant gonadotrophins, it is clear that FSH alone is capable of promoting follicular growth and development. This has been demonstrated in a number of species, including mice, rats, primates and humans.[42–45] In clinical situations, recombinant FSH has been used to treat women with Kallmann syndrome and hypogonadotrophic disorders. In these studies, stimulation produced multiple pre-ovulatory follicles but with inadequate oestrogen synthesis, resulting in poor-quality oocytes and lack of endometrial development.[44,46]

While there is little doubt that LH augments steroidogenesis and plays a critical role in the ovulatory process,[6] follicular growth is not dependent on its actions.[43,45,47] It has been suggested that follicular maturation is optimal when LH levels are kept below a 'ceiling' which, when exceeded, leads to an arrest in follicular development.[48] Furthermore there is controversy as to whether overstimulation with LH during the follicular growth phase might impact directly on oocyte viability, giving rise to poor fertilisation and implantation rates.[43,49] Studies from our laboratory have indicated that LH confers no advantage to oocyte maturation and that excessive levels may prove detrimental to the fertilised oocyte's ability to develop to the blastocyst stage.[50]

Ovarian steroidogenesis occurs as a result of FSH and LH stimulation. LH stimulation of the thecal cells results in the production of androgens that are subsequently metabolised to oestrogens in the granulosa cells by FSH-induced aromatase.[51] It has been suggested that an alteration in the sequence and pattern of steroid secretion, such as occurs during ovulation induction, might lead to incorrect molecular programming of the oocyte, which may in turn compromise fertilisation and further development.[52]

Apart from serving as substrates for oestrogen synthesis, androgens have been implicated in promoting follicular development,[53,54] upregulating FSH receptor expression[55]and enhancing FSH-stimulated follicular development.[56] Female mice with a conditional knockout that deletes androgen receptor function are subfertile and the granulosa cells of pre-ovulatory follicles undergo extensive atresia.[57] However, excess androgen levels have also been associated with inducing follicular atresia, and high androgen to oestrogen ratios within follicular fluid have been associated with poor fertilisation and development rates.[58,59]

Oestrogens have been shown to facilitate the proliferation of granulosa cells[60] and the actions of FSH and LH,[61] and also to inhibit follicular atresia.[62] However, there are a number of reports demonstrating that the role of oestrogen within the ovary is not obligatory.[43–45] It is now known that more than one oestrogen receptor (ER) exists in the mammalian ovary, which makes determining a role for this steroid in follicular and oocyte maturation more complicated to establish. Oestrogen receptor α (ERα) was first cloned by Green et al.,[63] while the second receptor, oestrogen receptor β (ERβ), was cloned by Kuiper et al.[64] Both ERs have been identified in the ovaries of a number of species.[65–67] In order to try to elucidate the role of each of these receptors, transgenic animals have been generated with deletions in ERα (ERKO), ERβ (BERKO) or both (αβERKO), and each exhibits different phenotypes.[68–70] As a consequence of ER deletion, circulating gonadotrophins and steroids are perturbed, which can account for the ovarian pathologies seen. Mice lacking the ERβ receptor are fertile although they have fewer and smaller litters,[69] while those lacking ERα develop ovarian haemorrhagic cysts and are infertile.[68] This phenotype is similar to that of mice engineered to overexpress the LHβ subunit[71] and it has been shown that by reducing serum LH the cystic ovarian phenotype can be alleviated in the ERKO mouse.[72] It was, therefore, still unclear from these studies whether ERα had any direct effect on follicular growth and development. Using an *in vitro* system we have found that isolated follicles from the ERKO mouse are capable of growth and development at the same rate as their wild-type counterparts.[73] In addition, it has been demonstrated that lack of this receptor does not impair the oocyte's ability to fertilise and complete development at least until the pre-implantation stage.[72] These results and the finding that the BERKO mouse is fertile support the notion that oestrogen is not an obligatory requirement for either follicular development or oocyte developmental competence, although it may play a role in maintaining the follicular somatic cell phenotype.[74] Further evidence to support the idea that oestrogen is not necessary in promoting oocyte developmental competence has come from studies in animals that have been rendered incapable of producing this steroid.[75]

The nature of how gonadotrophins and steroids influence oocyte maturation has yet to be elucidated. Within the ovarian follicle, FSH receptors are confined to the granulosa cells while LH receptors are found in the thecal cells during preantral growth. As follicles proceed through the antral stages, LH receptors are also found in the mural granulosa cell layers.[76] Both FSH and LH receptors, when activated, result in the generation of cyclic adenosine monophosphate (cAMP). Downstream events result in the production of protein kinase A, which mediates intracellular signalling events including gene transcription.[77] It has been shown that LH generates a much higher level of cAMP compared with FSH, resulting in the differential regulation of the genes responsible for steroidogenesis.[78] While it is most likely that the effects of LH and FSH are manifest as a result of their actions on granulosa cells, it is also possible that they may act directly on the oocyte as there are some reports suggesting that receptors for the gonadotrophins are present on the oocyte.[79–81]

Androgen and oestrogen receptors are found in the granulosa cells of growing follicles and their pattern of expression is developmentally regulated.[56,82,83] This changing pattern of receptor activity could influence the oocyte indirectly by altering the synthesis and transfer of molecules necessary for oocyte growth and maturation. Steroids could also have direct effects on the oocyte, as oestrogen receptors have been described in mouse and human oocytes,[84–86] and recently androgen receptors in rodent and pig oocytes.[87–89] Androgens have been shown to promote meiotic maturation in mouse oocytes.[89] These findings are in good agreement with studies we have been conducting. Using an *in vitro* system to manipulate steroid concentration during the antral growth phase of follicular development, we have found that elevating androgens led to a greater number of oocytes undergoing fertilisation while high oestrogen levels had the opposite effect.[90] As discussed above, oestrogen does not seem to be obligatory for oocyte developmental competence but few studies have investigated whether inappropriate exposure to this steroid during the follicle enclosed period has an effect on the oocyte. Our findings support the proposal that the oocyte needs to be exposed to the correct pattern of steroids in order to mature correctly.[91]

Role of other factors in oocyte competence

While gonadotrophins and steroids have been the focus of much research into follicular development, numerous other growth factors and cytokines have been identified as also having a role in oocyte developmental competence. Some of these factors affect the selection of follicles that proceed to the ovulatory stages while others directly enhance oocyte maturation. Most of the investigations into factors that have an effect on oocyte maturation have been conducted using *in vitro* systems. Whether these findings apply to all species or indeed are of physiological relevance has yet to be elucidated.

Members of the transforming growth factor β (TGFβ) superfamily of growth factors are clearly one such group. Some of these, such as GDF9 and BMP15, have been identified as oocyte-specific factors (see above), while other BMPs have been implicated in the control of FSH-induced steroidogenesis.[92] BMP receptors have also been identified in the oocytes of rodent follicles[92] and BMP receptor type II implicated in mediating GDF9 action in granulosa cells.[93] While the expression patterns of BMPs and their receptors alter as follicle and oocyte growth progresses,[92] little is understood about the factors controlling and regulating this pattern. Activins and inhibins exhibit a developmentally regulated pattern of expression throughout follicular development,[94,95] with activins being predominant in early antral follicles and the inhibins becoming more abundant as the follicle approaches the ovulatory stages. Four activin receptor subtypes have been identified in oocytes and have been shown to be differentially regulated during nuclear maturation,[96] implying a role for activin in oocyte maturation. Activin has also been shown to promote meiotic maturation in rats,[97] to increase the proportion of cleaved oocytes that complete pre-implantation development in the cow,[98] and to be associated with morphologically good-quality oocytes in humans.[99] Follistatin, although structurally unrelated to the TGFβ family, is a high-affinity binding protein for activin and has also been shown to bind BMPs,[100] thereby adding another layer of complexity in the elucidation of the pathway that the TGFβ family members play in optimising oocyte maturation.

Numerous other molecules have also been implicated in follicular development and oocyte maturation. The addition of epidermal growth factor (EGF) to culture media during oocyte *in vitro* maturation (IVM) stimulates cumulus expansion and meiotic maturation of the oocyte.[101,102] EGF-related ligands have been proposed as mediators of the ovulatory LH surge.[103] TGFα has been proposed as a promoter of oocyte meiotic maturation by exerting its effects via the cumulus granulosa cells[104] and it has also been reported in the nuclei of rat oocytes.[105]

The insulin-like growth factor (IGF) family and the associated binding proteins (IGFBPs) have been the subject of much research. Most of these studies have concentrated in the role of these factors in the selection of follicles destined for ovulation. The bioavailability of IGFs and changes in the secretion of IGFBPs are likely to play an important role. However, some of these factors may also impact directly on the oocyte. In the mouse IGF1 enhances the blastocyst development rate after exposure during the follicular growth stage[106] and in humans oocyte maturation is positively correlated with levels of IGF1 and IGFBP3 in follicular fluid.[107]

Genomic imprinting

Another aspect of oocyte maturation that needs to be considered is the epigenetic phenomenon of genomic imprinting. Nuclear transplantation studies performed during the 1980s revealed that uniparental embryos that contain two haploid sets of either maternal or paternal genomes are unable to develop beyond the early implantation stage.[108] These experiments revealed that the expression of some genes is differentially controlled and is dependent upon which parent the allele was inherited from. To date, several dozen genes have been found to be imprinted.[109] Of these it has been found that several play roles in embryo development, tumorigenesis and genetic diseases.[110] Kono *et al.*[111] have now produced a parthenogenetic mouse, but this required one oocyte to be obtained from the non-growing follicle of a transgenic mouse with the usual paternal expression of *H19* and *Igf2*.

When primordial germ cells (PGCs) migrate in the developing embryo, they still carry their maternal and paternal genomic imprints. These imprints are erased prior to follicle formation. Each oocyte then needs to lay down a maternal set of imprints, a process that is known to take place during follicle growth, with different genes imprinted at different stages of follicle development.[112,113]

Given that imprints are imposed at different time points during oocyte growth, it is possible that the gonadotrophin or steroidal milieu of the follicular environment has the potential to influence the imprinting process. Results from our laboratory have indicated that this may be the case.[114]

In vitro systems

Much of our information on follicular development and oocyte maturation has arisen as the result of *in vitro* examination of whole ovaries, isolated follicles, or cells of the follicle (Figure 9.3). Although *in vitro* systems have been developed for domestic species, most research carried out has used the mouse as a model.

Techniques for the *in vitro* development of whole ovaries have been described for 70 years,[115] and have been used to investigate gonadotrophin function and ovulatory processes.[116,117] This technique is now being used to investigate primordial follicle initiation and growth,[118–120] and has been applied to human tissue both to evaluate growth mechanisms[121] and as a means of reinstating fertility after cancer treatment.[122]

A number of *in vitro* systems have evolved that support the preantral to ovulatory stages of follicle development. Such techniques use either mechanical dissection of follicles, which ensures that the unit stays intact, or isolation of follicles by enzymatic digestion of whole or pieces of ovary.[123] It is these systems in particular that have yielded much information on the effects of gonadotrophins, steroids and other growth factors on follicular development although very few studies have used oocyte competence as an endpoint. While isolation and *in vitro* development of human follicles has been attempted,[124] it is only in rodents that these methods have produced mature oocytes capable of fertilisation and where live young have been born.[120] Despite a better understanding of the factors that affect follicular development arising from these *in vitro* studies, the success rates for the production of viable offspring after *in vitro* follicular development remain very low.

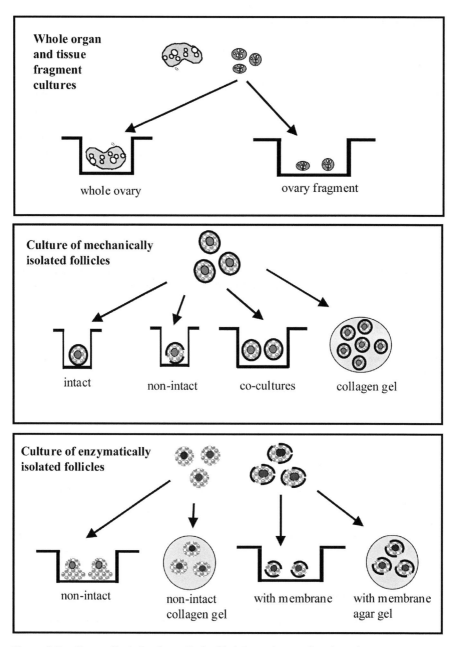

Figure 9.3. Diagram illustrating the methods of isolation and types of ovarian culture systems; reproduced with permission from Murray and Spears[123]

The complete *in vitro* maturation of oocytes from the primordial stage resulting in the birth of live young has only been achieved in the mouse,[120] where a combination of organ culture and isolated oocyte–somatic cell culture techniques was necessary. These studies have clearly demonstrated that the complete *in vitro* maturation of oocytes is a possibility. In humans, this approach has been used with cryopreserved tissue and the *in vitro* development of follicles to the antral stage has been achieved but we are still a long way from achieving complete *in vitro* maturation of a human follicle or oocyte.[125] Unlike rodents, the development of a human primordial follicle to the point of ovulation takes months rather than weeks and will require the development of long multi-stage protocols that induce the correct signalling between oocyte and somatic cells in order to be successful.

Conclusion

We are still some way from fully understanding the factors that produce viable and fully competent oocytes and it is only comparatively recently that the importance of some aspects of this process, such as imprinting, have come to light. Recent studies have indicated that ART may increase the risk of some congenital disorders such as Beckwith–Wiedemann syndrome.[126] Despite this, the number of techniques offered in clinical practice is continually increasing. For example, by early 2004 more than 300 children had been born after IVM of immature oocytes.[127] While this technique may offer an alternative to superovulatory techniques and the risks associated with gonadotrophin stimulation,[128,129] IVM itself has been implicated in alteration to normal embryonic development.[130] With this increasing interest in ART, further basic research into what makes a good egg is clearly vital.

References

1. Steptoe PC, Edwards RG. Birth after the reimplantation of a human embryo. *Lancet* 1978;2:366.
2. Hardy K, Wright C, Rice S, Tachataki M, Roberts R, Morgan D, *et al*. Future developments in assisted reproduction in humans. *Reproduction* 2002;123:171–83.
3. Gougeon A. Regulation of ovarian follicular development in primates: facts and hypotheses. *Endocr Rev* 1996;17:121–55.
4. Oelsner G, Serr DM, Maschiach S, Blankstein S, Snyder M, Lunefield B. The study of induction of ovulation with menotropins; analysis of 1897 treatment cycles. *Fertil Steril* 1978;30:538–44.
5. Baker TG. Gametogenesis. *Acta Endocrinol Suppl (Copenh)* 1972;166:18–41.
6. Hillier SG. Current concepts of the role of FSH and LH in folliculogenesis. *Hum Reprod* 1994;9:188–91.
7. Gosden RG. Ovulation 1: Oocyte development throughout life. In: Grudzinskas JG and Yovich JL, editors. *Gametes: the Oocyte*. Cambridge: Cambridge University Press; 1995. p. 119–49.
8. Lintern-Moore S, Moor GMP. The initiation of follicle and oocyte growth in the mouse ovary. *Biol Reprod* 1979;20:773–8.
9. Richards JS. Hormonal control of gene expression in the ovary. *Endocr Rev* 1994;15:725–51.
10. Gosden RG, Hunter RHF, Telfer EE, Torrance C, Brown N. Physiological factors underlying the formation of ovarian follicular fluid. *J Reprod Fertil* 1988;82:813–25.
11. Amsterdam A, Koch Y, Lieberman ME, Lindner HR. Distribution of binding sites for human chorionic gonadotropin in the preovulatory follicle of the rat. *J Cell Biol* 1975;67:894–900.
12. Gosden RG, Bownes M. Cellular and molecular aspects of oocyte development. In: Grudzinskas JG and Yovich JL, editors. *Gametes: the Oocyte*. Cambridge: Cambridge University Press; 1995. p. 23–53.
13. Wassarman PM. The mammalian ovum. In: Knobil E, Neill J, editors. *The Physiology of Reproduction*. New York: Raven Press; 1988. p. 69–102.
14. Fair T, Hulshof SC, Hyttel P, Greve T, Boland M. Oocyte ultrastructure in bovine primordial to early tertiary follicles. *Anat Embryol (Berl)* 1997;195:327–36.
15. Carroll J, Jones KT, Whittingham DG. Ca2+ release and the development of Ca2+ release mechanisms during oocyte maturation: a prelude to fertilization. *Rev Reprod* 1996;1:137–43.

16. Pico L, Clegg KB. Quantitative changes in total RNA, total poly(A) and ribosomes in early mouse embryos. *Dev Biol* 1982;89:362–78.

17. Bachvarova R, De Leon V, Johnson A, Kaplan G, Paynton BV. Changes in total RNA, polyadenylated RNA, and actin mRNA during meiotic maturation of mouse oocytes. *Dev Biol* 1985;108:325–31.

18. Gandolfi TA, Gandolfi F. The maternal legacy to the embryo: cytoplasmic components and their effects on early development. *Theriogenology* 2001;55:1255–76.

19. Yu J, Deng M, Medvedev S, Yang J, Hecht NB, Schultz RM. Transgenic RNAi-mediated reduction of MSY2 in mouse oocytes results in reduced fertility. *Dev Biol* 2004;268:195–206.

20. Tong ZB, Gold L, De Pol A, Vanevski K, Dorward H, Sena P, *et al.* Developmental expression and subcellular localization of mouse MATER, an oocyte-specific protein essential for early development. *Endocrinology* 2004;145:1427–34.

21. Wu X, Viveiros MM, Eppig JJ, Bai Y, Fitzpatrick SL, Matzuk MM. Zygote arrest 1 (Zar1) is a novel maternal-effect gene critical for the oocyte-to-embryo transition. *Nat Genet* 2003;33:187–91.

22. Eppig JJ. Coordination of nuclear and cytoplasmic oocyte maturation in eutherian mammals. *Reprod Fertil Dev* 1996;8:485–9.

23. Sorensen RA, Wassarmen DM. Relationship between growth and meiotic maturation of the mouse oocyte. *Dev Biol* 1976;50:531–6.

24. Su YQ, Wigglesworth K, Pendola FL, O'Brien MJ, Eppig JJ. Mitogen-activated protein kinase activity in cumulus cells is essential for gonadotropin-induced oocyte meiotic resumption and cumulus expansion in the mouse. *Endocrinology* 2002;143:2221–32.

25. Eppig JJ, Schroeder AC. Capacity of mouse oocytes from preantral follicles to undergo embryogenesis and development to live young after growth, maturation and fertilization *in vitro*. *Biol Reprod* 1989;41:268–76.

26. Latham KE, Wigglesworth K, McMenamin M, Eppig JJ. Stage-dependent effects of oocytes and growth differentiation factor 9 on mouse granulosa cell development: advance programming and subsequent control of the transition from preantral secondary follicles to early antral tertiary follicles. *Biol Reprod* 2004;70:1253–62.

27. McGrath SA, Esquela AF, Lee SJ. Oocyte-specific expression of growth/differentiation factor-9. *Mol Endocrinol* 1995;9:131–6.

28. Elvin JA, Yan C, Matzuk MM. Oocyte-expressed TGF-beta superfamily members in female fertility. *Mol Cell Endocrinol* 2000;159:1–5.

29. Wu X, Chen L, Brown CA, Yan C, Matzuk MM. Interrelationship of growth differentiation factor 9 and inhibin in early folliculogenesis and ovarian tumorigenesis in mice. *Mol Endocrinol* 2004;18:1509–19.

30. Solovyeva EV, Hayashi M, Margi K, Barkats C, Klein C, Amsterdam A, *et al.* Growth differentiation factor-9 stimulates rat theca-interstitial cell androgen biosynthesis. *Biol Reprod* 2000;63:1214–8.

31. Vitt UA, Hsueh AJ. Stage-dependent role of growth differentiation factor-9 in ovarian follicle development. *Mol Cell Endocrinol* 2002;186:211–17.

32. Vanderhyden BC, Macdonald EA, Nagyova E, Dhawan A. Evaluation of members of the TGFbeta superfamily as candidates for the oocyte factors that control mouse cumulus expansion and steroidogenesis. *Reprod Suppl* 2004;61:55–70.

33. Yan C, Wang P, DeMayo J, DeMayo FJ, Elvin JA, Carino C, *et al.* Synergistic roles of bone morphogenetic protein 15 and growth differentiation factor 9 in ovarian function. *Mol Endocrinol* 2001;15:854–66.

34. Montgomery GW, Galloway SM, Davis GH, McNatty KP. Genes controlling ovulation rate in sheep. *Reproduction* 2001;121:843–52.

35. Hanrahan JP, Gregan SM, Mulsant P, Mullen M, Davis GH, Powell R, *et al.* Mutations in the genes for oocyte-derived growth factors GDF9 and BMP15 are associated with both increased ovulation rate and sterility in Cambridge and Belclare sheep (*Ovis aries*). *Biol Reprod* 2004;70:900–9.

36. Di Pasquale E, Beck-Peccoz P, Persani L. Hypergonadotropic ovarian failure associated with an inherited mutation of human bone morphogenetic protein-15 (BMP15) gene. *Am J Hum Genet* 2004;75:106–11.

37. Simon AM, Goodenough PA, Li E, Paul DL, Goodenough DA. Female infertility in mice lacking connexin 37. *Nature* 1997;385:525–9.

38. Cecconi S, Rossi G, De Felici M, Colonna R. Mammalian oocyte growth *in vitro* is stimulated by soluble factor(s) produced by preantral granulosa cells and by Sertoli cells. *Mol Reprod Dev* 1996;44:540–6.

39. Elvin JA, Clark AT, Wang P, Wolfman NM, Matzuk MM. Paracrine actions of growth differentiation factor-9 in the mammalian ovary. *Mol Endocrinol* 1999;13:1035–48.

40. Antczak M,Van Blerkom J. Oocyte influences on early development: the regulatory proteins leptin and STAT3 are polarized in mouse and human oocytes and differentially distributed within the cells of the preimplantation stage embryo. *Mol Hum Reprod* 1997;3:1067–86.

41. Eppig JJ, Downs SM. Gonadotropin-induced murine oocyte maturation *in vivo* is not associated with decreased cyclic adenosine monophosphate in the oocyte-cumulus cell complex. *Gamete Res* 1988;20:125–31.

42. Mannaerts B, Uilenbroek J, Schot P, de Leeuw R. Folliculogenesis in hypophysectomised rats after treatment with r. h. FSH. *Biol Reprod* 1994;51:72–81.

43. Zelinski-Wooten MB, Hutchison JS, Hess DL,Wolf DP, Stouffer RL. FSH alone supports follicle growth and oocyte development in GnRH antagonist-treated monkeys. *Hum Reprod* 1995;10:1658–66.

44. Balasch J, Miro F, Burzaco I.The role of LH in human follicle development and oocyte fertility; evidence from IVF in a woman with long-standing hypogonadotrophic hypogonadism and using rhFSH. *Hum Reprod* 1995;10:1678–83.

45. Spears N, Murray AA,Allison V, Boland NI, Gosden RG. Role of gonadotrophins and ovarian steroids in the development of mouse follicles *in vitro. J Reprod Fertil* 1998;113:19–26.

46. Shoham Z, Jacobs HS, Insler V. LH increase leads to infertility and increased miscarriages. *Fertil Steril* 1993;58:1153–61.

47. Fauser BC. Follicular development and oocyte maturation in hypogonadotrophic women employing recombinant follicle-stimulating hormone: the role of oestradiol. *Hum Reprod Update* 1997;3:101–8.

48. Loumaye E, Engrand P, Shoham Z, Hillier SG, Baird DT. Clinical evidence for an LH ceiling? *Hum Reprod* 2003;18:2719–20.

49. Regan L, Owen EJ, Jacobs HS. Hypersecretion of LH, infertility and miscarriage. *Lancet* 1990;336:1141–4.

50. Murray A, Molinek M, Hillier SG, Spears N. unpublished results.

51. Armstrong DT, Dorrington JH. Estrogen biosynthesis in the ovaries and testes. *Adv Sex Horm Res* 1977;3:217–58.

52. Moor RM, Dai Y, Lee C, Fulka J Jr. Oocyte maturation and embryonic failure. *Hum Reprod Update* 1998;4:223–36.

53. Murray AA, Gosden RG,Allison V, Spears N. Effect of androgens on the development of mouse follicles growing *in vitro. J Reprod Fertil* 1998;113:27–33.

54. Vendola K, Zhou J,Wang J, Famuyiwa OA, Bievre M, Bondy CA. Androgens promote oocyte insulin-like growth factor I expression and initiation of follicle development in the primate ovary. *Biol Reprod* 1999;61:353–7.

55. Weil S,Vendola K, Zhou J, Bondy CA. Androgen and follicle-stimulating hormone interactions in primate ovarian follicle development. *J Clin Endocrinol Metab* 1999;84:2951–6.

56. Tetsuka M, Hillier SG. Differential regulation of aromatase and androgen receptor in granulosa cells. *J Steroid Biochem Mol Biol* 1997;61:233–9.

57. Hu YC,Wang PH,Yeh S,Wang RS, Xie C, Xu Q, *et al.* Subfertility and defective folliculogenesis in female mice lacking androgen receptor. *Proc Natl Acad Sci U S A* 2004;3:11209–14.

58. Anderiesz C,Trounson AO.The effect of testosterone on the maturation and developmental capacity of murine oocytes *in vitro. Hum Reprod* 1995;10:2377–81.

59. Xia P,Younglai EV. Relationship between steroid concentrations in ovarian follicular fluid and oocyte morphology in patients undergoing intracytoplasmic sperm injection (ICSI) treatment. *J Reprod Fertil* 2000;118:229–33.

60. Robker RL, Richards JS. Hormonal control of the cell cycle in ovarian cells: proliferation versus differentiation. *Biol Reprod* 1998;59:476–82.

61. Bley MA, Saragueta PE, Baranao JL. Concerted stimulation of rat granulosa cell deoxyribonucleic acid synthesis by sex steroids and follicle-stimulating hormone. *J Steroid Biochem Mol Biol* 1997;62:11–19.

62. Billig H, Furuta I, Hsueh AJ. Estrogens inhibit and androgens enhance ovarian granulosa cell apoptosis. *Endocrinol* 1993;133:2204–12.

63. Green S,Walter P, Kumar V, Krust A, Bornert JM, Argos P, *et al.* Human oestrogen receptor cDNA: sequence, expression and homology to v-erb-A. *Nature* 1986;19:134–9.

64. Kuiper GG, Enmark E, Pelto-Huikko M, Nilsson S, Gustafsson JA. Cloning of a novel receptor expressed in rat prostate and ovary. *Proc Natl Acad Sci U S A* 1996;93:5925–30.

65. Couse JF, Lindzey J, Grandien K, Gustafsson JA, Korach KS.Tissue distribution and quantitative analysis of estrogen receptor-alpha (ERalpha) and estrogen receptor-beta (ERbeta) messenger ribonucleic acid in the wild-type and ERalpha-knockout mouse. *Endocrinology* 1997;138:4613–21.

66. Sar M, Welsch F. Differential expression of estrogen receptor-beta and estrogen receptor-alpha in the rat ovary. *Endocrinol* 1999;140:963–71.

67. Saunders PT, Millar MR, Williams K, Macpherson S, Harkiss D, Anderson RA, *et al.* Differential expression of estrogen receptor-alpha and -beta and androgen receptor in the ovaries of marmosets and humans. *Biol Reprod* 2000;63:1098–105.

68. Lubahn DB, Moyer JS, Goldug TS, Couse JF, Korach KS, Smithies O. Alteration of reproductive function but not prenatal sexual development after insertional disruption of the mouse estrogen receptor gene. *Proc Natl Acad Sci U S A* 1993;90:11162–6.

69. Krege JH, Hodgin JB, Couse JF, Enmark E, Warner M, Mahler JF, *et al.* Generation and reproductive phenotypes of mice lacking estrogen receptor beta. *Proc Natl Acad Sci U S A* 1998;95:15677–82.

70. Dupont S, Krust A, Gansmuller A, Dierich A, Chambon P, Mark M. Effect of single and compound knockouts of estrogen receptors alpha (ERalpha) and beta (ERbeta) on mouse reproductive phenotypes. *Development* 2000;127:4277–91.

71. Risma KA, Clay CM, Nett TM, Wagner T, Yun J, Nilson JH. Targeted overexpression of luteinizing hormone in transgenic mice leads to infertility, polycystic ovaries, and ovarian tumors. *Proc Natl Acad Sci U S A* 1995;92:1322–6.

72. Couse JF, Bunch DO, Lindzey J, Schomberg DW, Korach KS. Prevention of the polycystic ovarian phenotype and characterization of ovulatory capacity in the estrogen receptor- alpha knockout mouse. *Endocrinol* 1999;140:5855–65.

73. Murray A, Rosenfeld C, Smith R, Lubahn D, Hillier S, Spears N. Unpublished results.

74. Britt KL, Findlay JK. Regulation of the phenotype of ovarian somatic cells by estrogen. *Mol Cell Endocrinol* 2003;28:11–7.

75. Huynh K, Jones G, Thouas G, Britt KL, Simpson ER, Jones ME. Estrogen is not directly required for oocyte developmental competence. *Biol Reprod* 2004;70:1263–9.

76. Eppig JJ, Pendola FL, Wigglesworth K. Mouse oocytes suppress cAMP-induced expression of LH receptor mRNA by granulosa cells *in vitro*. *Mol Reprod Dev* 1998;49:327–32.

77. Richards JS. The ovarian follicle – a perspective in 2001. *Endocrinol* 2001;142:2184–93.

78. Yong EL, Hillier SG, Turner M, Baird DT, Ng SC, Bongso A, *et al.* Differential regulation of cholesterol side-chain cleavage (P450scc) and aromatase (P450arom) enzyme mRNA expression by gonadotrophins and cyclic AMP in human granulosa cells. *J Mol Endocrinol* 1994;12:239–49.

79. Meduri G, Charnaux N, Driancourt M, Combettes L, Granet P, Vannier B, *et al.* Follicle-stimulating hormone receptors in oocytes? *Clin Endocrinol Metab* 2002;87:2266–76.

80. Patsoula E, Loutradis D, Drakakis P, Kallianidis K, Bletsa R, Michalas S. Expression of mRNA for the LH and FSH receptors in mouse oocytes and preimplantation embryos. *Reproduction* 2001;121:455–61.

81. Patsoula E, Loutradis D, Drakakis P, Michalas L, Bletsa R, Michalas S. Messenger RNA expression for the follicle-stimulating hormone receptor and luteinizing hormone receptor in human oocytes and preimplantation-stage embryos. *Fertil Steril* 2003;79:1187–93.

82. Duffy DM, Abdelgadir SE, Stott KR, Resko JA, Stouffer RL, Zelinski-Wooten MB. Androgen receptor mRNA expression in the rhesus monkey ovary. *Endocrine* 1999;11:23–30.

83. Szoltys M, Slomczynska M. Changes in distribution of androgen receptor during maturation of rat ovarian follicles. *Exp Clin Endocrinol Diabetes* 2000;108:228–34.

84. Wu TC, Wang L, Wan YJ. Expression of estrogen receptor gene in mouse oocyte and during embryogenesis. *Mol Reprod Dev* 1992;33:407–12.

85. Wu TC, Wang L, Wan YJ. Detection of estrogen receptor messenger ribonucleic acid in human oocytes and cumulus-oocyte complexes using reverse transcriptase-polymerase chain reaction. *Fertil Steril* 1993;59:54–9.

86. Hiroi H, Momoeda M, Inoue S, Tsuchiya F, Matsumi H, Tsutsumi O, *et al.* Stage-specific expression of estrogen receptor subtypes and estrogen responsive finger protein in preimplantational mouse embryos. *Endocr J* 1999;46:153–8.

87. Szoltys M, Slomczynska M, Tabarowski Z. Immunohistochemical localization of androgen receptor in rat oocytes. *Folia Histochem Cytobiol* 200341:59–64.

88. Cardenas H, Pope WF. Androgen receptor and follicle-stimulating hormone receptor in the pig ovary during the follicular phase of the estrous cycle. *Mol Reprod Dev* 2002;62:92–8.

89. Gill A, Jamnongjit M, Hammes SR. Androgens promote maturation and signaling in mouse oocytes independent of transcription: a release of inhibition model for mammalian oocyte meiosis. *Mol Endocrinol* 2004;18:97–104.

90. Murray A, Swales A, Smith R, Hillier S, Spears N. Unpublished results.

91. Osborn JC, Moor RM. The role of steroid signals in the maturation of mammalian oocytes. *J Steroid Biochem* 1983;19:133–7.

92. Shimasaki S, Zachow RJ, Li D, Kim H, Iemura S, Ueno N, *et al*. A functional bone morphogenetic protein system in the ovary. *Proc Natl Acad Sci U S A* 1999;96:7282–7.
93. Vitt UA, Hayashi M, Klein C, Hsueh AJ. Growth differentiation factor-9 stimulates proliferation but suppresses the follicle-stimulating hormone-induced differentiation of cultured granulosa cells from small antral and preovulatory rat follicles. *Biol Reprod* 2000;62:370–7.
94. Miro F, Hillier SG. Modulation of granulosa cell DNA synthesis and differentiation by activin. *Endocrinol* 1996;137:464–8.
95. Newton H, Wang Y, Groome NP, Illingworth P. Inhibin and activin secretion during murine preantral follicle culture and following HCG stimulation. *Hum Reprod* 2002;17:38–43.
96. Sidis Y, Fujiwara T, Leykin L, Isaacson K, Tom T, Schneyer A. Characterisation of inhibin/activin subunit, activin receptor and follistatin mRNA in human and mouse oocytes: evidence for activins paracrine signaling from granulosa cells to oocytes. *Biol Reprod* 1998;59:807–12.
97. Sadatsuki M, Tsutsumi O, Yamada R, Muramatsu M, Taketani Y. Local regulatory effects of activin A and follistatin on meiotic maturation of rat oocytes. *Biochem Biophys Res Commun* 1993;15:388–95.
98. Silva CC, Knight PG. Modulatory actions of activin-A and follistatin on the developmental competence of *in vitro*-matured bovine oocytes. *Biol Reprod* 1998;58:558–65.
99. Lau CP, Ledger WL, Groome NP, Barlow DH, Muttukrishna S. Dimeric inhibins and activin A in human follicular fluid and oocyte-cumulus culture medium. *Hum Reprod* 1999;14:2525–30.
100. Otsuka F, Moore RK, Iemura S, Ueno N, Shimasaki S. Follistatin inhibits the function of the oocyte-derived factor BMP-15. *Biochem Biophys Res Commun* 2001;289:961–6.
101. Boland NI, Gosden RG. Effects of EGF on the growth and differentiation of cultured mouse ovarian follicles. *J Reprod Fertil* 1994;101:369–74.
102. De La Fuente R, O'Brien MJ, Eppig JJ. Epidermal growth factor enhances preimplantation developmental competence of maturing mouse oocytes. *Hum Reprod* 1999;14:3060–8.
103. Park JY, Su YQ, Ariga M, Law E, Jin SL, Conti M. EGF-like growth factors as mediators of LH action in the ovulatory follicle. *Science* 2004;303:682–4.
104. Brucker C, Alexander NJ, Hodgen GD, Sandow BA. Transforming growth factor-alpha augments meiotic maturation of cumulus cell-enclosed mouse oocytes. *Mol Reprod Dev* 1991;28:94–8.
105. Akkoyunlu G, Demir R, Ustunel I. Distribution patterns of TGF-alpha, laminin and fibronectin and their relationship with folliculogenesis in rat ovary. *Acta Histochem* 2003;105:295–301.
106. Demeestere I, Gervy C, Centner J, Devreker F, Englert Y, Delbaere A. Effect of insulin-like growth factor-I during preantral follicular culture on steroidogenesis, *in vitro* oocyte maturation, and embryo development in mice. *Biol Reprod* 2004;70:1664–9.
107. Nardo LG, Bellanca SA, Burrello N, Longo G, D'Agata R, Nardo F, *et al*. Concentrations of insulin-like growth factor (IGF)-I and IGF binding protein-3 in the follicular fluid of women undergoing ovarian hyperstimulation with different gonadotropin preparations. *Gynecol Endocrinol* 2001;15:413–20.
108. Surani MA, Barton SC, Norris ML. Development of reconstituted mouse eggs suggests imprinting of the genome during gametogenesis. *Nature* 1984;308:548–50.
109. Reik W, Dean W, Walter J. Epigenetic reprogramming in mammalian development. *Science* 2001;293:1089–93.
110. Paulsen M, Ferguson-Smith AC. DNA methylation in genomic imprinting, development, and disease. *J Pathol* 2001;195:97–110.
111. Kono T, Obata Y, Wu Q, Niwa K, Ono Y, Yamamoto Y, *et al*. Birth of parthenogenetic mice that can develop to adulthood. *Nature* 2004;428:860–4.
112. Obata Y, Kono T. Maternal primary imprinting is established at a specific time for each gene throughout oocyte growth. *J Biol Chem* 2001;15:5285–9.
113. Lucifero D, Mann MR, Bartolomei MS, Trasler JM. Gene-specific timing and epigenetic memory in oocyte imprinting. *Hum Mol Genet* 2004;13:839–49.
114. Swales A, Spears N. Mouse oocytes exposed to raised androgen and estrogen levels *in vitro* exhibit increased DNA methylation. 37th Annual Meeting, Society for the Study of Reproduction, 1–4 August 2004, Vancouver, Canada. Abstract.
115. Martinovitch PN. The development in-vitro of the mammalian gonad-ovary and ovogenesis. *Proc R Soc Lond (Biol)* 1938;125:232–49.
116. Ryle M. Morphological responses to pituitary gonadotrophins by mouse ovaries *in vitro*. *J Reprod Fertil* 1969;20:307–12.
117. Neal P, Baker TG. Response of mouse ovaries *in vivo* and in organ culture to pregnant mare's serum gonadotrophin and human chorionic gonadotrophin. *J Reprod Fertil* 1973;33:399–401.
118. Kezele P, Skinner MK. Regulation of ovarian primordial follicle assembly and development by estrogen and progesterone: endocrine model of follicle assembly. *Endocrinol* 2003;144:3329–37.

119. Spears N, Molinek MD, Robinson LL, Fulton N, Cameron H, Shimoda K, *et al.* The role of neurotrophin receptors in female germ-cell survival in mouse and human. *Dev* 2003;130:5481–91.

120. O'Brien MJ, Pendola JK, Eppig JJ. A revised protocol for *in vitro* development of mouse oocytes from primordial follicles dramatically improves their developmental competence. *Biol Reprod* 2003;68:1682–6.

121. Hreinsson JG, Scott JE, Rasmussen C, Swahn ML, Hsueh AJ, Hovatta O. Growth differentiation factor-9 promotes the growth, development, and survival of human ovarian follicles in organ culture. *J Clin Endocrinol Metab* 2002;87:316–21.

122. Hovatta O. Cryopreservation and culture of human primordial and primary ovarian follicles. *Mol Cell Endocrinol* 2000;169:95–7.

123. Murray A, Spears N. Follicular development *in vitro*. *Semin Reprod Med* 2001;18:109–22.

124. Roy SK, Treacy BJ. Isolation and long-term culture of human preantral follicles. *Fertil Steril* 1993;59:783–90.

125. Hovatta O. Cryopreservation and culture of human ovarian cortical tissue containing early follicles. *Eur J Obstet Gynecol Reprod Biol* 200;113 Suppl 1:S50–4.

126. Gosden R, Trasler J, Lucifero D, Faddy M. Rare congenital disorders, imprinted genes, and assisted reproductive technology. *Lancet* 2003;7:1975–7.

127. Chian RC, Lim JH, Tan SL. State of the art in in-vitro oocyte maturation. *Curr Opin Obstet Gynecol* 2004;16:211–9.

128. Child TJ, Phillips SJ, Abdul-Jalil AK, Gulekli B, Tan SL. A comparison of *in vitro* maturation and *in vitro* fertilization for women with polycystic ovaries. *Obstet Gynecol* 2002;100:665–70.

129. Son WY, Park SJ, Hyun CS, Lee WD, Yoon SH, Lim JH. Successful birth after transfer of blastocysts derived from oocytes of unstimulated woman with regular menstrual cycle after IVM approach. *J Assist Reprod Genet* 2002;19:541–3.

130. Sinclair KD, Young LE, Wilmut I, McEvoy TG. In-utero overgrowth in ruminants following embryo culture: lessons from mice and a warning to men. *Hum Reprod* 2000;15 Suppl 5:68–86.

131. Gosden RG, Boland NI, Spears N, Murray AA, Chapman M, Wade JC, *et al.* The biology and technology of follicular oocyte development *in vitro*. *Reprod Med Rev* 1994;2:129–52.

Chapter 10
What makes 'good sperm'?

Allan Pacey

Introduction

Spermatozoa have but one purpose: to deliver the male genome to the egg and fertilise it. In order to achieve this, the fertilising sperm must undergo a number of discrete, sequential and appropriately timed functions that are largely determined by the environment in which fertilising is taking place. These are summarised in Table 10.1. Considering sperm functions in this way shows the functional demands required by the fertilising sperm following an act of coitus at midcycle are, for example, undoubtedly much greater than those for sperm following a simple insemination procedure, such as intrauterine insemination (IUI). In turn, these are generally thought to be more demanding than those required for successful fertilisation by *in vitro* fertilisation (IVF), with sperm that fertilise following intracytoplasmic sperm injection (ICSI) (where the only requirement is for sperm to have competent DNA capable of successfully decondensing) having the least number of demands placed upon them. Therefore, to be able to define simply what makes 'good sperm' is not as straightforward as it first might seem. However, for the purpose of this article, sperm function following unassisted conception will be considered as the starting point from which appropriate references to assisted conception techniques will be made, where relevant.

Defining 'good sperm'

While the semen analysis[1] is still considered the best yardstick by which semen quality (and thus male fertility) is defined, in terms of attempting to identify the 'good sperm' within an ejaculate it is generally considered to be a relatively blunt instrument. Although there is broad correlation between independent measures of sperm concentration, motility and morphology and the probability of conception within a given period of time,[2] this relationship probably exists because with increasing numbers of sperm within an ejaculate the probability of there being sufficient numbers of functional sperm (with the correct physiological competence to cope with the hostility of the female reproductive tract and also deploy the appropriate strategy *en route* to the site of fertilisation) also increases. For example, we know that

Table 10.1. Summary of sperm functions required to achieve successful fertilisation of an oocyte during unassisted (natural) conception (coitus), intracervical (IC) or intrauterine (IUI) insemination, gamete intrafallopian transfer (GIFT), in vitro fertilisation (IVF) or intracytoplasmic sperm injection (ICSI); a tick indicates that a sperm must be able to undergo each functional step listed whereas a cross indicates that this aspect of sperm function is not required

Sperm function	Mode of fertilisation/conception					
	Coitus	IC	IUI	GIFT	IVF	ICSI
Passage through cervical mucus	✔	✘	✘	✘	✘	✘
Transport through the uterus	✔	✔	✘	✘	✘	✘
Passage through the uterotubal junction	✔	✔	✔	✘	✘	✘
Sperm–epithelial contact	✔	✔	✔	?[a]	✘	✘
Capacitation	✔	✔	✔	✔	✔	✘
Binding to the egg	✔	✔	✔	✔	✔	✘
Passage through the zona pellucida	✔	✔	✔	✔	✔	✘
Decondensation of sperm DNA	✔	✔	✔	✔	✔	✔

[a] In the case of GIFT, it is unclear whether sperm–epithelial contact will play an important role given that sperm are inseminated into the uterine (fallopian) tube at the distal (ovarian) end whereas during insemination procedures (including natural coitus) sperm enter at the proximal (uterine) end

there is a broad correlation between the proportion of motile sperm within an ejaculate and the quality of nuclear DNA,[3] but this does not mean that all motile sperm are functionally competent. Similarly, the quality of motility as observed at semen analysis may bear little resemblance to the ability of a sperm to become hyperactivated at the appropriate time within the female reproductive tract or to be able to respond to the correct chemical or physical cues (see below). Therefore, it is clear that if 'good sperm' are to be identified in the laboratory more sophisticated tests need to be used and, in many cases, still need to be developed.

There have over the years been many putative sperm function tests developed that have attempted to better define in the laboratory aspects of sperm function (reviewed by Mortimer[4]). These are listed in Table 10.2 and range from relatively simple sperm migration tests to detailed assessments of the ability to acrosome react or bind to the zona pellucida. Although many of these tests have often shown good independent correlations with successful conception, they have had limited general appeal and often remain the preserve of research studies rather than being useful in a clinical environment. Moreover, there is no single test that examines all of the critical aspects of sperm function listed in Table 10.1 and none are able to consider multiple or sequential aspects such as the ability of sperm that have passed through cervical mucus to acrosome react and/or bind to the oolemma, for example. Moreover, for many of the sperm functions listed in Table 10.1, there are no suitable *in vitro* tests to assess them (Table 10.2).

So what are the important measurable aspects of sperm function that define a 'good sperm'? From a functional standpoint these can be divided into four broad categories as outlined below.

Table 10.2. Summary of sperm function tests currently available and their relationship to the sperm functions listed in Table 10.1; a tick indicates that the test actually provides relevant information for the given aspect of sperm function, whereas a cross indicates that no relevant information is provided by the test; a question mark indicates that there is too little information to be clear about what physiologically relevant aspect of sperm function is being tested

Sperm function	Sperm function test					
	Sperm kinematic analysis	Sperm migration tests	Sperm mucus interaction	Sperm zona binding	Ability to acrosome react	Tests of DNA quality
Passage through cervical mucus	✔	?	✔	✗	✗	✗
Transport through the uterus	?	?	✗	✗	✗	✗
Passage through the uterotubal junction	?	?	✗	✗	✗	✗
Sperm–epithelial contact	✗	✗	✗	✗	✗	✗
Capacitation	✗	✗	✗	✗	✔	✗
Binding to the egg	✗	✗	✗	✔	✔	✗
Passage through the zona pellucida	✗	✗	✗	✗	✗	✗
Decondensation of sperm DNA	✗	✗	✗	✗	✗	✔

Sperm transport

Although we have known for some time that the appropriate motility pattern[5] and sperm head morphology[6] are required to allow penetration through midcycle cervical mucus, it is only in recent years that the complexity of the sperm transport mechanism within the female reproductive tract has become apparent. For example, there is now strong evidence to suggest that sperm may play very little role in reaching the uterine tubes but are transported there by inherent muscular contractions of the female reproductive tract.[7] Moreover, this mechanism seems highly directional and experiments have shown that around midcycle the female tract preferentially moves material to the side of the developing follicle, presumably in anticipation of ovulation.

Within the isthmic region of the uterine tube it is thought that sperm–epithelial contact (see Figure 10.1(a)) is a crucial part of pre-ovulatory events,[8] the significance of which will be discussed below. However, prior to fertilisation sperm must become detached from their association with the epithelium if they are to move to the tubal ampulla and take part in fertilisation. In achieving this, sperm hyperactivation is thought to play a crucial role[9] – in addition to assisting sperm to move around in the labyrinthine lumen of the oviduct, to penetrate mucous substances and, finally, to penetrate the zona pellucida of the oocyte. Although the precise signals that lead to epithelial-bound sperm becoming hyperactivated and detaching from the tubal isthmus are unknown, it should be considered that any failure in this mechanism may lead to sperm remaining bound to the epithelium and therefore unavailable for fertilisation. In this context, it is interesting to note that the sperm of some men seem unable to hyperactivate *in vitro* in response to known inducers such as follicular fluid,[10] although it is unknown whether they respond under more physiological conditions

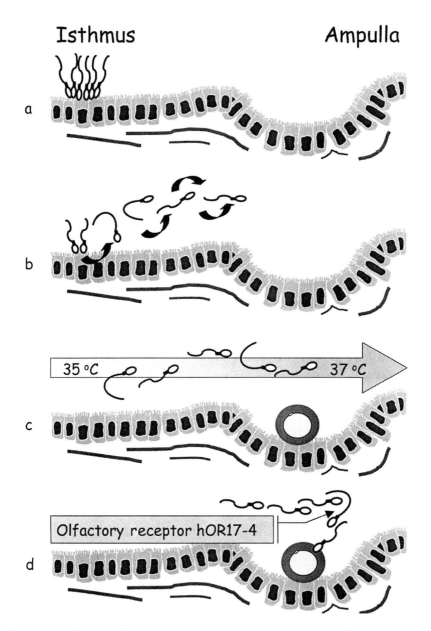

Isthmus   **Ampulla**

Figure 10.1. Diagrammatic representation of sperm behaviour and functions within the uterine tube immediately prior to fertilisation: briefly, (a) shows the formation of a sperm reservoir in the isthmic region of the tube with sperm attached to the endosalpinx by their heads (see Baillie *et al.*[43]); (b) shows the detachment of sperm from the endosalpinx through the forces generated by hyperactivated motility (see Pacey *et al.*[9]); (c) the long-range mechanism by which sperm are directed to the tubal ampulla according to temperature gradients (see Bahat *et al.*[27]); and (d) the short-range mechanism by which sperm are attracted by chemotaxis to the unfertilised oocyte (see Eisenbach[28]) *in vivo*. In addition, if sperm hyperactivate too early, then there is evidence from animal studies that sperm could fail to pass through the uterotubal junction.[11] Therefore, changes in sperm motility patterns – such as the onset of hyperactivated motility – need to be both timely and coordinated if sperm are to reach the site of fertilisation at the appropriate moment (see Figure 10.1(b)). However, we currently have no methodology that allows us to assess both the nature of movement within individual sperm and, more importantly, their ability to change in response to relevant physiological cues and within conditions that appropriately mimic the complexity of the female reproductive tract.

Survival, capacitation and sperm–epithelial dialogue

One of the important aspects of sperm transport to emerge over the past ten years is the role of sperm–epithelial contact in regulating sperm physiology during the pre-ovulatory period.[8] For example, it has been shown that co-culture of sperm with epithelium from the human endosalpinx prolongs sperm viability,[12,13] increases motility[14–16] and delays the process of sperm capacitation.[17] This is thought to be critical in maintaining a functional population of sperm within the uterine (fallopian) tube for as long as possible should coitus (or insemination) occur a long time before ovulation. In addition, it has also been suggested that only 'functionally superior' sperm are able to attach to the endosalpinx,[18] raising the possibility that 'good sperm' can be recognised by the female reproductive tract and be preferentially sequestered prior to ovulation in a tubal reservoir.

Unfortunately, we know very little about the molecular basis of sperm attachment to the endosalpinx. Work in non-human mammals has suggested that the interaction between surface-associated sperm lectins and oligosaccharides present on the epithelial surface are important mediators.[19] However, work from my own laboratory[20] has indicated a role for the Arg-Gly-Asp (RGD) adhesion sequence in human tissues. In either case, once these details have been worked out, this could form the basis of an *in vitro* sperm function test to assess how sperm from different men may bind to the endosalpinx and respond appropriately to that interaction. For example, there is good evidence in horses that there are significant differences between stallions in the ability of their sperm to bind to monolayers of oviductal epithelium, which may be related to differences in their fertility.[21] Clearly, if we could identify those sperm within the human ejaculate that have the appropriate epithelial-binding mechanisms, then we may be able to make better predictions about the probability of a man's fertility following natural coitus or simple insemination procedures.

In addition to regulating sperm physiology, sperm contact with the epithelium may play an important role in affecting the physiology of the epithelium itself. This is evidenced by changes in the calcium levels of epithelial cells seen to bind sperm,[22] as well as noticeable changes in the protein composition of conditioned medium following co-culture experiments as analysed by sodium dodecyl sulphate polyacrylamide gel electrophoresis (SDS-PAGE).[23,24] More recently, it has been shown using microarray technology that the gene expression profile of oviductal epithelium in mice can be significantly altered in the endosalpinx following natural insemination.[25]

Therefore, 'good sperm' may be those that are both able to bind to the endosalpinx and modulate their own physiology appropriately, but are also able to trigger appropriate signal transduction in the epithelium and influence epithelial physiology (be that changes in calcium levels, triggering transcription of genes and/or the secretion of proteins). While it is possible that in doing this spermatozoa may be able to elicit a favourable environment for themselves, it is equally possible that epithelial-derived secretions may be able to influence other processes, such as embryo development by stimulating the secretion of proteins or other aspects of epithelial physiology that alter the environment of the uterine tube. Moreover, this also raises the tantalising possibility that the female reproductive tract can interpret sperm surface proteins in terms of male genetic quality and fitness. This is could be useful both in choosing subpopulations of sperm within an ejaculate and in choosing between sperm from different males that may be present within the female reproductive tract at the same time.[26]

Sperm–egg recognition and fertilisation

There are thought to be two complementary mechanisms responsible for guiding mammalian sperm to the site of fertilisation. The first (long-range) mechanism is where capacitated sperm – released from intimate contact with the endosalpinx (see above) – are guided by thermotaxis towards the site of fertilisation.[27] This results from a temperature difference of up to 2°C between the (cooler) tubal isthmus and the (warmer) tubal ampulla (see Figure 10.1(c)). It has been proposed that, once the sperm are in the tubal ampulla, and at a closer proximity to the egg, a second (short-range) mechanism whereby capacitated sperm become chemotactically responsive to follicular factor(s) guides sperm closer to the unfertilised egg[28] (see Figure 10.1(d)). The molecular mechanism by which chemotaxis is mediated is becoming clearer and has made progress with the recent discovery of an olfactory receptor (hOR17-4) associated with the sperm mid-piece[29] that is coupled to a cyclic adenosine monophosphate (cAMP)-mediated signalling cascade.[30] While further studies need to be carried out, it is clear that this mechanism could become an important target for future pharmacological treatment for infertility or contraception. Clearly, in unassisted reproduction, 'good sperm' are those that can respond appropriately to these directional signals, and in time it may be possible to screen for the absence or presence of the receptor as a diagnostic test during infertility investigations.

Given the complex series of events that occur inside the female reproductive tract prior to fertilisation following natural coitus or an insemination procedure such as IUI, it is interesting to compare this with the relatively simplicity of the conditions that prevail during fertilisation *in vitro*. For example, however complex we may think that IVF has become it is still common practice to incubate oocytes with many tens of thousands of sperm in order to achieve successful fertilisation.[31] This is in comparison with the situation *in vivo* where it is thought that there are only a relatively small number of sperm (perhaps less than ten) around the oocyte at the time of fertilisation.[28] This staggering difference almost certainly reflects our inability to adequately mimic *in vitro* the environment and sperm selection mechanisms of the female reproductive tract during natural (unassisted) conception.

Whether fertilisation occurs *in vitro* or *in vivo*, however, it is almost certain that the cellular and molecular processes of sperm–egg recognition and fertilisation are identical. As such, a 'good sperm' is one that can:

1. successfully penetrate the cumulus
2. interact and bind with the zona pellucida
3. undergo the acrosome reaction and penetrate the zona pellucida
4. bind and fuse with egg plasma membrane.

We have made significant progress in understanding the biology of these steps (presumably by virtue of the fact that it is much easier to study *in vitro* than other parts of the reproductive process) and they have recently been reviewed.[32]

Interestingly, however, one remaining area of uncertainty in sperm–zona interaction is the identification and characterisation of the sperm surface protein that binds to the zona protein ZP3 and enables acrosome-intact sperm to bind to the zona pellucida. Although many candidates have been put forward, none have yet found wide acceptance. This is unfortunate, as we know that defective sperm–zona interaction can be a major contributor to the infertility of men with severe teratozoospermia[33] or oligozoospermia.[34] Although there has been some success in developing *in vitro* sperm function tests that adequately mimic the interaction between human sperm and human zona pellucida,[35] such tests rely upon the incubation of sperm with intact, dissected or solubilised human oocytes and then subsequently assessing ability of sperm to acrosome react. It is difficult to see how this can gain more widespread acceptance as a routine test given that it requires access to large numbers of human oocytes in order to be performed routinely. This is because human sperm generally do not bind to the zona pellucida of other mammalian species and also because there has been limited success in producing biologically active human zona proteins recombinantly. Clearly, if we could make progress in identifying those 'good sperm' that possess the necessary receptors and intracellular mechanisms to interact with the zona pellucida appropriately, then we could better advise patients of their need for assisted conception and make a more informed decision between the need for conventional IVF or ICSI.

DNA quality

The final measurable aspect of sperm function that defines a 'good sperm' is the quality of the DNA contained within the sperm head. In many respects this could be considered the single most important property of sperm in as much as even if a sperm is able to be successfully transported to the site of fertilisation and bind/penetrate an egg (or be selected and injected into an egg during an ICSI procedure) a sperm with damaged or fragmented DNA may lead to fertilisation failure or poor embryo development.

Sperm DNA is uniquely packaged. This is both to allow the sperm to fit inside what is a relatively small sperm nucleus and to protect it from damage prior to fertilisation. Yet, at the time of fertilisation, sperm nuclear DNA must be transferred to the egg but also be delivered in a physical and chemical form that allows the developing embryo access to the genetic material. While it may seem obvious that 'good sperm' should contain undamaged genetic material or have appropriately robust mechanisms to protect its DNA component from damage, it is only recently that appropriate techniques have been developed and applied to measure the integrity of sperm DNA.[36]

Studies of sperm DNA quality have shown that DNA integrity is directly related to the probability of conception, both in the general population (attempting to conceive naturally) and in couples attending for assisted conception treatment. For example, Spano *et al.*[37] used the sperm chromatin structure assay to investigate the DNA integrity of men entering a two-year follow-up study with their partners, and who were attempting to conceive for the first time. This study found that poor-quality chromatin structure, assessed by this technique, was highly predictive of male subfertility regardless of the number, motility or morphology of spermatozoa.

Moreover, no pregnancies were reported when more than 30–40% of spermatozoa were seen to contain damaged DNA. This has subsequently been confirmed by other studies. It is, therefore, perhaps not entirely surprising to find that men attending infertility clinics have higher levels of DNA damage in their sperm.[3] Indeed, several studies have shown that DNA integrity is directly related to IVF outcomes.[38,39] Furthermore, a recent study[40] was able to show that blastocyst development was indirectly correlated to DNA damage as assessed using the terminal deoxynucleotidyl transferase-mediated deoxyuridine triphosphate (dUTP) *in situ* DNA nick end labelling (TUNEL) technique.

It is, therefore, perhaps ironic that some methods by which sperm are prepared for use in assisted conception techniques, such as IVF, may themselves lead to DNA damage by removing sperm from the protective environment of seminal plasma and then exposing the sperm to reactive oxygen species generated from seminal leucocytes.[41] In addition, it is known that sperm cryopreservation can significantly damage the DNA of infertile men – but not fertile men – putting them at a significant disadvantage if samples provided as a backup for treatment are actually used.[42]

Concluding remarks

Spermatozoa are clearly complex cells that must display many different functions – in the correct sequence – in order to successfully navigate the female reproductive tract and reach the site of fertilisation. Clearly, 'good sperm' are those that successfully make that journey and that are able to fertilise any oocytes found there. In addition, not only should a 'good sperm' be able to fertilise an oocyte, but its DNA should be of sufficient quality to allow embryo development and implantation to occur.

An interesting question is whether sperm that do not have the capacity to reach the site of fertilisation are therefore necessarily 'bad sperm'. For example, if it were possible to collect from the female reproductive tract those sperm that failed to pass through the uterotubal junction or that failed to bind to the endosalpinx in the tubal isthmus, would it be possible to create viable embryos with them? The answer is almost certainly yes, but a more sophisticated technique would need to be used: some of the sperm would almost certainly achieve fertilisations at IVF whereas others would only do so if they were injected into oocytes by ICSI (assuming their DNA was suitably competent). So what does that mean for our definition of 'good sperm'? Does it undermine it? No, it simply reminds us that for some men their sperm can only successfully achieve fertilisation following the use of more sophisticated techniques. The problem remains how we can efficiently identify men with poorly functioning sperm and therefore provide the most appropriate treatment.

There has been some progress over the years in developing putative tests of sperm function and, while some have gained some credibility, none have received universally popular appeal over and above routine semen analysis. In addition, by listing the physiological sperm functions required for successful fertilisation alongside available sperm function tests (Table 10.2), it can be seen that there exist no tests which examine some of the critical aspects of sperm function within the female reproductive tract. These include tests to predict the ability of sperm to pass through the uterine cavity, or through the uterotubal junction and their subsequent inter-action with the endosalpinx. This is a significant shortfall in our ability to both understand and assess what defines 'good sperm' and should be one of the foci of future research projects in this area.

References

1. World Health Organization. *WHO Laboratory Manual for the Examination of Human Semen and Sperm–Cervical Mucus Interaction.* Cambridge: Cambridge University Press; 1999.
2. Bonde JP, Ernst E, Jensen TK, Hjollund NH, Kolstad H, Henriksen TB, *et al.* Relation between semen quality and fertility: a population-based study of 430 first-pregnancy planners. *Lancet* 1998;352:1172–7.
3. Irvine DS, Twigg JP, Gordon EL, Fulton N, Milne PA, Aitken RJ. DNA integrity in human spermatozoa: relationships with semen quality. *J Androl* 2000;21:33–44.
4. Mortimer D. *Practical Laboratory Andrology.* Oxford: Oxford University Press; 1994.
5. Aitken RJ, Sutton M, Warner P, Richardson DW. Relationship between the movement characteristics of human spermatozoa and their ability to penetrate cervical mucus and zona-free hamster oocytes. *J Reprod Fertil* 1985;73:441–9.
6. Katz DF, Morales P, Samuels SJ, Overstreet JW. Mechanisms of filtration of morphologically abnormal human sperm by cervical mucus. *Fertil Steril* 1990;54:513–16.
7. Kunz G, Beil D, Deininger H, Wildt L, Leyendecker G. The dynamics of rapid sperm transport through the female genital tract: evidence from vaginal sonography of uterine peristalsis and hysterosalpingoscintigraphy. *Hum Reprod* 1996;11:627–32.
8. Scott MA. A glimpse at sperm function *in vivo*: sperm transport and epithelial interaction in the female reproductive tract. *Anim Reprod Sci* 2000;60–1:337–48.
9. Pacey AA, Davies N, Warren MA, Barratt CLR, Cooke ID. Hyperactivation may assist human spermatozoa to detach from intimate association with the endosalpinx. *Hum Reprod* 1995;10:2603–9.
10. Mackenna A, Barratt CLR, Kessopoulou E, Cooke ID. The contribution of a hidden male factor to unexplained infertility. *Fertil Steril* 1993;59:405–11.
11. Shalgi R, Smith T, Yanagimachi R. A quantitative comparison of the passage of uncapacitated hamster spermatozoa through the uterotubal junction. *Biol Reprod* 1991;46:419–24.
12. Ellington JE, Jones AE, Davitt CM, Schneider CS, Brisbois RS, Hiss GA, *et al.* Human sperm function in coculture with human macaque or bovine oviduct epithelial cell monolayers. *Hum Reprod* 1998;13:2797–804.
13. Morales P, Palma V, Salgado AM, Villalon M. Sperm interaction with human oviductal cells *in vitro*. *Hum Reprod* 1996;11:1504–9.
14. Guerin JF, Ouhibi N, Regnier-Vigouroux G, Menezo Y. Movement characteristics and hyperactivation of human sperm on different epithelial cell monolayers. *Int J Androl* 1991;14:412–22.
15. Yeung WSB, Ng VKH, Lau EYL, Ho PC. Human oviductal cells and their conditioned medium maintain the motility and hyperactivation of human spermatozoa *in vitro*. *Hum Reprod* 1994;9:656–60.
16. Yao Y, Ho P, Yeung WSB. Human oviductal cells produce a factor(s) that maintains the motility of human spermatozoa *in vitro*. *Fertil Steril* 2000;73:479–86.
17. Murray SC, Smith TT. Sperm interaction with fallopian tube apical membrane enhances sperm motility and delays capacitation. *Fertil Steril* 1997;68:351–7.
18. Ellington JE, Evenson DP, Wright RW, Jones AE, Schneider CS, Hiss GA, *et al.* Higher quality human sperm in a sample selectively attach to oviduct (fallopian tube) epithelial cells *in vitro*. *Fertil Steril* 1999;71:924–9.
19. Suarez SS. Formation of a reservoir of sperm in the oviduct. *Reprod Domest Anim* 2002;37:140–3.
20. Reeve L, Ledger WL, Pacey AA. Does the Arg-Gly-Asp (RGD) adhesion sequence play a role in mediating sperm interaction with the human endosalpinx? *Hum Reprod* 2003;18:1461–8.
21. Thomas PG, Ball BA. Cytofluorescent assay to quantify adhesion of equine spermatozoa to oviduct epithelial cells *in vitro*. *Mol Reprod Dev* 1996;43:55–61.
22. Ellington JE, Varner DD, Burghardt RC, Meyers-Wallen R, Barhoumi SP, Brinsko SP, *et al.* Cell-to-cell communication of equine uterine tube (oviduct) cells as determined by anchored cell analysis in culture. *Anim Reprod Sci* 1993;30:313–24.
23. Ellington JE, Ignoz GG, Ball BA, Meyers-Wallen VN, Currie WB. *De novo* protein synthesis by bovine uterine tube (oviduct) epithelial cells changes during co-culture with bull spermatozoa. *Biol Reprod* 1995;48:851–6.
24. Thomas PGA, Ignoz GG, Ball BA, Brinsko SP. Effect of coculture with stallion spermatozoa on *de novo* protein synthesis and secretion by equine oviductal epithelial cells. *Am J Vet Res* 1995;56:1657–62.
25. Fazeli A, Affara N, Hubank M, Holt WV. Sperm-induced modification of the oviductal gene expression profile after natural insemination in mice. *Biol Reprod* 2004;71:60–5.

26. Birkhead TR. Cryptic female choice: criteria for establishing female sperm choice. *Evolution* 1998;52:1212–18.

27. Bahat A, Tur-Kaspa I, Gakamsky A, Giojalas LC, Breitbart H, Eisenbach M. Thermotaxis of mammalian sperm cells: a potential navigation mechanism in the female genital tract. *Nat Med* 2003;9:149–50.

28. Eisenbach M. Mammalian sperm chemotaxis and its association with capacitation. *Dev Genet* 1999;25:87–94.

29. Spehr M, Gisselmann G, Poplawski A, Riffell JA, Wetzel CH, Zimmer RK, *et al.* Identification of a testicular odorant receptor mediating human sperm chemotaxis. *Science* 2003;299:2054–8.

30. Spehr M, Schwane K, Riffell JA, Barbour J, Zimmer RK, Neuhaus EM, *et al.* Particulate adenylate cyclase plays a key role in human sperm olfactory receptor-mediated chemotaxis. *J Biol Chem* 2004;279:40194–203.

31. Elder K, Dale B. In Vitro *Fertilisation*. Cambridge: Cambridge University Press; 2000.

32. Primakoff P, Myles DG. Penetration, adhesion and fusion in mammalian sperm–egg interaction. *Science* 2002;296:2183–5.

33. Liu DY, Baker HWG. Frequency of defective sperm–zona interaction in severely teratozoospermic infertile men. *Hum Reprod* 2003;18:802–7.

34. Liu DY, Baker HWG. High frequency of defective sperm–zona interaction in oligozoospermic infertile men. *Hum Reprod* 2004;19:228–33.

35. Bastiaan HS, Windt ML, Menkveld R, Kruger TF, Oehninger S, Franken DR. Relationship between zona pellucida-induced acrosome reaction, sperm morphology, sperm–zona pellucida binding, and *in vitro* fertilization. *Fertil Steril* 2003;79:49–55.

36. Perreault SD, Aitken RJ, Baker HW, Evenson DP, Huszar G, Irvine DS, *et al.* Integrating new tests of sperm genetic integrity into semen analysis: breakout group discussion. *Adv Exp Med Biol* 2003;518:253–68.

37. Spano M, Bonde JP, Hjøllund HI, Kolstad HA, Cordelli E, Leter G, and The Danish First Pregnancy Planner Study Team. Sperm chromatin damage impairs human fertility. *Fertil Steril* 2000;73:43–50.

38. Tomsu M, Sharma V, Miller D. Embryo quality and IVF treatment outcome may correlate with different sperm comet assay parameters. *Hum Reprod* 2002;17:1856–62.

39. Morris ID, Ilott S, Dixon L, Brison DR. Spectrum of DNA damage in human sperm assessed by single cell gel electrophoresis (Comet assay) and its relationship to fertilisation and embryo development. *Hum Reprod* 2002;17:990–8.

40. Seli E, Gardner DK, Schoolcraft WB, Moffatt O, Sakkas D. Extent of nuclear DNA damage in ejaculated spermatozoa impacts on blastocyst development after *in vitro* fertilisation. *Fertil Steril* 2004;82:378–83.

41. Zalta A, Hafez T, Comhaire F. Evaluation of the role of reactive oxygen species in male infertility. *Hum Reprod* 1995;10:1444–51.

42. Donnelly ET, Steele EK, McClure N, Lewis SE. Assessment of DNA integrity and morphology of ejaculated spermatozoa from fertile and infertile men before and after cryopreservation. *Hum Reprod* 2001;16:1191–9.

43. Baillie HS, Pacey AA, Warren MA, Scudamore IW, Barratt CL. Greater numbers of human spermatozoa associate with endosalpingeal cells derived from the isthmus compared with those from the ampulla. *Hum Reprod* 1997;12:1985–92.

Chapter 11

Morphogenesis of the early mammalian embryo: cell lineage heterogeneity and developmental potential

Tom P Fleming, Judith J Eckert, Fay C Thomas and Bhavwanti Sheth

Introduction

The predominant morphological event occurring during mammalian pre-implantation development is the generation of a blastocyst with distinct cell lineages and with differing cell fates.[1] This cell heterogeneity is an essential component of early morphogenesis and is associated with the maintenance of developmental potential for the embryo. Thus, as cleavage proceeds, cells either differentiate into an epithelium, the trophectoderm, which resides on the embryo surface, or remain relatively undifferentiated and occupy the central region of the embryo, forming the inner cell mass (ICM). The trophectoderm is responsible for active transport processes which collectively regulate exchange of ions, nutrients, metabolites, growth factors and other developmentally important molecules between the maternal tract and the embryo interior.[1] It also generates the blastocoelic cavity of the blastocyst by transepithelial transport driven by Na,K-ATPase enzyme located on trophectoderm basolateral membranes.[2] During blastocyst expansion, the ICM, located to one side of the blastocoel beneath the trophectoderm, segregates into epiblast (primary ectoderm) and hypoblast (primary endoderm) lineages, the latter forming adjacent to the blastocoel. After implantation, the trophectoderm and hypoblast give rise to extra-embryonic lineages while the epiblast is the progenitor of the entire fetus.

In the current era of embryonic stem (ES) cell technologies and their prospective application to reproductive and clinical treatments,[3] it is important to understand from where ES cells derive, what factors are critical in maintaining their potential, and, significantly, what biological mechanisms influence their activity within the intact embryo. Indeed, appreciation of the factors regulating the decision-making processes of pluripotential cells *in vivo* will be informative for maximising the proliferative and differentiative capacity of ES cells *in vitro*. In this paper, we consider how embryonic blastomeres emerge with differing phenotypes and fates during early morphogenesis, what molecular processes regulate cellular heterogeneity, and how the embryo develops in a *dynamic* environment by which intrinsic and extrinsic conditions can modulate these basic mechanisms of lineage diversification. Most of the biological mechanisms involved have been studied in the mouse model upon which this review will focus.

Origin of fetal and extra-embryonic cell lineages

During cleavage in the mouse (around 4 days), all blastomeres acquire intercellular membrane adhesion mediated by the calcium-dependent E-cadherin/catenin adhesion complex.[1,4] This is achieved at the 8-cell stage, called embryonic compaction, resulting in close cellular apposition, loss of distinct cellular outlines, and formation of the morula stage of development. Compaction heralds the first step in cellular differentiation in the embryo because all blastomeres concomitantly undergo cell polarisation in a manner typical of epithelial cells, generating a microvillous, non-adhesive, apical membrane facing the outside environment and a non-microvillous, adhesive, basolateral membrane at remaining cell contact sites.[5,6] These surface features coincide with major reorganisation of the cytoskeletal and endocytic systems within the cytoplasm, such that cellular polarity embraces not only morphological but also functional criteria such as enhanced endocytic uptake at the apical domain.[7–10]

All blastomeres in the embryo, therefore, initiate differentiation along the trophectoderm epithelial pathway. E-cadherin-mediated adhesion plays a central role in coordinating epithelial polarisation. If compaction is inhibited experimentally, cellular polarisation is delayed or absent and, if present, occurs along random axes.[6] The molecular processes controlling the onset of compaction have been investigated in detail.[1,4] Significantly, this switch in embryonic phenotype does not appear to be regulated by timed expression of specific components of the E-cadherin complex; indeed, biosynthesis and membrane association of the major constituents of the complex take place from early cleavage after activation of the zygotic genome.[11,12] Post-translational control of E-cadherin adhesion appears to be primarily regulated by the activity of intracellular Ca^{2+} mobilisation[13] and protein kinase C (PKC) signalling. $PKC\alpha$ relocates to the membrane at the time of compaction, and stimulation of conventional PKCs by phorbol ester treatment both advances the onset of compaction and $PKC\alpha$ relocalisation.[14–16] Evidence to date suggests that β-catenin serine/threonine phosphorylation may be a target of PKC, permitting cytoskeletal anchorage of the E-cadherin/catenin complex to activate the adhesive state.[15] Tyrosine dephosphorylation of β-catenin is upregulated at compaction and may also contribute to its inception.[17]

The polarised epithelial character of 8-cell blastomeres at compaction leads directly to cell diversification in the embryo through asymmetric cell divisions (Figure 11.1).[18] The polarised state is stable[19] and persists into mitosis and, in a proportion of blastomeres, division planes are orthogonal to the axis of polarity, resulting in daughter cells at the 16-cell stage inheriting distinct apico-basal domains of the parental cytoplasm. Those cells inheriting the apical microvillous pole domain remain on the embryo surface and maintain a polarised epithelial phenotype while those cells inheriting the adhesive basal domain become enclosed within the embryo interior and display a nonpolarised state. In remaining 8-cell blastomeres, division planes are parallel to the axis of polarity, with both daughter cells inheriting approximately half of the parental apical pole; these cells also remain on the embryo surface with a polarised phenotype. The origin of outer polar and inner nonpolar cell types following asymmetric division of polarised 8-cell blastomeres represents the major pathway by which trophectoderm and ICM lineages are established, respectively.[1]

Consequently, the embryo engages in a separation of cellular activities during the 16-cell stage whereby outer polar cells continue to upregulate epithelial differentiation

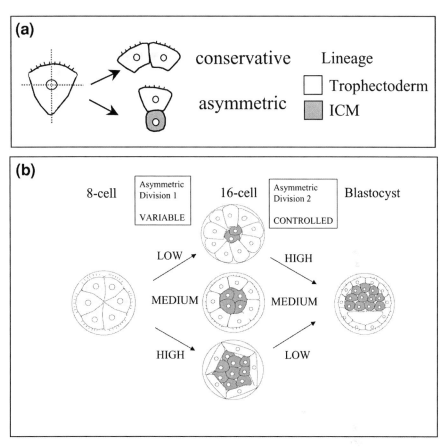

Figure 11.1. (a) Cell division orientation within 8-cell blastomere; (b) Relationship between proportion of asymmetric divisions at 8- and 16-cell stages leads to blastocyst with trophectoderm and ICM cell numbers within relatively narrow limits

and inner nonpolar cells suppress this activity and maintain a pluripotent state. At the time of division to the 32-cell stage, outer blastomeres again engage in either differentiative or conservative divisions, with daughter cells inheriting all or part of the parental apical domain remaining in the outer trophectoderm lineage while those that do not enter the internal ICM lineage.[20,21] These two rounds of cytokinesis effectively complete the process of lineage segregation within the embryo; in subsequent divisions, trophectoderm and ICM lineages remain separate except in exceptional circumstances.[22] Mouse embryos also coordinate in quantitative terms the extent of asymmetric divisions occurring within the 8- and 16-cell division cycles (Figure 11.1(b)). Thus, while a variable number of 8-cell blastomeres divide asymmetrically in different embryos, an inverse relationship exists between this number and that

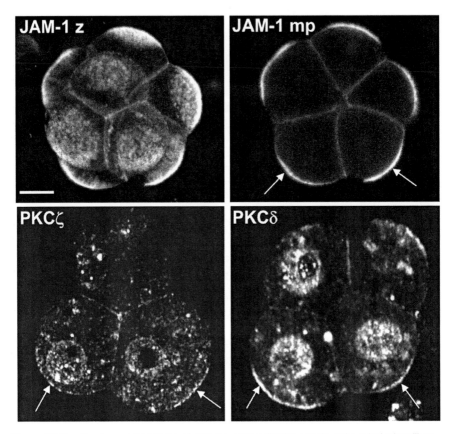

Figure 11.2. Top: immunolocalisation of JAM-1 junction adhesion protein at the apical microvillous pole at the time of compaction, shown as confocal microscope z-series or single midplane (mp) optical section; Bottom: immunolocalisation of PKCζ and PKCδ at apical membrane sites (arrows) of compact 8-cell embryos confocal sections; bar = 20 μm.

occurring at the next cycle.[21] This mechanism appears to reside in the impact of cell interactions on cell shape and spindle orientation, and ensures that the relative pools of trophectoderm and ICM cells within individual embryos are maintained within narrow limits. The capacity of the embryo to regulate closely the relative size of early cell lineages has implications for later development. Thus, experimental manipulations by which trophectoderm and ICM cell numbers or ratio are altered *in vitro* result in delayed or abnormal development after embryo transfer into pseudopregnant recipients.[23] In addition, suboptimal environmental conditions during pre-implantation development, such as reduced growth factor or amino acid composition *in vitro* or maternal undernutrition *in vivo*, using different animal models, are associated with both reduced trophectoderm and/or ICM cell numbers, reduced fetal and postnatal growth rates, and an adverse physiological or metabolic phenotype, such as relative hypertension.[23]

Molecular mechanisms controlling lineage diversification by asymmetric division have been examined, in particular, in invertebrate model organisms such as the nematode *Caenorhabditis elegans* and the fly *Drosophila*. In these models, the *Par* gene complex including atypical PKCs is implicated in the generation of cell lineage diversity and is localised asymmetrically during differentiative divisions.[24] Cell fate diversification in these models can occur by atypical PKC phosphorylation of cytoskeletal components resulting in differential inheritance of determinant proteins.[25] We[26] have investigated the expression in the embryo of JAM-1, an epithelial tight junction (TJ) transmembrane protein (see below for discussion of TJ biogenesis in the embryo) which also recruits mammalian ASIP/PAR3 and atypical PKC to junction sites for establishment of cell polarity in cultured epithelial cells and JAM-1 transfected fibroblasts and Chinese hamster ovary (CHO) cells.[27,28] We have found that JAM-1 associates transiently with the apical microvillous pole during compaction, and co-localises at this site with atypical PKCζ and novel PKCδ isotypes.[26] (Figure 11.2). Similarly, atypical PKC is localised to the apical membrane of blastomeres during cleavage of *Xenopus* embryos where a role in asymmetric cell division has been proposed.[29] These data on the *Par* gene complex indicate that apical membrane PKCζ at compaction may similarly contribute to the process of early lineage diversification in the mouse embryo through cytoskeletal reorganisation and cell polarity. Novel PKCδ is known to bind F-actin in neutrophils and epithelial cells and appears to function in dynamic restructuring of the membrane–associated actin cytoskeleton.[30,31] Thus, this isotype of PKC may contribute to the cytoskeletal reorganisation of blastomeres at compaction.

Trophectoderm differentiation: progressive maturation of an epithelial phenotype

As indicated above, following compaction, outer cells gradually acquire a fully functional epithelial phenotype such that during the 32-cell stage the trophectoderm engages in transepithelial transport to form the blastocoel. Analysis of gene and protein expression associated with key aspects of the epithelial phenotype reveal a progressive maturation process during the 24-hour period separating compaction and cavitation. For example, this can be seen in the Na,K-ATPase enzyme which localises to basolateral membranes and is responsible for ATP-dependent ion transport necessary to drive apico-basal transport of other metabolites and the generation of the blastocoel cavity by movement of water down its osmotic gradient. Maturation in Na,K-ATPase activity occurs as cleavage proceeds such that delayed expression of the β-subunit required for membrane delivery relative to the catalytic α-subunit provides a means to coordinate the timing of trophectoderm transport activity.[2] Similarly, the adhesive and junctional complexes present between trophectoderm cells and necessary for cohesion and integrity of the epithelial layer for cavitation to occur also mature gradually during the interval between compaction and cavitation. Our laboratory has focused attention particularly on the biogenesis of the apico-lateral TJ, the belt-like intercellular complex which forms the permeability seal required to prevent leakage of blastocoelic fluid.

The TJ proteins which form the sealing complex comprise transmembrane and peripheral cytoplasmic plaque constituents that link to the actin cytoskeleton.[32] In the mouse embryo, these proteins are expressed and assemble at the membrane in three waves, corresponding to 8-, 16- and 32-cell stages.[1,4] Thus, at the 8-cell stage, the transmembrane constituent, JAM-1,[26] and the cytoplasmic proteins ZO-1α-[33] and RAB13[34] assemble at the junction site; at the 16-cell stage the plaque proteins cingulin[35] and ZO-2 assemble, while at the early 32-cell stage other key constituents including the transmembrane adhesive proteins claudins and occludin[33,36] localise to the junction for the first time. This final step switches the TJ from inactive to active states and is followed rapidly by blastocoel fluid accumulation. While the progressive nature of sequential membrane assembly of TJ constituents reflects a temporal programme of junctional gene and protein expression, the final maturation step at the 32-cell stage appears to be mediated by transcriptional regulation. At this time, the ZO-1α+ isoform is transcribed *de novo*, is immediately translated and associates intracellularly with pre-existing occludin protein to facilitate its delivery to the membrane.[33,36] Thus, biosynthetic control mechanisms appear to be critical in regulating the timing of trophectoderm differentiation and transport function to a precise cell cycle.

We have evaluated potential post-translational mechanisms that may additionally regulate trophectoderm differentiation. Analysis of occludin biochemistry at the time of membrane assembly in the 32-cell stage mouse embryo has shown that the protein becomes phosphorylated prior to assembly.[36] Other studies have shown that release of intracellular calcium, partly mediated via G-protein-coupled receptors, is a major regulator of blastocoel formation.[37–40] We have investigated the role of PKC signalling in blastocyst formation and, using PKC isoform-specific inhibitory and stimulatory peptides, demonstrated a role for PKCδ and PKCζ in stimulating the time of blastocoel formation.[41] At a mechanistic level, modulating the activity of these isoforms caused the Na,K-ATPase enzyme to be internalised from trophectoderm basolateral membranes as one causative pathway by which blastocoel cavitation is PKC-mediated. PKC regulation of trophectoderm differentiation also acts via the TJ. Using the 'ICM immunosurgery' model described below, inhibition of either PKCδ or PKCζ specifically by peptide treatment inhibited membrane assembly of ZO-2 TJ protein while PKCζ alone regulated ZO-1α+ isoform assembly.[42] Both of these PKC isoforms partially co-localise with the TJ during trophectoderm differentiation (Figure 11.3), further supporting their involvement in TJ biogenesis.[41]

Cell contacts and the dynamic regulation of cell lineage allocation

The mammalian embryo has long been considered to exhibit remarkable regulative capacity, presumably reflecting a plasticity in developmental potential to combat different environmental conditions. Cell contact patterns between blastomeres have a major influence on this dynamic state. While compaction and epithelial cell polarisation at the 8-cell stage is mediated by cell adhesion (see earlier), contact patterns remain effective in steering developmental pathways throughout the cleavage period. Thus, the progressive maturation of epithelial differentiation in the outside lineage is maintained and upregulated by the cell contact asymmetry that these cells experience. Similarly, inside cells suppress epithelial differentiation by virtue of the cell contact symmetry (total enclosure) that they experience during cleavage. The dynamic nature of these interactive processes can be demonstrated by blastocyst immunosurgery. This method allows the ICM to be removed and cultured separately by lysing the outer trophectoderm layer. The change in cell contacts experienced by

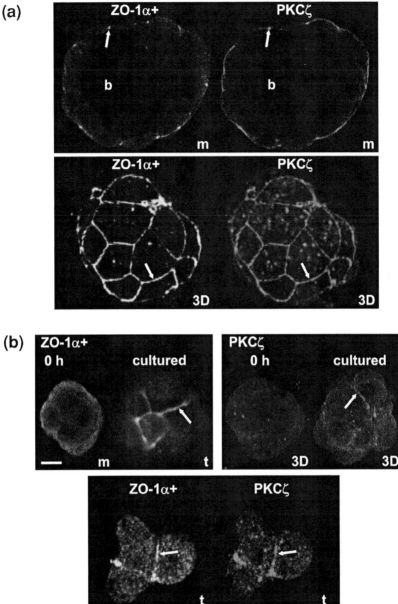

Figure 11.3. (a) Blastocysts double-labelled for tight junction protein ZO-1α+ and PKCζ; in midplane (m) sections, both localise to tight junctions appearing as spot-like contact sites (arrows) between trophectoderm cells; in z-series 3D reconstructions, the belt-like staining pattern around each trophectoderm cell is evident (arrows); (b) ICMs after immunosurgery shown in midplane (m) or tangential (t) planes or as z-series (3D), following immunolocalisation for ZO-1α+ and PKCζ, either immediately after isolation or after culture; arrows indicate junctional localisation of both proteins; bar = 20 μm

the ICM after isolation, now with its outer cells experiencing a contact-free surface, results in a gradual change in cell fate for these outer cells with epithelial differentiation upregulated. As a consequence, these cells change fate from ICM to trophectoderm-like, resulting in transepithelial transport and reformation of a blastocoel cavity within 9–12 hours of culture.[43–46] Upon transfer to pseudopregnant foster mothers, these 'mini blastocysts' can induce a decidual reaction, further confirming the trophectodermal identity of the outer cells.[44] The capacity to re-cavitate and re-form trophectoderm-like outer cells is progressively lost when ICMs are isolated from older, more expanded blastocysts which then form predominantly primary endoderm-like structures.[45,47] Isolated ICMs also have the capacity to develop into offspring when injected into host blastocysts,[48] indicating their authenticity and developmental competence.

We have investigated how cell fate can be so tightly regulated by cell contact patterns within the embryo. At the biosynthetic level, transcription of genes important in trophectoderm differentiation, such as those encoding TJ constituents, do not appear to be controlled by cell contact patterns. Thus, for example, transcription of ZO-1 isoforms, RAB13, cingulin and occludin occur within both trophectoderm and ICM lineages during normal development[34,36] although protein translation and detection of proteins either by immunofluorescence or biochemical means is restricted to the trophectoderm lineage, upregulated by cell contact asymmetry.[46,49] Consequently, expression and membrane assembly of TJ proteins in ICMs following immunosurgery is independent of new transcription but can be inhibited by suppression of protein synthesis.[46]

The cell contact pattern, either asymmetric or symmetric, maintaining trophectoderm and ICM lineage pathways respectively, acts upstream of signal transduction mechanisms regulating phenotypic status. Thus, imposing cell contact asymmetry on the ICM by immunosurgery causes relocation of PKC isoforms, including δ and ζ, from cytoplasmic to membrane domains as they become critically involved in membrane delivery of newly synthesised TJ proteins (Figure 11.3).[50] However, if cell contact asymmetry is incompletely provided, for example by leaving the ICM within the lysed trophectoderm layer during immunosurgery, mobilisation of PKCs and TJ assembly within the ICM is inhibited.[42] Specificity also exists in the signalling pathways activated and regulated by cell contact patterns. Thus, while PKC-mediated pathways are clearly responsive and functional with respect to cell contact pattern, gap junctional intercellular communication appears not to be involved in phenotypic decision making following changes in contact pattern.[42]

Transcriptional factors and cell lineage diversification

Surprisingly few transcription factors have been identified as having a role in regulating cell lineage diversification during early mouse development. The POU-domain factor, OCT4, is expressed during oogenesis and early cleavage and localises to the ICM and subsequently epiblast lineage in expanding blastocysts.[51,52] OCT4, in concert with the HMG box factor SOX2, acts to maintain ICM and ES cell pluripotency, inducing upregulation of ICM-specific genes such as FGF4, a mitogen active in trophectoderm proliferation.[53] OCT4 also represses trophectoderm differentiation within the ICM and in *Oct4*-null embryos inner cells exhibit epithelial characteristics and express trophectoderm genes.[54,55] Nanog homeobox gene is also differentially expressed in the ICM lineage of the embryo and is required for its determination and repression of hypoblast differentiation.[56,57] *Cdx2*, the caudal-related homeobox gene, has a reciprocal role in controlling trophectoderm differentiation. It becomes differentially expressed within this lineage in the blastocyst[58] and, in mutant condition, trophoblast differentiation cannot be maintained.[59]

Analysis of transcription factor expression and differentiative potential of mutant embryos tends to show that the appropriate transcription factor complexes act secondarily to maintain lineage diversification rather than actively inducing it. Thus, in the *Oct4-* and *Cdx2*-null embryo, a distinct blastocyst is formed with overt trophectoderm and ICM lineages and blastocoel cavity prior to developmental failure.[54,60] These characteristics indicate that cell polarisation, asymmetric cell divisions and continued cell interactions during cleavage as discussed above are responsible for initiating lineage diversification within the embryo which then becomes reinforced by upregulation of appropriate transcription factor families. Moreover, since changes in cell contact patterns by, for example, immunosurgery can exert rapid changes in cellular phenotype in the absence of transcriptional activation,[46] the distinction in lineage transcription factor patterns would appear to consolidate contact-mediated, dynamic decisions imposed by environmental cues.

Egg polarity, cell polarity and cell interactions

While the regulative capacity and inherent asynchrony of cleavage in the early embryo have been recognised for many years, recent research has demonstrated that in relatively undisturbed embryos a relationship exists between the animal–vegetal (AV) polarity of the egg and the orientation of the blastocyst.[61,62] By careful lineage marking analyses, it has been shown that the embryonic–abembryonic axis of the blastocyst tends to form perpendicular to the AV axis of the egg. Moreover, these data indicate that, as cleavage initiates, the earliest dividing 2-cell blastomere tends to contribute preferentially to the embryonic pole of the blastocyst comprising the polar trophectoderm and ICM.[63] How might these new data on egg polarity and axis determination relate to the cellular properties of blastomeres, reviewed above, concerning cell polarity, asymmetric divisions and trophectoderm/ICM lineage segregation? It would appear that these two aspects of early development may derive from common mechanisms mediated by cell interactions to guide cell fate. In support of the egg polarity data, it has been established from experimental studies that temporally more advanced blastomeres tend to contribute disproportionately to the ICM.[64] Thus, the 2-cell blastomere undergoing division ahead of its sister is likely to maintain this temporal advantage such that its progeny will enter embryo compaction and acquire adhesive properties slightly ahead of other blastomeres. Experimental manipulation of compaction has indicated that cells vary in the relative size of the apical microvillous pole domain and that those cells with smaller apical poles tend to divide asymmetrically more frequently to yield one daughter cell within the ICM lineage.[65] Consequently, as early acquisition of an adhesive state is likely to lead to more intercellular adhesive contacts and a deeper position for a cell during compaction, this in turn would likely result in a smaller apical pole domain and increased frequency of asymmetric division. What appears critically important, therefore, in the relationship linking egg polarity with blastocyst axis is the mechanism inducing cell cycle heterogeneity at the 2-cell stage, a factor which is as yet unexplained.

Conclusions

The origin of early cell lineages within the mammalian embryo is largely dependent upon the pattern and nature of blastomere intercellular contacts. Such contacts regulate cell polarisation at compaction to generate divergent lineages by asymmetric division and then maintain those lineages on their distinct developmental pathways as the blastocyst is formed. They most likely underlie a secondary process whereby distinct transcription factor expression consolidates lineage diversification. Some but not all of the molecular signalling pathways critical in phenotype specification by cell contact patterns have been identified and will be an area of intense interest in the future. Such cell contact patterns are also likely to contribute to the temporal relationships recently discovered between the organisation of the egg and axes present within the blastocyst. The importance of cell interactions should not be underestimated, therefore, both in human embryo development *in vitro* and in the derivation and potential of human embryonic stem cells.

Acknowledgements

We are grateful to the Medical Research Council, the Biotechnology and Biological Research Council, The Wellcome Trust, the National Institutes of Health (USA) and University of Southampton funding for research within the first author's laboratory.

References

1. Fleming TP, Wilkins A, Mears A, Miller DJ, Thomas F, Ghassemifar MR, *et al.* The making of an embryo: short-term goals and long-term implications. *Reprod Fertil Dev* 2004;16:325–37.
2. Watson AJ, Barcroft LC. Regulation of blastocyst formation. *Front Biosci* 2001;6:708–30.
3. Murray P, Edgar D. The topographical regulation of embryonic stem cell differentiation. *Philos Trans R Soc Lond B Biol Sci* 2004;359:1009–20.
4. Fleming TP, Sheth B, Fesenko I. Cell adhesion in the preimplantation mammalian embryo and its role in trophectoderm differentiation and blastocyst morphogenesis. *Front Biosci* 2001;6:1000–7.
5. Ziomek CA, Johnson MH. Cell surface interactions induce polarisation of mouse 8-cell blastomeres at compaction. *Cell* 1980;21:935–42.
6. Johnson MH, Maro B, Takeichi M. The role of cell adhesion in the synchronization and orientation of polarization in 8-cell mouse blastomeres. *J Embryol Exp Morphol* 1986;93:239–55.
7. Reeve WJD. Cytoplasmic polarity develops at compaction in rat and mouse embryos. *J Embryol Exp Morphol* 1981;62:351–67.
8. Johnson MH, Maro B. The distribution of cytoplasmic actin in mouse 8-cell blastomeres. *J Embryol Exp Morphol* 1984;82:97–117.
9. Fleming TP, Pickering SJ. Maturation and polarisation of the endocytotic system in outside blastomeres during mouse preimplantation development. *J Embryol Exp Morphol* 1985;89:175–208.
10. Houliston E, Pickering SJ, Maro B. Redistribution of microtubules and pericentriolar material during the development of polarity in mouse blastomeres. *J Cell Biol* 1987;104:1299–308.
11. Sefton M, Johnson MH, Clayton L. Synthesis and phosphorylation of uvomorulin during mouse early development. *Development* 1992;115:313–18.
12. Ohsugi M, Hwang SY, Butz S, Knowles BB, Solter D, Kemler R. Expression and cell membrane localization of catenins during mouse preimplantation development. *Dev Dyn* 1996;206:391–402.
13. Pey R, Vial C, Schatten G, Hafner M. Increase in intracellular Ca2+ and relocation of E-cadherin during experimental decompaction of mouse embryos. *Proc Natl Acad Sci U S A* 1998;95:12977–82.
14. Winkel GK, Ferguson JE, Takeichi M, Nuccitelli R. Activation of protein kinase C triggers premature compaction in the four-cell stage mouse embryo. *Dev Biol* 1990;138:1–15.
15. Pauken CM, Capco DG. Regulation of cell adhesion during embryonic compaction of mammalian embryos: roles for PKC and beta-catenin. *Mol Reprod Dev* 1999;54:135–44.
16. Kawai Y, Yamaguchi T, Yoden T, Hanada M, Miyake M. Effect of protein phosphatase inhibitors on

the development of mouse embryos: protein phosphorylation is involved in the E-cadherin distribution in mouse two-cell embryos. *Biol Pharm Bull* 2002;25:179–83.

17. Ohsugi M, Butz S, Kemler R. Beta-catenin is a major tyrosine-phosphorylated protein during mouse oocyte maturation and preimplantation development. *Dev Dyn* 1999;216:168–76.

18. Johnson MH, Ziomek CA. The foundation of two distinct cell lineages within mouse morula. *Cell* 1981;24:71–80.

19. Fleming TP, Pickering SJ, Qasim F, Maro B. The generation of cell surface polarity in mouse 8-cell blastomeres: the role of cortical microfilaments analysed using cytochalasin D. *J Embryol Exp Morphol* 1986;95:169–91.

20. Johnson MH, Ziomek CA. Cell interactions influence the fate of mouse blastomeres undergoing the transition from the 16- to the 32-cell stage. *Dev Biol* 1983;95:211–8.

21. Fleming TP. A quantitative analysis of cell allocation to trophectoderm and inner cell mass in the mouse blastocyst. *Dev Biol* 1987;119:520–31.

22. Dyce J, George M, Goodall H, Fleming TP. Do trophectoderm and inner cell mass cells in the mouse blastocyst maintain discrete lineages? *Development* 1987;100:685–98.

23. Fleming TP, Kwong WY, Porter R, Ursell E, Fesenko I, Wilkins A, *et al.* The embryo and its future. *Biol Reprod* 2004;71:1046–54.

24. Knoblich JA. Asymmetric cell division during animal development. *Nat Rev Mol Cell Biol* 2001;2:11–20.

25. Betschinger J, Mechtler K, Knoblich JA. The Par complex directs asymmetric cell division by phosphorylating the cytoskeletal protein Lgl. *Nature* 2003;422:326–30.

26. Thomas FC, Sheth B, Eckert JJ, Bazzoni G, Dejana E, Fleming TP. Contribution of JAM-1 to epithelial differentiation and tight-junction biogenesis in the mouse preimplantation embryo. *J Cell Sci* 2004;117:5599–608.

27. Itoh M, Sasaki H, Furuse M, Ozaki H, Kita T, Tsukita S. Junctional adhesion molecule (JAM) binds to PAR-3: a possible mechanism for the recruitment of PAR-3 to tight junctions. *J Cell Biol* 2001;154:491–7.

28. Ebnet K, Suzuki A, Horikoshi Y, Hirose T, Meyer Z, Brickwedde MK, *et al.* The cell polarity protein ASIP/PAR-3 directly associates with junctional adhesion molecule (JAM). *EMBO J* 2001;20:3738–48.

29. Chalmers AD, Strauss B, Papalopulu N. Oriented cell divisions asymmetrically segregate aPKC and generate cell fate diversity in the early Xenopus embryo. *Development* 2003;130:2657–68.

30. Lopez-Lluch G, Bird MM, Canas B, Godovac-Zimmerman J, Ridley A, Segal AW, *et al.* Protein kinase C-delta C2-like domain is a binding site for actin and enables actin redistribution in neutrophils. *Biochem J* 2001;357:39–47.

31. Liedtke CM, Hubbard M, Wang X. Stability of actin cytoskeleton and PKC-delta binding to actin regulate NKCC1 function in airway epithelial cells. *Am J Physiol Cell Physiol* 2003;284:C487–96.

32. Gonzalez-Mariscal L, Betanzos A, Nava P, Jaramillo BE. Tight junction proteins. *Prog Biophys Mol Biol* 2003;81:1–44.

33. Sheth B, Fesenko I, Collins JE, Moran B, Wild AE, Anderson JM, *et al.* Tight junction assembly during mouse blastocyst formation is regulated by late expression of ZO-1 alpha+ isoform. *Development* 1997;124:2027–37.

34. Sheth B, Fontaine JJ, Ponza E, McCallum A, Page A, Citi S, *et al.* Differentiation of the epithelial apical junctional complex during mouse preimplantation development: a role for rab13 in the early maturation of the tight junction. *Mech Dev* 2000;97:93–104.

35. Fleming TP, Hay M, Javed Q, Citi S. Localisation of tight junction protein cingulin is temporally and spatially regulated during early mouse development. *Development* 1993;117:1135–44.

36. Sheth B, Moran B, Anderson JM, Fleming TP. Post-translational control of occludin membrane assembly in mouse trophectoderm: a mechanism to regulate timing of tight junction biogenesis and blastocyst formation. *Development* 2000;127:831–40.

37. Stachecki JJ, Yelian FD, Schultz JF, Leach RE, Armant DR. Blastocyst cavitation is accelerated by ethanol- or ionophore-induced elevation of intracellular calcium. *Biol Reprod* 1994;50:1–9.

38. Stachecki JJ, Armant DR. Regulation of blastocoele formation by intracellular calcium release is mediated through a phospholipase C-dependent pathway in mice. *Biol Reprod* 1996;55:1292–8.

39. Stachecki JJ, Armant DR. Transient release of calcium from inositol 1,4,5-trisphosphate-specific stores regulates mouse preimplantation development. *Development* 1996;122:2485–96.

40. Wang J, Rout UK, Bagchi IC, Armant DR. Expression of calcitonin receptors in mouse preimplantation embryos and their function in the regulation of blastocyst differentiation by calcitonin. *Development* 1998;125:4293–302.

41. Eckert JJ, McCallum A, Mears A, Rumsby MG, Cameron IT, Fleming TP. Specific PKC isoforms

regulate blastocoel formation during mouse preimplantation development. *Dev Biol* 2004;274:384–401.

42. Eckert JJ, McCallum A, Mears A, Rumsby MG, Cameron IT, Fleming TP. Unpublished data.
43. Handyside AH. Time of commitment of inside cells isolated from preimplantation mouse embryos. *J Embryol Exp Morphol* 1978;45:37–53.
44. Rossant J, Lis WT. Potential of isolated mouse inner cell masses to form trophectoderm derivatives *in vivo*. *Dev Biol* 1979;70:255–61.
45. Fleming TP, Warren PD, Chisholm JC, Johnson MH. Trophectodermal processes regulate the expression of totipotency within the inner cell mass of the mouse expanding blastocyst. *J Embryol Exp Morphol* 1984;84:63–90.
46. Fleming TP, Hay MJ. Tissue-specific control of expression of the tight junction polypeptide ZO-1 in the mouse early embryo. *Development* 1991;113:295–304.
47. Chisholm JC, Johnson MH, Warren PD, Fleming TP, Pickering SJ. Developmental variability within and between mouse expanding blastocysts and their ICMs. *J Embryol Exp Morphol* 1985;86:311–36.
48. Azim M, Surani H, Torchiana D, Barton SC. Isolation and development of the inner cell mass after exposure of mouse embryos to calcium ionophore A23187. *J Embryol Exp Morphol* 1978;45:237–47.
49. Javed Q, Fleming TP, Hay M, Citi S. Tight junction protein cingulin is expressed by maternal and embryonic genomes during early mouse development. *Development* 1993;117:1145–51.
50. Eckert JJ, McCallum A, Mears A, Rumsby MG, Cameron IT, Fleming TP. PKC signalling regulates tight junction membrane assembly in the pre-implantation mouse embryo. *Reproduction* 2004;127:653–67.
51. Scholer HR, Hatzopoulos AK, Balling R, Suzuki N, Gruss P. A family of octamer-specific proteins present during mouse embryogenesis: evidence for germline-specific expression of an Oct factor. *EMBO J* 1989;8:2543–50.
52. Palmieri SL, Peter W, Hess H, Scholer HR. Oct-4 transcription factor is differentially expressed in the mouse embryo during establishment of the first two extraembryonic cell lineages involved in implantation. *Dev Biol* 1994;166:259–67.
53. Ambrosetti DC, Basilico C, Dailey L. Synergistic activation of the fibroblast growth factor 4 enhancer by Sox2 and Oct-3 depends on protein–protein interactions facilitated by a specific spatial arrangement of factor binding sites. *Mol Cell Biol* 1997;17:6321–9.
54. Nichols J, Zevnik B, Anastassiadis K, Niwa H, Klewe-Nebenius D, Chambers I, *et al.* Formation of pluripotent stem cells in the mammalian embryo depends on the POU transcription factor Oct4. *Cell* 1998;95:379–91.
55. Liu L, Roberts RM. Silencing of the gene for the beta subunit of human chorionic gonadotropin by the embryonic transcription factor Oct-3/4. *J Biol Chem* 1996;271:16683–9.
56. Chambers I, Colby D, Robertson M, Nichols J, Lee S, Tweedie S, *et al.* Functional expression cloning of Nanog, a pluripotency sustaining factor in embryonic stem cells. *Cell* 2003;113:643–55.
57. Mitsui K, Tokuzawa Y, Itoh H, Segawa K, Murakami M, Takahashi K, *et al.* The homeoprotein Nanog is required for maintenance of pluripotency in mouse epiblast and ES cells. *Cell* 2003;113:631–42.
58. Beck F, Erler T, Russell A, James, R. Expression of Cdx-2 in the mouse embryo and placenta: possible role in patterning of the extra-embryonic membranes. *Dev Dyn* 1995;204:219–27.
59. Chawengsaksophak K, James R, Hammond VE, Kontgen F, Beck F. Homeosis and intestinal tumours in Cdx2 mutant mice. *Nature* 1997;386:84–7.
60. Kunath T, Strumpf D, Rossant J. Early trophoblast determination and stem cell maintenance in the mouse – a review. *Placenta* 2004;25 Suppl A:S32–8.
61. Gardner RL. Patterning is initiated before cleavage in the mouse. *Ann Anat* 2002;184:577–81.
62. Zernicka-Goetz M. Patterning of the embryo: the first spatial decisions in the life of a mouse. *Development* 2002;129:815–29.
63. Piotrowska K, Wianny F, Pedersen RA, Zernicka-Goetz M. Blastomeres arising from the first cleavage division have distinguishable fates in normal mouse development. *Development* 2001;128:3739–48.
64. Surani MA, Barton SC. Spatial distribution of blastomeres is dependent on cell division order and interactions in mouse morulae. *Dev Biol* 1984;102:335–43.
65. Pickering SJ, Maro B, Johnson MH, Skepper JN. The influence of cell contact on the division of mouse 8-cell blastomeres. *Development* 1988;103:353–63.

Chapter 12
Epigenetics in development and cloning by nuclear transfer: alternative approaches to nuclear reprogramming

Keith HS Campbell and Ramiro Alberio

Summary

The mechanisms by which a cell attains and maintains a differentiated phenotype is fundamental to the process of animal development. During development and differentiation, cells undergo spatial and temporal patterns of gene expression. The mechanisms controlling such events do not, in the majority of cases, involve alterations in DNA sequence; rather, modifications to DNA and chromatin structure have been implicated. Such modifications, which include methylation of the DNA and post-translational modification of core histones, have been termed 'epigenetic' and are heritable through mitotic division. Epigenetic 'reprogramming' occurs at all stages of development but is becoming well characterised during germ cell and early embryo development. The technique of somatic cell nuclear transfer (SCNT) has demonstrated that oocyte cytoplasmic components are able to interact with somatic nuclear genetic material and result in the production of viable offspring. The mechanisms involved in these de-differentiation or re-differentiation events are unknown but have been broadly termed 'nuclear reprogramming' and are thought to involve 'epigenetic reprogramming' of the genome. The fact that SCNT techniques have proved that the egg cytoplasm is able to 'reprogramme' the genetic material from differentiated nuclei raises the possibility that the differentiated phenotype of a cell may be manipulated by other means in order to de-differentiate or trans-differentiate cell function. This paper will briefly review 'epigenetic reprogramming' during early development, describe the background to the technique of NT, and discuss the present knowledge on 'reprogramming' in cloned embryos. Finally, novel proposals for the 'reprogramming' of somatic cells in order to improve the efficiency of SCNT or change the phenotype of somatic cells *in vitro* will be discussed.

Introduction

Eukaryotic DNA is assembled into chromatin and chromosomes by association with histones. Briefly, the DNA helix is wrapped around core histones to form a simple bead-like structure (nucleosome) that is then folded into higher order chromatin. Higher order chromatin contains other proteins that are required for a range of functions, including assembly and maintenance of structure, and DNA replication, repair, transcription and recombination. By means of nucleosomal DNA, the genome is organised into functional regions that are transcriptionally active or transcriptionally repressive. However, the transcriptional state is not fixed and the covalent modification of nucleosomal DNA or the core histones is important in the control of many biological processes, including transcription and DNA replication. This epigenetic regulation of gene expression by modification of DNA and chromatin structure has been implicated in the processes controlling development, differentiation and disease. In this chapter we will not give a detailed account of the present knowledge on epigenetic regulation, but will rather try to integrate present knowledge with the ability to 'reprogramme' gene expression by NT. For more detailed discussions on epigenetic regulation, a number of excellent reviews are available.[1-7]

Animal cloning following the transfer of embryonic or somatic nuclei into enucleated oocytes has demonstrated the remarkable ability of the oocyte to reprogramme nuclei and give rise to offspring. Cloning with embryonic nuclei was first demonstrated in amphibians[8] and later in mammals.[9,10] As nuclei from later developmental stages were used for cloning, obtaining development to term proved difficult, suggesting a biological restriction to the reprogramming of fully differentiated cells.[11,12] The more contemporary cloning of a mammal using an adult somatic cell[13] demonstrated that such genetic information can be reprogrammed in oocyte cytoplasm. The development of cloning technology in mammals has opened a new view in the understanding of how nuclei acquire differentiated functions and how epigenetic regulatory mechanisms determine the expression and repression of genes. The possible clonal propagation of individuals has important economic implications in biotechnology and biomedicine as shown by the generation of numerous cloned transgenic animals with the ability to produce valuable proteins in their body fluids (blood, milk, etc.), being resistant to disease, or with altered composition of their productive traits.

A deeper understanding of how this remarkable fully differentiated cell, the oocyte/egg, mediates the reversal of cell differentiation will contribute to the elucidation of important mechanisms of gene regulation, lineage commitment and differentiation programming, and may also provide tools for the development of more efficient techniques for the reprogramming of somatic cell nuclei and the production of stem cells for human cell therapies.

Factors associated with epigenetic remodelling

The mammalian genome is composed of coding and non-coding regions: active genes or coding regions represent only a small proportion of the genome and mechanisms must exist that control their expression against a background of non-coding DNA that contains introns, repetitive elements and transposable elements. In recent years, two of the mechanisms that have been identified in these processes are DNA methylation and histone modification.

DNA can be methylated on cytosine residues by the enzyme DNA cytosine methyltransferase, of which three known isoforms have so far been isolated and characterised. Methylation of cytosine residues occurs at so-called CpG islands, which are currently defined as regions of > 200 nucleotides with a high GC content ($> 60\%$). Methylation at CpG islands has been implicated in both the repression/

silencing of gene expression and also in transcriptional activation, dependent upon whether methylation inactivates a positive or negative regulatory element (for reviews see Reik et al.[2,14] and Ferguson-Smith and Surani[6]).

A second group of mechanisms involves the covalent modification of core histones. The N-termini of histones can undergo a range of modifications including, acetylation, phosphorylation, methylation, ubiquitination and ADP ribosylation (for a review see Lachner et al.[5]). Such modifications of the core histones have been implicated in transcriptional activation, repression, cell cycle progression and chromatin condensation, and overall are associated with facilitating chromosome organisation and epigenetic control which may be involved in lineage determination and maintenance.

DNA methylation during development

The maternal and paternal genomes in mammals exhibit differential gene expression during development. This phenomenon, known as genomic imprinting and which is implicated in cell lineage determination, fetal growth and human diseases, is associated with DNA methylation. In the mouse, during development of the germ cells, the primordial germ cells undergo genome-wide demethylation prior to entering a mitotic (male) or meiotic (female) arrest. Prior to exiting this arrest phase the genomes become remethylated in a sex-dependent manner. In males remethylation occurs at the prospermatogonia stage while in females it occurs during oocyte growth following birth. Following fertilisation both the maternal and paternal chromatin undergo a second reprogramming of methylation status. In the mouse, rapid demethylation of the sperm DNA occurs by an active mechanism immediately after fertilisation. On formation of the pronuclei, both paternal and maternal DNA are then demethylated by a passive mechanism that continues through development erasing methylation on all but the imprinted genes by the blastocyst stage. Embryonic remethylation in a lineage-specific manner then occurs following implantation.

This remodelling of DNA methylation patterns varies between species. In cattle, for instance, demethylation of both maternal and paternal genomes occurs between the 2- and 4-cell stages, followed by de novo methylation at the 8-cell stage onwards with a characteristic hypermethylation of the inner cell mass (ICM) at the blastocyst stage. However, such observations based on fluorescence intensity may be misleading, as exemplified by studies in the sheep. Beaujean and colleagues[15] demonstrated that in sheep demethylation occurred slowly up to the 8-cell stage and then remained almost constant. However, the apparent intensity of methylation increased owing to reducing nuclear size.

The role of demethylation in development is unknown. However, as stated above, the maintenance of imprinted marks seems to occur, suggesting that demethylation is not genome-wide and not random. The differences observed between species may reflect differences in chromatin organisation rather than demethylating activities in oocyte cytoplasm, as mouse sperm were demethylated when injected into ovine oocyte (for a review see Young and Beaujean[16]).

Histone H4 acetylation during early embryo development

The acetylation of core histones has been implicated in transcriptional activation and repression: acetylated histones are transcriptionally active and unacetylated ones are transcriptionally repressed. Histone H4 can be acetylated on lysine residues at positions 5, 8, 12 and 16. In the mouse, both the maternal and paternal chromatin are unacetylated at the time of fertilisation. In the zygote the paternal chromatin becomes rapidly hyperacetylated, and this is followed by a slower acetylation of the female chromatin. However, both pronuclei become acetylated, which may correlate with the onset of zygotic transcription that occurs at the 1- to 2-cell stage.[17] In cattle, we have examined acetylation of histone H4: as in the mouse, both gametes are unacetylated. Following fertilisation, both pronuclei become transiently hyperacetylated during the first cell cycle, acetylation then declines until the 8- to 16-cell stage, at which time a slow increase is observed. Again, this correlates with the onset of zygotic transcription (8–16 cells in bovine embryos). By the blastocyst stage, the pattern is more complicated, with differential acetylation observed between the ICM and trophectoderm (TE) cells. With the ICM being hypoacetylated on lysine residues 5 and 12, this observation was less frequent for lysine 16 and not observed for lysine 8.[18] The role of this differential acetylation of both cell types and lysines is unknown but may reflect differential patterns of gene expression between the two cell types.

Nuclear reprogramming in cloned embryos

Embryo reconstruction by SCNT has been used to demonstrate that mammalian somatic cells can de-differentiate into a totipotent nucleus when introduced into an oocyte. This process of de-differentiation of somatic cells after nuclear transplantation is defined as 'nuclear reprogramming',[19] although this terminology gives little information on the molecular events that characterise this process. Overall, the frequency of development to term of so-called cloned embryos is low, although difficulties arise in comparing the results from different laboratories, and in different species estimates of approximately 2–3% of fused couplets have been reported.[20] Losses during early pregnancy account for up to 40% in ruminants (cattle, sheep and goats). It has been reported that failure to form a normal placenta is the main cause of miscarriage at this stage.[21]

Lack of normal placentome development and vascularisation is also accountable for growth deficiencies as well as for the frequent observation of hydrops later in gestation.[22,23] Similar placental abnormalities have been observed in mouse and sheep, although not in goats and pigs. Postnatal development is characterised by a higher mortality rate in the first week after birth. This can be the result of dystocia, related to the increased body size of the fetuses, immature lungs, general weakness, predisposition to infections, and weight loss.[24]

Despite the high rate of losses, normal cloned animals have been reported in the literature,[25,26] although some authors have shown that gene expression of all cloned mice is altered.[27] Owing to the stochastic pattern in the occurrence of abnormalities, an incomplete or abnormal 'reprogramming' is suggested as the main reason for the altered gene expression and phenotypic aberrations. The consequences of such alterations are unpredictable and may be far-reaching.

The next part of this review will focus on nuclear modifications related to SCNT and the strategies that have been developed to improve the efficiency of nuclear reprogramming. When planning on strategies for nuclear reprogramming by NT, one may suggest that converting the somatic nuclear configuration into an embryonic state is highly desirable, so this may promote a succession of events similar to those occurring during early embryo development. We will discuss the results of many studies that have investigated various aspects of nuclear remodelling after SCNT.

Nuclear architecture

After fusion of a somatic cell with an enucleated oocyte, the changes observed in the donor cell will depend on the maturation-promoting factor (MPF) activity of the recipient egg. One aspect that has been investigated in cloned embryos reconstructed with embryonic or somatic cells is the nucleolar assembly and its relationship with resumption of transcription. Nucleolar disassembly, as defined by the dissolution of some of the nucleolar components, is observed in embryonic and somatic clones produced after fusion into aged pre-activated oocytes. The dissociation of nucleolar components was observed from the 1-cell to the early 8-cell stage. However, by the late 8- to 16-cell embryos, normal nucleolar structures were observed in embryonic clones. In contrast, somatic clones fail in many cases to form normal nucleoli. In this case, the failure accounts for the low development to blastocyst reported with this protocol.[28] Another study found that somatic clones reconstructed with granulosa cells into metaphase II (MII) oocytes showed a clear dissolution of nucleolar structures from the first cell cycle, together with absence of transcriptional activity. Cloned embryos reassembled nucleoli a cell cycle earlier than *in vitro* produced embryos. However, more than 50% did not stain for upstream binding factor, which is required for the binding of RNA polymerase I to DNA, suggesting that these embryos may have limited developmental potential.[29]

A further analysis of nuclear structure remodelling has been made by the analysis of the structure of the nuclear envelope. Nuclear lamins are part of the intermediate filament superfamily of proteins that in mammals are classified as A/C-type (present in differentiated cells) and B-type (present in all cells) and they are localised in the inner nuclear membrane of the nucleus conforming the nuclear lamina.[30] During mouse embryogenesis, lamin A/C is not present in the nuclei of early cleavage stage embryos[31] and ICM cells, although it is expressed in TE cells of blastocysts.[32] In contrast, in the bovine we have found no lamin A/C expression in TE cells, indicating that the appearance of the somatic-type lamins is delayed compared with the mouse.[33] Lamin B is detected in undifferentiated teratocarcinoma cells, whereas lamin A/C reappears in teratocarcinoma cells undergoing differentiation and during cell lineage determination in the embryo.[34] Therefore, it is suggested that pluripotent cells undergo a major reorganisation of the nucleus during differentiation that has a direct role in gene regulation.[34] The removal of somatic lamin A/C from the donor nucleus has been implicated as a barrier to 'reprogramming' and development in murine NT embryos.[31] Further evidence on the replacement of somatic variants of proteins following NT has recently been provided by studies in mouse. Rapid exchange of histone H1 with H1oo occurs after a somatic cell is fused with an MII oocyte. H1oo has greater mobility than somatic H1, suggesting instability of the nucleosomes in early embryonic nuclei, a situation that could be important in nuclear reprogramming.[35,36] These results suggest that replacement of somatic cell components after transfer into an egg environment is necessary for complete nuclear reprogramming and that modification of the nuclear lamina structure in somatic cells may provide a way of altering gene expression and reverse differentiation of somatic cells.

Chromatin condensation

Components of the oocyte cytoplasm are capable of inducing changes in nuclear architecture as well as modifications of the DNA and DNA-associated molecules, rendering the somatic chromatin amenable for reprogramming its gene expression. The specific factors involved in the remodelling process remain unknown. However, early studies aiming to find out what makes a suitable oocyte for mammalian NT have led to the discovery that cell cycle coordination between the donor and recipient cells is an essential step to ensure normal ploidy of cloned embryos (for a review see Campbell *et al.*[37]). These findings opened the way for the development of reconstruction protocols that preserve DNA integrity.[38,39]

It has been suggested that MPF activity is beneficial for nuclear reprogramming because it induces nuclear envelope breakdown of the donor cell and facilitates the access of oocyte components to the donor chromatin. Indeed, most successful attempts of SCNT in species cloned so far use cytoplast with high MPF activity, suggesting that the MII arrested oocyte promotes better somatic cell nuclear reprogramming. Studies carried out in mice[40] and bovine[41–44] have directly compared the efficiency of development of SCNT embryos produced in both high and low MPF activity cytoplasts. Development is obtained only when high MPF activity cytoplasts are used, indicating that reprogramming activity is present in young matured oocytes. In contrast to these studies, other reports in sheep,[45] goats[46] and bovine[47–50] show that embryos can also develop and give offspring when pre-activated recipients (with low MPF activity) are used for SCNT. The discrepancy between studies is difficult to interpret and, considering the variations in the manipulation protocols used and the assessment of the oocyte status as well as the remodelling of the transferred nuclei in the different studies, makes it difficult to draw a final conclusion.

Determination of a high or low MPF activity in the recipient oocyte is used as the main indicator of a pre-activated or non-activated state. However, it is also well known that mitogen-activated protein kinase (MAPK) undergoes dephosphorylation after oocyte activation and its inactivation is correlated with pronuclear formation although this occurs at a much slower rate than the MPF inactivation.[51–54] It has also been shown that MPF and MAPK activities have no influence in chromatin condensation, since condensed chromosomes are observed prior to germinal vesicle breakdown (GVBD) in butyrolactone I arrested oocytes, which have no active MPF or MAPK.[55] Moreover, when somatic cells are transferred into low MPF cytoplasts with active MAPK activity, development to blastocysts is reduced, indicating that MAPK activity is not involved in nuclear reprogramming.[42] This evidence strongly suggests that MPF and MAPK are not reprogramming molecules themselves. However, the remodelling of the somatic nucleus is more efficient when it is transferred into an oocyte with both kinase activities. The modifications induced may contribute to expose the chromatin to factors involved in the removal of epigenetic marks from the somatic cell, modification of the histones and the DNA and reshaping nuclear structure to an embryonic configuration.

Remodelling epigenetic marks of somatic chromatin

Early embryo development and cell differentiation is characterised by a series of chromatin modifications that modulate gene expression patterns in both a spatial and temporal manner. These chromatin modifications, also called epigenetic modifications of the genome, are heritable and regulate the access of factors to the DNA, thereby modulating transcriptionally active or silent chromatin states. The epigenetic marks include differential DNA methylation and post-translational modifications on histone amino termini.[2,7] It has been suggested that the epigenetic marking system is a fundamental regulatory mechanism with consequences for cell fate determination and development.[7] SCNT provides evidence of how epigenetic reprogramming is exerted by egg components. In contrast to what is observed after fertilisation, abnormal DNA methylation has been reported in SCNT-produced embryos.[56,57] The abnormal demethylation/remethylation patterns observed may explain the high rate of loss of such embryos after implantation. However, it is still unknown whether the failure to erase those epigenetic marks is due to oocyte quality or whether the methods for embryo reconstruction do not permit such events to occur properly. For instance, normal demethylation at specific sequences occurs in porcine embryos reconstructed by serial NT.[58] In contrast, bovine embryos produced by transfer of a somatic cell into an MII oocyte show abnormal DNA methylation.[56,59] These experiments clearly demonstrate that, although the egg is able to reprogramme somatic chromatin, the process is very inefficient, possibly owing to selection of 'incompetent' recipient eggs, inappropriate reconstruction methods, or alternatively owing to the use of donor cells that have been highly epigenetically modified. In fact, differences in methylation patterns have been observed in cattle embryos reconstructed using different donor cell types, suggesting that some somatic cell types may be more able to be reprogrammed.[60]

In addition to DNA modifications, histone H3 and H4 are subject to differential methylation and acetylation in zygotes and 2- to 4-cell stage embryos.[61,62] Localisation of acetylated histones at specific lysine residues is indicative of a permissive state for transcription, and this is dependent on DNA replication during the first cell cycle.[62] These observations lead to the hypothesis that access of transcription factors is facilitated in the periphery of the nucleus and therefore establishment of appropriate gene expression in early embryos is spatially determined.[62] Our experiments in bovine embryos show similar differential acetylation of H4 at lysine residues as reported in the mouse during early embryo development.[18] However, when specific lysine residues are analysed, striking differences have been observed. In contrast to the mouse, bovine embryos show a steady increase of acetylated histone H4 lysine 5 from the 2-cell to the 16-cell stage, whereas histone H4 lysine 8 is acetylated at the 1- and 2-cell stage, followed by a significant reduction by the 8- and 16-cell stage.[18] These observations point to a clear epigenetic difference in the organisation of the chromatin during early embryogenesis in bovine embryos. In mouse NT embryos, deacetylation of histones occurs in the donor chromatin after transfer into an MII enucleated oocyte.[17] The epigenetic characterisation of chromatin structure in early embryos may help to explain whether in bovine (and other non-murine species such as farm animals and human embryos), where the zygotic gene activation (ZGA) occurs later (4–16 cell) than in the mouse, gene repression is mediated by constitutive association of protein complexes (such as histone acetylases, etc.) with the chromatin. These species differences are particularly important when one envisages the derivation of human embryonic stem (ES) cells on the basis of mouse embryology.

It is possible that many of the oocytes currently used for SCNT are not fully competent to reprogramme a somatic nucleus; this may be related to qualitative or quantitative effects of oocyte proteins or to the period of time for which the somatic chromatin is exposed. This would suggest that priming the chromatin of somatic cells by egg components prior to embryo development may facilitate a better nuclear reprogramming. This approach has been taken by performing SCNT twice, resulting in both pigs[63] and mice[64] with apparently fewer developmental abnormalities, suggesting an improvement in reprogramming. Another attempt to erase epigenetic marks from somatic cells has been taken by using pharmacological agents on cells prior to NT. Treatment of adult fibroblasts with low doses of trichostatin A, a histone deacetylase inhibitor, increases embryo development in bovine somatic NT. However, addition of 5-aza-2'-deoxycytidine, a DNA demethylation agent, proved to be detrimental in bovine clones.[65] When sodium butyrate, a nonspecific histone deacetylase inhibitor, was used in fetal fibroblasts prior to NT, a two-fold increase in blastocyst development was obtained.[66]

Enucleation of the MII oocyte may itself be detrimental to development. Experiments in the mouse showed that the majority of MPF activity remained associated with the enucleated karyoplast.[67] In contrast, experiments in pigs[68] and sheep[69] have shown that MPF levels are not reduced by enucleation. However, other proteins which may be involved in the control of early development, chromatin or nuclear structure may be removed by the enucleation process. To examine this possibility, we have used two-dimensional polyacrylamide gel electrophoresis (2D-PAGE) to examine the distribution of proteins in cytoplast and karyoplast. Preliminary experiments have shown an unequal distribution of proteins between these two compartments and experiments are now underway to identify the proteins.[70] The mechanisms by which 'reprogramming' of the somatic nucleus occurs and the proteins involved are unknown. However, as described above, use of MII oocytes containing active MPF appears to be beneficial. We have developed a system to increase MPF and MAPK kinase activities in MII oocytes. The use of such oocytes as cytoplast recipients increases the quality of embryos produced by NT, in terms of total cell number,[69] and further experiments are underway to monitor development of these embryos to term.

Cellular 'plasticity': can we 'reprogramme' the somatic nucleus?

How restricted are somatic cells in their differentiation potential?

In the adult, stem cell populations are found in a number of tissues, including blood, skin, the central nervous system, liver and gastrointestinal tract.[71] Traditionally, their differentiation potential was thought to be lineage restricted. However, more recent data have suggested that they can differentiate into cell types outside their developmental lineage.[71] The ability of somatic cells to trans-differentiate has been demonstrated in a number of systems. Transplantation experiments in *Drosophila* demonstrated that imaginal disc cells can switch fates, i.e. leg cells to antenna or antenna to wing, a process termed transdetermination.[72] In amphibians and birds, corneal cells can form a new retina after surgical ablation.[73] In mammals, injection of endothelial cells into damaged heart tissue results in generation of beating cardiomyocytes,[74] and similarly pancreatic epithelial precursors have been reported to differentiate into hepatocytes.[75] *In vitro*, co-culture of embryonic or neonatal umbilical vein endothelial cells with neonatal cardiomyocytes causes trans-differentiation into beating cardiomyocytes.[74] Ectopic expression of adipogenic transcription factors can cause trans-differentiation of myoblasts into mature adipocytes,[76] and expression of a hepatic transcription factor in pancreatic cells can cause conversion into hepatocytes.[77]

Can somatic cells be de-differentiated into ES cells or pluripotent intermediates?

SCNT experiments in mammals demonstrated that the genome of a differentiated cell could be modified by exposure to oocyte cytoplasm and the resultant embryo could give rise to viable offspring.[45] The production of an embryo and then offspring by NT involves the de-differentiation and re-differentiation of the somatic genome; in mice this has allowed the isolation and culture of ES cells from embryos created using somatic cells as nuclear donors. The possibility of converting a somatic genome to that of an ES cell has also been suggested by cell hybridisation experiments. Fusion of lymphocytes with ES cells has resulted in the reactivation of an ES-specific silent transgene (*Oct4*) present in the lymphocyte,[78] suggesting that the somatic nucleus is at least partially reprogrammed to the undifferentiated state. In a similar manner, trans-differentiation of somatic cells has also been demonstrated: treatment of permeabilised murine 3T3 fibroblasts with cytoplasmic extracts prepared from T lymphocytes was reported to reprogramme gene expression of the fibroblast to express T lymphocyte-specific genes. Furthermore, the 3T3 cells adopted a lymphocyte-like morphology and the effects lasted for several weeks after treatment.[79] Although as yet undefined, the mechanisms involved in these processes have been termed 'nuclear reprogramming'.

Together, these observations have altered our views on the plasticity of the differentiated state, suggesting that de-differentiation or trans-differentiation may be induced in somatic cells. The nuclear reprogramming events in cell nuclear replacement (CNR) and cell hybridisation which result in de-differentiation are linked to cytoplasmic factors in the oocyte or ES cell. Therefore, reprogramming should be possible with cytoplasmic extracts prepared from these cell types.

Can cytoplasmic extracts from undifferentiated cells de-differentiate the somatic phenotype?

The evidence presented above suggests that cytoplasmic factors from certain cells can reprogramme gene expression in somatic nuclei. Characterisation of the mechanisms involved in these 'reprogramming' events would provide defined methods for controlling cell phenotype. In mammals, oocytes, primordial germ cells (PGCs), ES, embryonic germ (EG) and embryonic carcinoma (EC) cells are all potential candidates for the production of reprogramming extracts. However, a limitation to their use is the extractable cell volume of these cell types and the volumes required for reliable treatment of somatic cells. An alternative is to identify extracts from other cell types or other species that could recapitulate the reprogramming events. One possibility is the use of amphibian oocytes and eggs, which provide a large cytoplasmic volume. Amphibian models have provided a wealth of information on early development and nuclear reprogramming;[19] similarly, cytoplasmic extracts (see below) have been extensively studied as a means of nuclear reprogramming. The major species used for these studies has been *Xenopus laevis,* primarily owing to the ease of animal husbandry. Using *Xenopus* eggs we have developed and partially characterised a cell-free cytoplasmic extract for the reprogramming of somatic cells.

Reprogramming of somatic nuclei by Xenopus laevis oocyte/egg cytoplasmic extracts

Experiments have demonstrated that the cytoplasm of oocytes and activated eggs as well as cytoplasmic extracts can induce multiple changes in somatic nuclei. Although differences occur between oocytes and activated eggs, these observations include nuclear swelling, incorporation of oocyte proteins, loss of nuclear proteins, induction of oocyte-specific transcripts, dissolution of nucleoli, DNA synthesis[19,80] and expression of pluripotency genes.[81] In fact, expression of the pluripotency gene *Oct4* has been reported in permeabilised cells exposed to *Xenopus* egg and embryo extracts.[82] These examples show to what extent nuclear remodelling can be induced using egg components. Part of the remodelling events may consist of the replacement of somatic variants of proteins with oocyte-specific counterparts, which may lead to structural changes in nuclear configuration. Several oocyte-specific proteins have an essential role during early embryo development (e.g. histone H1o, DNMT1o, etc.). Therefore, with the evidence that oocyte-specific molecules may be determinant for the totipotent state, we wish to develop a system for the identification of egg-specific remodelling components.

A heterologous system has been established in our laboratory using bovine fetal fibroblasts and *Xenopus laevis* egg extracts. This system allows incubation of whole permeabilised cells in egg extracts. We investigated whether somatic cell nuclei, which contain lamin A/C, when exposed to an amphibian egg environment, undergo nuclear envelope remodelling, and whether failure to do so restricts normal cellular and developmental events in an egg cytoplasmic extract. We found that somatic lamin A/C is removed from the somatic nuclei by an active process that requires both permeable nuclear pores and ATP. In egg extracts, incorporation of embryonic type lamin B3, specific to *Xenopus laevis* eggs, occurred; however, this was not observed in oocyte extracts, which contain no free lamin B3. Moreover, transcription mediated by RNA polymerases I and II was abolished in egg extracts but continued in oocyte extracts. We also observed a redistribution of nucleolar proteins in cells exposed to *Xenopus* egg extracts for 2 h, which may in part explain why transcription of ribosomal genes decreases.

Conclusions

The ability of the egg to 'reprogramme' the genome of a somatic cell, as occurs in animal cloning, is helping to define the role of epigenetic control during embryonic development and cellular differentiation. Although cloning technology has now been applied across a range of species, increases in the frequency of successful development have been small. The use of some of the alternative or additional steps to the cloning procedure described here coupled with a greater knowledge of epigenetic control of early development may help to unlock the secrets of development and differentiation and allow control over cell specialisation.

References

1. Li E. Chromatin modification and epigenetic reprogramming in mammalian development. *Nat Rev Genet* 2002;3:662–73.
2. Reik W, Dean W, Walter J. Epigenetic reprogramming in mammalian development. *Science* 2001;293:1089–93.

3. Jones PA, Takai D. The role of DNA methylation in mammalian epigenetics. *Science* 2001;293:1068–70.
4. Aalfs JD, Kingston RE. What does 'chromatin remodeling' mean? *Trends Biochem Sci* 2000;25:548–55.
5. Lachner M, O'Sullivan RJ, Jenuwein T. An epigenetic road map for histone lysine methylation. *J Cell Sci* 2003;116:2117–24.
6. Ferguson-Smith AC, Surani MA. Imprinting and the epigenetic asymmetry between parental genomes. *Science* 2001;293:1086–9.
7. Jenuwein T, Allis CD. Translating the histone code. *Science* 2001;293:1074–80.
8. Briggs R, King TJ. Transplantation of living nuclei from blastula cells into enucleated frog's eggs. *Proc Natl Acad Sci U S A* 1952;38:455–61.
9. Illmensee K, Hoppe PC. Nuclear transplantation in *Mus musculus*: developmental potential of nuclei from preimplantation embryos. *Cell* 1981;23:9–18.
10. Willadsen SM. Nuclear transplantation in sheep embryos. *Nature* 1986;320:63–5.
11. Gurdon JB, Laskey RA, Reeves OR. The developmental capacity of nuclei transplanted from keratinized skin cells of adult frogs. *J Embryol Exp Morphol* 1975;34:93–112.
12. Campbell KHS, Wilmut I. Recent advances on *in vitro* culture and cloning of ungulate embryos. *Vth World Congress on Genetics as Applied to Livestock* 1994;20:180–7.
13. Wilmut I, Schnieke AE, McWhir J, Kind AJ, Campbell KH. Viable offspring derived from fetal and adult mammalian cells. *Nature* 1997;385:810–13.
14. Reik W, Santos F, Dean W. Mammalian epigenomics: reprogramming the genome for development and therapy. *Theriogenology* 2003;59:21–32.
15. Beaujean N, Taylor JE, McGarry M, Gardner JO, Wilmut I, Loi P, *et al*. The effect of interspecific oocytes on demethylation of sperm DNA. *Proc Natl Acad Sci U S A* 2004;101:7636–40.
16. Young LE, Beaujean N. DNA methylation in the preimplantation embryo: the differing stories of the mouse and sheep. *Anim Reprod Sci* 2004;82–3:61–78.
17. Kim JM, Liu H, Tazaki M, Nagata M, Aoki F. Changes in histone acetylation during mouse oocyte meiosis. *J Cell Biol* 2003;162:37–46.
18. Maalouf WE, Alberio R, Campbell KH. Acetylation of histone H4 lysine −5 and lysine −8 during development of *in vitro* produced bovine embryos. *Reprod Fertil Dev* 2004;16:125.
19. Gurdon JB, Laskey RA, De Robertis EM, Partington GA. Reprogramming of transplanted nuclei in amphibia. *Int Rev Cytol Suppl* 1979;(9):161–78.
20. Gurdon JB, Colman A. The future of cloning. *Nature* 1999;402:743–6.
21. Hill JR, Burghardt RC, Jones K, Long CR, Looney CR, Shin T, *et al*. Evidence for placental abnormality as the major cause of mortality in first-trimester somatic cell cloned bovine fetuses. *Biol Reprod* 2000;63:1787–94.
22. Heyman Y, Chavatte-Palmer P, LeBourhis D, Camous S, Vignon X, Renard JP. Frequency and occurrence of late-gestation losses from cattle cloned embryos. *Biol Reprod* 2002;66:6–13.
23. Hill JR, Roussel AJ, Cibelli JB, Edwards JF, Hooper NL, Miller MW, *et al*. Clinical and pathologic features of cloned transgenic calves and fetuses (13 case studies). *Theriogenology* 1999;51:1451–65.
24. Zakhartchenko V, Mueller S, Alberio R, Schernthaner WG, Stojkovic M, Wenigerkind H, *et al*. Nuclear transfer in cattle with non-transfected and transfected fetal or cloned transgenic fetal and postnatal fibroblasts. *Mol Reprod Dev* 2001;60:362–9.
25. Cibelli JB, Campbell KH, Seidel GE, West MD, Lanza RP. The health profile of cloned animals. *Nat Biotechnol* 2002;20:13–14.
26. Chavatte-Palmer P, Heyman Y, Richard C, Monget P, LeBourhis D, Kann G, *et al*. Clinical, hormonal, and hematologic characteristics of bovine calves derived from nuclei from somatic cells. *Biol Reprod* 2002;66:1596–603.
27. Humpherys D, Eggan K, Akutsu H, Friedman A, Hochedlinger K, Lander ES, *et al*. Abnormal gene expression in cloned mice derived from embryonic stem cell and cumulus cell nuclei. *Dev Biol* 2002;99:12889–94.
28. Baran V, Vignon X, LeBourhis D, Renard JP, Flechon JE. Nucleolar changes in bovine nucleotransferred embryos. *Biol Reprod* 2002;66:534–43.
29. Laurincik J, Zakhartchenko V, Stojkovic M, Brem G, Wolf E, Muller M, *et al*. Nucleolar protein allocation and ultrastructure in bovine embryos produced by nuclear transfer from granulosa cells. *Mol Reprod Dev* 2002;61:477–87.
30. Fawcett DW. On the occurrence of a fibrous lamina on the inner aspect of the nuclear envelope in certain cells of vertebrates. *Am J Anat* 1966;119:129–45.
31. Moreira PN, Robl JM, Collas P. Architectural defects in pronuclei of mouse nuclear transplant embryos. *J Cell Sci* 2003;116:3713–20.

32. Schatten G, Maul G, Schatten H, Chaly N, Simerley C, Balczon R, *et al.* Nuclear lamins and peripheral nuclear antigens during fertilization and embryogenesis in mice and sea urchins. *Proc Natl Acad Sci U S A* 1985;82:4727–31.

33. Kelly R, Alberio A, Campbell KH. A comparative study of lamin A/C expression in bovine embryos using two different antibodies. *Reprod Fertil Dev* 2004;17:205.

34. Stewart C, Burke B. Teratocarcinoma stem cells and early mouse embryos contain only a single major lamin polypeptide closely resembling lamin B. *Cell* 1987;51:383–92.

35. Gao S, Chung YG, Parseghian MH, King GJ, Adashi EY, Latham KE. Rapid H1 linker histone transitions following fertilization or somatic cell nuclear transfer: evidence for a uniform developmental program in mice. *Dev Biol* 2004;266:62–75.

36. Teranishi T, Tanaka M, Kimoto S, Ono Y, Miyakoshi K, Kono T, *et al.* Rapid replacement of somatic linker histones with the oocyte-specific linker histone H1foo in nuclear transfer. *Dev Biol* 2004;266:76–86.

37. Campbell KH, Loi P, Otaegui PJ, Wilmut I. Cloning mammals by nuclear transfer. Co-ordinating nuclear and cytoplasmic events. *Rev Reprod* 1996;1:40–6.

38. Collas P, Balise JJ, Robl JM. Influence of cell cycle stage of the donor nucleus on development of nuclear transplant rabbit embryos. *Biol Reprod* 1992;46:492–500.

39. Campbell KH, Loi P, Cappai P, Wilmut I. Improved development to blastocyst of ovine nuclear transfer embryos reconstructed during the presumptive S-phase of enucleated activated oocytes. *Biol Reprod* 1994;50:1385–393.

40. Kim JM, Ogura A, Nagata M, Aoki F. Analysis of the mechanism for chromatin remodeling in embryos reconstructed by somatic nuclear transfer. *Biol Reprod* 2002;67:760–6.

41. Tani T, Kato Y, Tsunoda Y. Direct exposure of chromosomes to nonactivated ovum cytoplasm is effective for bovine somatic cell nucleus reprogramming. *Biol Reprod* 2001;64:324–30.

42. Tani T, Kato Y, Tsunoda Y. Reprogramming of bovine somatic cell nuclei is not directly regulated by maturation promoting factor or mitogen-activated protein kinase activity. *Biol Reprod* 2003;69:1890–4.

43. Du F, Sung LY, Tian XC, Yang X. Differential cytoplast requirement for embryonic and somatic cell nuclear transfer in cattle. *Mol Reprod Dev* 2002;63:183–91.

44. Shin MR, Park SW, Shim H, Kim NH. Nuclear and microtubule reorganization in nuclear-transferred bovine embryos. *Mol Reprod Dev* 2002;62:74–82.

45. Campbell KH, Ritchie WA, McWhir J, Wilmut I. Sheep cloned by nuclear transfer from a cultured cell line. *Nature* 1996;380:64–6.

46. Baguisi A, Behboodi E, Melican DT, Pollock JS, Destrempes MM, Cammuso C, *et al.* Production of goats by somatic cell nuclear transfer. *Nat Biotechnol* 1999;17:456–61.

47. Liu JL, Wang MK, Sun QY, Xu Z, Chen DY. Effect of telophase enucleation on bovine somatic nuclear transfer. *Theriogenology* 2000;54:989–98.

48. Bordignon V, Keyston R, Lazaris A, Bilodeau AS, Pontes JH, Arnold D, *et al.* Transgene expression of green fluorescent protein and germ line transmission in cloned calves derived from in vitro-transfected somatic cells. *Biol Reprod* 2003;68:2013–23.

49. Kurosaka S, Nagao Y, Minami N, Yamada M, Imai H. Dependence of DNA synthesis and *in vitro* development of bovine nuclear transfer embryos on the stage of the cell cycle of donor cells and recipient cytoplasts. *Biol Reprod* 2002;67:643–7.

50. Vignon X, Chesne P, Le Bourhis D, Flechon JE, Heyman Y, Renard JP. Developmental potential of bovine embryos reconstructed from enucleated matured oocytes fused with cultured somatic cells. *C R Acad Sci III* 1998;321:735–45.

51. Liu L, Yang X. Interplay of maturation-promoting factor and mitogen-activated protein kinase inactivation during metaphase-to-interphase transition of activated bovine oocytes. *Biol Reprod* 1999;61:1–7.

52. Alberio R, Kubelka M, Zakhartchenko V, Hajduch M, Wolf E, Motlik J. Activation of bovine oocytes by specific inhibition of cyclin-dependent kinases. *Mol Reprod Dev* 2000;55:422–32.

53. Liu L, Ju JC, Yang X. Parthenogenetic development and protein patterns of newly matured bovine oocytes after chemical activation. *Mol Reprod Dev* 1998;49:298–307.

54. Liu L, Ju JC, Yang X. Differential inactivation of maturation-promoting factor and mitogen-activated protein kinase following parthenogenetic activation of bovine oocytes. *Biol Reprod* 1998;59:537–45.

55. Kubelka M, Motlik J, Schultz RM, Pavlok A. Butyrolactone I reversibly inhibits meiotic maturation of bovine oocytes, without influencing chromosome condensation activity. *Biol Reprod* 2000;62:292–302.

56. Dean W, Santos F, Stojkovic M, Zakhartchenko V, Walter J, Wolf E, *et al.* Conservation of

methylation reprogramming in mammalian development: aberrant reprogramming in cloned embryos. *Proc Natl Acad Sci U S A* 2001;98:13734–8.

57. Kang YK, Park JS, Koo DB, Choi YH, Kim SU, Lee KK, *et al.* Limited demethylation leaves mosaic-type methylation states in cloned bovine pre-implantation embryos. *EMBO J* 2002;21:1092–100.

58. Kang YK, Koo DB, Park JS, Choi YH, Kim HN, Chang WK, *et al.* Typical demethylation events in cloned pig embryos. Clues on species-specific differences in epigenetic reprogramming of a cloned donor genome. *J Biol Chem* 2001;276:39980–4.

59. Bourc'his D, Le Bourhis D, Patin D, Niveleau A, Comizzoli P, Renard JP, *et al.* Delayed and incomplete reprogramming of chromosome methylation patterns in bovine cloned embryos. *Curr Biol* 2001;11:1542–6.

60. Santos F, Zakhartchenko V, Stojkovic M, Peters A, Jenuwein T, Wolf E, *et al.* Epigenetic marking correlates with developmental potential in cloned bovine preimplantation embryos. *Curr Biol* 2003;13:1116–21.

61. Worrad DM, Turner BM, Schultz RM. Temporally restricted spatial localization of acetylated isoforms of histone H4 and RNA polymerase II in the 2-cell mouse embryo. *Dev* 1995;121:2949–59.

62. Stein P, Worrad DM, Belyaev ND, Turner BM, Schultz RM. Stage-dependent redistributions of acetylated histones in nuclei of the early preimplantation mouse embryo. *Mol Reprod Dev* 1997;47:421–9.

63. Polejaeva IA, Chen SH, Vaught TD, Page RL, Mullins J, Ball S, *et al.* Cloned pigs produced by nuclear transfer from adult somatic cells. *Nature* 2000;407:86–90.

64. Ono Y, Shimozawa N, Ito M, Kono T. Cloned mice from fetal fibroblast cells arrested at metaphase by a serial nuclear transfer. *Biol Reprod* 2001;64:44–50.

65. Enright BP, Kubota C, Yang X, Tian XC. Epigenetic characteristics and development of embryos cloned from donor cells treated by trichostatin A or 5-aza-2′-deoxycytidine. *Biol Reprod* 2003;69:896–901.

66. Shi W, Hoeflich A, Flaswinkel H, Stojkovic M, Wolf E, Zakhartchenko V. Induction of a senescent-like phenotype does not confer the ability of bovine immortal cells to support the development of nuclear transfer embryos. *Biol Reprod* 2003;69:301–9.

67. Fulka J Jr, Motlik J, Fulka J, Crozet N. Activity of maturation promoting factor in mammalian oocytes after its dilution by single and multiple fusions. *Dev Biol* 1986;118:176–81.

68. Goto S, Naito K, Ohashi S, Sugiura K, Naruoka H, Iwamori N, *et al.* Effects of spindle removal on MPF and MAP kinase activities in porcine matured oocytes. *Mol Reprod Dev* 2002;63:388–93.

69. Lee JH, Campbell KH. MPF and MAPK kinases in ovine oocytes: effects of enucleation and caffeine on activity and developmental competence of nuclear transfer embryos. *Reprod Fertil Dev* 2004;16:125.

70. Campbell KHS, Alberio R, Lee JH, Malouf W, Liddell S. Effects of enucleation on the proteome of metaphase II oocytes. Unpublished data.

71. Blau HM, Brazelton TR, Weimann JM. The evolving concept of a stem cell: entity or function? *Cell* 2001;105:829–41.

72. Wei G, Schubiger G, Harder F, Muller AM. Stem cell plasticity in mammals and transdetermination in *Drosophila*: common themes? *Stem Cells* 2000;18:409–14.

73. Henry JJ, Elkins MB. Cornea–lens transdifferentiation in the anuran, *Xenopus tropicalis. Dev Genes Evol* 2001;211:377–87.

74. Condorelli G, Borello U, De Angelis L, Latronico M, Sirabella D, Coletta M, *et al.* Cardiomyocytes induce endothelial cells to trans-differentiate into cardiac muscle: implications for myocardium regeneration. *Proc Natl Acad Sci U S A* 2001;98:10733–8.

75. Dabeva MD, Hwang SG, Vasa SR, Hurston E, Novikoff PM, Hixson DC, *et al.* Differentiation of pancreatic epithelial progenitor cells into hepatocytes following transplantation into rat liver. *Proc Natl Acad Sci U S A* 1997;94:7356–61.

76. Hu E, Tontonoz P, Spiegelman BM. Transdifferentiation of myoblasts by the adipogenic transcription factors PPAR gamma and C/EBP alpha. *Proc Natl Acad Sci U S A* 1995;92:9856–60.

77. Shen CN, Horb ME, Slack JM, Tosh D. Transdifferentiation of pancreas to liver. *Mech Dev* 2003;120:107–16.

78. Tada M, Takahama Y, Abe K, Nakatsuji N, Tada T. Nuclear reprogramming of somatic cells by *in vitro* hybridization with ES cells. *Curr Biol* 2001;11:1553–8.

79. Hakelien AM, Landsverk HB, Robl JM, Skalhegg BS, Collas P. Reprogramming fibroblasts to express T-cell functions using cell extracts. *Nat Biotechnol* 2002;20:460–6.

80. Kill IR, Bridger JM, Campbell KH, Maldonado-Codina G, Hutchison CJ. The timing of the formation and usage of replicase clusters in S-phase nuclei of human diploid fibroblasts. *J Cell Sci* 1991;100(Pt 4):869–76.

81. Byrne JA, Simonsson S, Western PS, Gurdon JB. Nuclei of adult mammalian somatic cells are directly reprogrammed to oct-4 stem cell gene expression by amphibian oocytes. *Curr Biol* 2003;13:1206–13.
82. Hansis C, Barreto G, Maltry N, Niehrs C. Nuclear reprogramming of human somatic cells by xenopus egg extract requires BRG1. *Curr Biol* 2004;14:1475–80.

Chapter 13

Risks associated with assisted reproduction: insights from animal studies

Kevin D Sinclair and Ravinder Singh

Introduction

The rapid evolution of assisted reproductive technologies (ART) over the past 30 years has completely revolutionised infertility treatment in humans, becoming a common and accepted form of clinical care benefiting an estimated one in ten people of reproductive age in developed countries who are subfertile or infertile. The success of these technologies can be credited as much to the remarkable plasticity and tolerance of mammalian gametes and the pre-implantation embryo to physical manipulations and alterations to their chemical environment as to any specific refinement that may have been introduced over the years as our understanding of early mammalian biology has evolved. This is perhaps best exemplified by the extraordinary early success enjoyed with the culture of human zygotes in simple balanced salt solutions or complex media formulated with somatic cell culture in mind. However, the empiricism with which refinements to these culture media subsequently arose together with the rather indiscriminate way in which procedures such as intracytoplasmic sperm injection (ICSI) were introduced and then adopted has led many commentators to question the safety of ART.[1-3]

These concerns were heightened a number of years ago when it emerged that the extended culture of animal zygotes (particularly ruminant zygotes) could lead to a high incidence of developmental abnormalities and congenital defects in offspring which are often associated with *in utero* overgrowth.[4] Many of the phenotypes associated with this 'large offspring syndrome' (LOS) have features reminiscent of some naturally occurring human overgrowth syndromes, such as the Beckwith–Wiedemann syndrome (BWS), that are associated with errors in an imprinted cluster of genes on human chromosome 11.[5] It was thus perhaps not surprising that, shortly thereafter, the same authors would report an associated loss of imprinting and expression of the gene encoding the type 2 insulin-like growth factor receptor (*IGF2R*) with LOS.[6] Reports of similar epigenetic alterations in genomic imprinting following ART in humans have since been published and these have fuelled the recent debate on the safety of procedures currently employed in human assisted reproduction.[7,8] Risk factors associated with some of these procedures are considered in this review and their relevance critically assessed, drawing from information gleaned from basic studies with rodents and large animal species.

Pregnancy outcomes following ART

The major obstetric challenges facing those involved with ART continue to be preterm deliveries, low-birthweight babies and additional complications associated with multiple births.[9–12] High-order multiple pregnancies, arising from the transfer of two or more embryos, is without doubt the single most important factor leading to poor perinatal outcomes following ART.[11,13] Residual complications, once the adverse effects of multiple gestations have been accounted for, are not solely attributable to ART. They are often confounded by female age and infertility which are, in their own right, recognised independent risk factors in the aetiology of perinatal morbidity following ART.[14] This raises a number of important issues with respect to the design and analysis of many of the large-scale retrospective observational studies published to date[10,12] which have been unable to completely discriminate between these independent risk factors and ART.[15] Furthermore, given the low natural incidence of imprinting-related disorders in humans (e.g. 1/13 700 to 1/14 300 for BWS; 1/200 000 to 1/400 000 for Angelman syndrome (AS)), it has been difficult to make a proper quantitative assessment of the risks of inducing and/or transmitting such defects by ART. This would require the assessment of significantly larger populations of ART children than has been possible to date.[16] Our inability to currently quantify these risks, however, should not lead us to trivialise their importance nor deny their existence. Where clinical observational studies fail to provide definitive answers regarding the safe use of ART, insight may be gained from the numerous animal studies conducted in recent years.

Risk factors

Age

The natural decline in fertility with increasing maternal age is well recognised and occurs largely as a consequence of defects in ovarian physiology and oocyte quality. Indeed, the pregnancy rate of women with age-related infertility who receive eggs from younger women is three to four times greater than that achieved when oocytes from older women are used during *in vitro* fertilisation (IVF) cycles.[17] The decline in oocyte quality is indicated by the increased incidence of oocyte aneuploidy. Chromosomal abnormalities account for approximately half of all miscarriages, with aneuploidies (mostly three copies of the same chromosome or a single copy of the X chromosome) accounting for roughly 60% of these.[18] Around 90% of all chromosomal abnormalities have a maternal origin, with most linked to a metaphase I (MI) error during female meiosis. The incidence of trisomies increases exponentially with age from around 2% of all clinically recognised pregnancies for women less than 25 years of age to around 35% in women over 40 years of age.[19] The 'double hit' theory[20] predicts that errors initiated during MI (in the fetal ovary) are subsequently confounded by errors that occur during metaphase II (MII) (in the adult ovary), thus leading to age-dependent nondisjunction. As the majority of women presented for fertility treatment tend to fall in the 35–40 year age category so the incidence of maternal age-related trisomies is greater in this group. Indeed, there are several reports in the literature of increased chromosome abnormalities and prevalent chromosome mosaics in spare or arrested pre-implantation stage human embryos following IVF.[21,22] However, as the earliest cleavage divisions of the mammalian embryo seem to be particularly vulnerable to chromosome missegregation,[23] so exposure to an artificial *in vitro* environment may lead to an additional increase in chromosomal abnormalities in pre-implantation embryos, as has been observed in both cattle[24] and mice.[25]

Infertility

Female infertility is itself a recognised risk factor associated with poor perinatal outcomes following ART. For example, one UK population-based case–control study demonstrated that, relative to fertile women, subfertile women who conceive spontaneously are at increased risk of having a perinatal death.[26] After adjustment for the effects of multiple pregnancies in that study, the risk of perinatal death following fertility treatment (i.e. IVF and gamete intrafallopian transfer (GIFT)) was found to be no greater than for untreated subfertile women. These observations were later confirmed by another British study which showed that, after adjustments for related factors, singletons conceived through ovulation induction and intrauterine insemination (OI/IUI) using partner's sperm were almost five times more likely to have low birthweights compared with the singletons conceived by OI/IUI using donor sperm or naturally conceived singletons.[27] This study was devised in such a way as to allow the authors to conclude that factors intrinsic to subfertile women predispose to preterm deliveries and smaller infants, and that reduced fetal birthweight is not necessarily a consequence of ovarian stimulation. These intrinsic factors, however, remain to be identified. Although higher incidences of pre-eclampsia, placental abruption and preterm labour, characteristic of such cases,[28] suggest suboptimal uterine conditions as the cause, genetic or epigenetic defects already present in the oocyte at the time of conception may also contribute to this problem. The transfer of embryos to surrogates could help address this issue. Although surrogacy is not widely practised, the limited data set of Schieve et al.[10] and the re-analysis by Serafini[29] of perinatal outcomes from a number of published studies suggest that the incidence of low-birthweight singletons is no greater following surrogate embryo transfer than following natural conception in fertile couples.

Superovulation

The risk of adverse perinatal outcomes following the use of high doses of gonadotrophins needed to stimulate follicular growth and to mature several eggs simultaneously is an area of some controversy.[30,31] Much of the debate has centred on the effects of the superovulatory drugs themselves, and the consequences that their use might have on the oviduct and uterus, with less attention given to their effects on oocyte growth and maturation within ovarian follicles. However, the observation that clomiphene citrate (a nonsteroidal synthetic oestrogen agonist-antagonist used for enhancing follicular development) could increase the incidence of miscarriages in humans[32] was later supported by some mouse data which showed an increase in the incidence of cytogenic abnormalities in mouse oocytes following clomiphene treatment.[33] More recent studies with mice have confirmed that superovulation with various combinations of pregnant mare's serum gonadotrophin and human chorionic gonadotrophin can indeed reduce implantation rates and impair the development of surviving pups, and that these effects arise as a consequence of impaired oocyte/embryo quality as well as an impaired uterine milieu.[34–36] Autotransplantation in superovulated large animal species is extremely rare, and it is more common for recovered zygotes/embryos to be transferred to surrogates. However, in sheep, progesterone supplementation and the temporary exposure of day 3 embryos to an advanced uterine environment have both been shown to increase fetal development and to alter fetal myogenesis.[5] Although these effects may be quite different to those reported above, they clearly indicate that the endocrine milieu around the time of conception is critical for the normal establishment and outcome of pregnancy.

In vitro maturation (IVM)

The retrieval of germinal vesicle-stage (GV) oocytes from small and medium-sized ovarian follicles offers several advantages over conventional IVF methods, including a reduction in pharmacological interventions and risks associated with ovarian hyperstimulation.[37] In spite of these advantages, the efficiency of IVM remains low and consequently the technique is not widely practised.[38] Statistics on pregnancy and perinatal outcomes are therefore limited and in many instances difficult to separate from the underlying causes of subfertility. For instance, the retrieval of GV oocytes and IVM is often carried out with women for whom polycystic ovary syndrome (PCOS) has been diagnosed. These women are at increased risk of developing hypertension and gestational diabetes mellitus and, in insulin-resistant patients, the frequency of pre-eclampsia is also greater.[39] Each of these factors can independently contribute to the complications that lead to the high incidence of neonatal care generally associated with PCOS pregnancies. Nevertheless, it is now becoming increasingly apparent that the developmental potential of embryos is largely determined by the time of fertilisation[40,41] so that factors that influence oocyte growth and/or maturation may be of paramount importance to the successful establishment of pregnancy with normal perinatal outcomes. A significant observation in this regard is the reduction in growth differentiation factor 9 (GDF9) mRNA levels in the primary oocytes of women with PCOS.[42] This member of the transforming growth factor beta (TGFβ) superfamily of growth and differentiation factors plays a key role in regulating follicle growth during the pre- and early antral stages of development. This observation confirms that oocytes from such women are already defective by the time of retrieval and fertilisation. It further suggests that these defects may have been 'programmed' at an earlier stage of development, including during intrauterine life. The precedent for this suggestion comes from the prenatally androgenised rhesus monkey, long heralded as a suitable non-human primate model of PCOS. Post-fertilisation development was found to be significantly impaired in oocytes from monkeys exposed prenatally to testosterone propionate.[43] However, at present it can not be claimed with certainty that defects present in these oocytes were programmed during prenatal life or arose as a consequence of the abnormal intrafollicular steroid milieu present during the early antral stages of follicle development.

Cytoplasmic transfer and mitochondrial DNA

Deletions and mutations to mitochondrial DNA (mtDNA) are associated with a number of degenerative diseases in humans, including the maternally inherited Leber's hereditary optic neuropathy and a number of neuromuscular diseases such as

Kearns–Sayre syndrome.[44] Given the metabolic function of the mitochondrion, its genome is particularly vulnerable to the damaging effects of reactive oxygen superoxides, a situation made worse by the fact that the mitochondrial genome is intronless, is devoid of protective histones and has limited DNA repair mechanisms. MtDNA mutations accumulate in post-mitotic tissues, such as skeletal muscle, at a rate that is significantly greater than that of nuclear DNA. However, these mutations also occur spontaneously during oogenesis, particularly in older women.[45] Normally, the atretic regulation of ageing oocytes containing such mutations would prevent their ovulation but the use of superovulation and follicular aspiration procedures within ART programmes promote their presence, so contributing to the poor and variable results that frequently accompany IVF. In some women, with a history of poor embryo development and implantation failure following frequent IVF attempts, cytoplasmic transfer has been conducted in an attempt to increase mitochondrial copy number and also to increase the presence of other potentially beneficial cytoplasmic factors.[46] While such interventions may improve pregnancy outcome in some women, a number of commentators[47] have cautioned its use. They have called for further work to better understand mitochondrial–mitochondrial and nucleo–mitochondrial interactions, both of which can affect cellular metabolism, mtDNA inheritance and embryo survival, and which may also lead to disease risks associated with mitochondrial heteroplasmy. However, following reports that the procedure can increase the risk of Turner syndrome, an X-chromosome defect that can cause miscarriage in early pregnancy, the US Food and Drug Administration (FDA) effectively banned its use within the USA in 2001.

Intracytoplasmic sperm injection (ICSI), IVF and *in vitro* culture (IVC)

As with many procedures in ART, the introduction and subsequent widespread adoption of assisted fertilisation techniques such as ICSI preceded, by several years, what many would consider to be the necessary steps of method development and refinement normally conducted in appropriate animal models. Although the risk of adverse perinatal outcomes following the use of this technique would seem low,[12,15] there are, nevertheless, several precedents for why such a procedure may be unsafe. Zona penetration and tail scoring may lead to cytoplasmic leakage and/or exposure of the cytoplasm to culture media, the constituent and ionic compositions of which are markedly different from that of the intracellular milieu of the spermatozoon.[48] Furthermore, in non-human primates ICSI has been shown to result in abnormal nuclear remodelling which is due in part to the persistence of vesicle-associated membrane protein, the acrosome and the perinuclear theca on the sperm head. These sperm components, which are normally removed during the natural process of fertilisation or IVF, may also contribute to the chromosomal anomalies observed following ICSI.[49,50] The risk that injected sperm may also serve as a vector of foreign (including viral) DNA in clinical ICSI is real, for sperm-mediated gene transfer has now been successfully used to create transgenic offspring in several species including mice, non-human primates and farm animals.[51] The very nature of the procedure, which means that the normal stringent selection pressures on the male gamete encountered during the natural course of conception are bypassed, may, in addition, contribute to the increased incidence of chromosomal anomalies observed in ICSI offspring.[52] Male-factor infertility is often associated with chromosome abnormalities and is known to account for around 10–15% of early recurrent abortions following either natural conception or IVF.[53] Experience to date indicates that early embryonic development and implantation rates are both inversely related to the severity of oligoasthenozoospermia and associated chromosomal anomalies in ICSI cycles.[54,55]

In contrast to pregnancies established by ICSI, there has been less concern expressed and, to a certain extent, less controversy regarding the perinatal outcome of IVF pregnancies. New and sequential media formulations, that more precisely match the evolving needs of the developing pre-implantation embryo, have now largely replaced the simple balanced salt solutions and complex media formulations which were often used in combination with serum and/or somatic support cells in human embryo culture.[56] These alterations have contributed to the significant improvement in post-fertilisation development and clinical pregnancies observed over the past decade following IVF and IVC.[57] The avoidance of serum and somatic support cells in culture is significant, for these culture components are known to contribute to the LOS in farm animals[5] and developmental defects in mice[58] leading to altered postnatal growth and physiology.[59] Extended culture (to the blastocyst stage) in the absence of such media components, however, is not without risk. Increased *in utero* growth associated with altered ovine fetal development[60,61] and calf birthweight[62] have been reported when zygotes were cultured in chemically defined and semi-defined (albumin supplemented) media in the absence of serum and somatic support cells. More subtle alterations to media composition, including alterations to the basic formulation and/or the presence or absence of components such as glucose, amino acids and ammonium, have also led to aberrant patterns of fetal growth and development in mice.[63-66]

To date, however, there is little evidence that extended culture to the blastocyst stage has had any detrimental effect on pregnancy establishment and perinatal outcomes in humans, although there is a tendency for the incidence of monozygotic twins and associated complications to be increased.[67-69] Other techniques associated with an increased incidence of monozygotic twins include ICSI[70] and assisted hatching.[71] On balance, however, the benefits of blastocyst culture would seem to outweigh any risks, both perceived and real. It presents the opportunity to transfer single embryos to a more synchronous uterine environment, thereby obviating complications associated with high-order pregnancies while maintaining acceptable clinical pregnancy rates.[72] A greater understanding of the aetiology of monozygotic twinning, however, is called for so that the benefits of single-embryo transfer, in terms of multiple gestations, are not negated.[73]

Cryopreservation

The cryopreservation of spermatozoa is a well-proven technology in both farm animal species and in artificial insemination (AI) programmes in humans. Pregnancy rates using frozen/thawed semen from fertile men are comparable to that following natural conception (around 28% in young women[74,75]) and, in long-term follow-up studies with children conceived by AI or IVF, there is no evidence of any adverse effects with its use.[76] Not surprisingly, therefore, the widespread perception among the scientific community is that semen freezing, storage and use for AI is highly reliable and safe. However, it is noteworthy that only a very small proportion (< 1%) of fresh mammalian ejaculated spermatozoa contain all of the attributes necessary for fertilisation, and cryopreservation reduces this proportion even further.[77] Cryopreservation can also increase the incidence of DNA fragmentation in spermatozoa and this is negatively correlated with both pre-implantation embryo development[78,79] and pregnancy establishment[80] after IVF or ICSI. In ICSI cycles there is no opportunity for 'natural' sperm selection – the spermatozoon to be injected must be identified by manual inspection. Although the selection of frozen/thawed spermatozoa on the basis of motility can, to a certain extent, overcome the problem of poor fertilisation and pregnancy rates,[81] recent computerised karyometric image analysis has highlighted our inability to select sperm with normal condensed nuclei purely on morphological criteria.[82]

Embryo cryopreservation is also commonly practised and is a convenient way to handle supernumerary embryos following ovarian stimulation and IVF. It has the added advantages of allowing storage of cryopreserved donated embryos while facilitating synchronisation between donors and recipients. Although embryo cryopreservation is known to adversely affect implantation rates there is no evidence to date of any adverse effects on perinatal outcomes or early infant development.[83,84] Similarly, although there are reports of cytotoxic effects of cryoprotectants leading to alterations in gene expression, concerns regarding their safe use remain hypothetical.[85] The situation with regard to oocyte cryopreservation is not dissimilar. Here, however, too few embryos derived from frozen/thawed oocytes have been transferred to provide any meaningful assessment of pregnancy outcome. Storage of human mature oocytes by conventional slow-rate programmable (equilibrium) freezing is known to result in low post-thaw survival and low post-fertilisation developmental rates,[86] the causes of which are thought to include meiotic spindle defects leading to numerical chromosome disorders,[87] and loss of mitochondrial polarity and calcium signalling.[88] The large size of the mammalian oocyte, together with species-specific differences in the permeability of the plasmalemma to cryoprotectants, are thought to lead to variable and inefficient cellular protection during slow-rate freezing.[89] Research efforts have consequently turned to vitrification as an alternative means of cryopreservation. Vitrification involves ultra-rapid rates of cooling in the presence of high concentrations of cryoprotectants. It has been shown to result in increased post-thaw survival and cleavage rates following ICSI in human oocytes.[90,91] However, the very high concentrations of cytotoxic chemicals employed are potentially teratogenic, early experience with mice indicating an increased incidence of aneuploidy in zygotes and developmental defects of the central nervous system in fetuses derived from vitrified oocytes.[92]

Epigenetic modifications and genomic imprinting

Evidence of a direct link between early embryonic manipulations and epigenetic modifications to DNA, leading to altered imprinted gene expression, has now been established in both the mouse[58,64,93] and sheep,[6,94] two species that exhibit strikingly different changes in DNA methylation during syngamy and early pre-implantation development,[95] the significance of which will be discussed later. These alterations in genomic imprinting correlate with a varied range of aberrant fetal phenotypes that depend on the species in question, the type of insult during oocyte and/or pre-implantation development, the gene(s) affected and the nature of the epigenetic modification. In sheep, we[6] observed a loss of imprinting (loss of methylation on the second intron differentially methylated region (DMR)) of the normally active maternal allele of *IGF2R* which resulted in a significant reduction in its expression in all affected tissues within LOS fetuses. This occurred following the five-day culture of *in vivo* derived zygotes from follicle-stimulating hormone (FSH)-stimulated cycles in the presence of serum. Many of the phenotypes observed in that and other[96] studies by our group showed remarkable similarities to a number of naturally occurring overgrowth syndromes, most notably BWS, in humans associated with abnormalities in an imprinted cluster of genes on chromosome 11 (11p15.5), which include paternally expressed *Igf2* and maternal expressed *H19*, *p57KIP2* and *KvLQT1*.[5] The expression of equivalent genes (*Igf2*, *H19*) and maternally expressed *Grb10* was altered following the culture of mouse embryos in M16 with 10% fetal calf serum (FCS), resulting in a reduction in *in utero* growth.[58]

By considering several imprinted genes, these[58] and other authors[93,97] highlighted the rather stochastic nature of dysregulated gene expression when early embryos are manipulated or cultured in an artificial environment, illustrating the complexity with which the imprinted status of these genes is regulated. Part of this complexity may be due to the asynchronous nature of methylation acquisition at the DMRs of imprinted genes during oocyte growth,[98] together with the variable stages of oocyte development at the point of follicular aspiration. Such variability may be compounded by the extensive chromatin remodelling that takes place during fertilisation. This process is known to involve active demethylation of paternal chromatin prior to syngamy in some (e.g. mouse, cow and human) but not all (e.g. rabbit and sheep) species,[95] and may go some way to explain interspecies variation in imprinted gene expression following IVF or ICSI.

Under normal circumstances, imprinted loci are thought to retain characteristic methylation differences during pre-implantation development. However, immuno-flourescent staining with an antibody against 5-methylcytosine showed that the methylation patterns of mouse embryos differed between superovulated and nonsuperovulated females and between different *in vitro* culture systems.[99] In contrast, no differences in global DNA methylation were detected between *in vivo* derived and *in vitro* cultured sheep embryos throughout pre-implantation development.[95] These apparent differences between species and/or studies may indicate that (1) alterations to DNA methylation of only a subset of the genome is important at this time and/or (2) the immunodetection method used is generally not sensitive enough to detect subtle temporal changes in DNA methylation at specific loci.

Imprinting disorders in humans conceived by ART have now been reported and these also vary both in terms of phenotypes observed and the loci affected.[100–104] At present, however, the development of a unifying hypothesis that could link an environmental insult to a specific epigenetic modification is beyond our reach. Maher et al.[105] pointed out that, of the 19 ART-related BWS cases reported in the studies cited above, only nine involved ICSI and also that most of the ART-associated epimutations linked to cases of BWS and AS involved a loss of methylation on the maternal allele. Similarly, all of our LOS cases in sheep involved a loss of methylation on the maternal allele of *IGF2R*. However, although the biallelic expression of H19 reported in mouse blastocysts cultured in Whitten's medium was also associated with a loss of methylation, on this occasion this loss of imprinting occurred on an imprinting control region (ICR) 2 kbp upstream of the H19 promoter on the paternal allele.[64] In contrast to this study, the addition of FCS to M16 media in the mouse study of Khosla et al.[58] resulted in an increase in methylation at this ICR.

Other species-specific differences exist rendering it difficult to extrapolate from animals to humans. For example, although the gene for IGF2R is imprinted in both the mouse and sheep, and the dosage control of this gene is crucial for development in these species,[106] its imprinted status in humans remains ambiguous[107] and epigenetic modifications of this gene are not commonly found in human overgrowth syndromes.[108] In contrast, the majority of the sporadic cases of BWS discussed previously occur as a consequence of a loss of maternal allelic methylation within an intronic region of *KCNQ1*. Consequently, although the genes affected may differ, the principle that imprinted genes are susceptible to adverse environmental factors would seem to hold true across the species.

Conclusions

Given the fundamental nature of the intracellular events that occur during the final stages of oocyte growth and maturation, leading to syngamy and early post-fertilisation development, and, given the type and level of insult that these gametes and early embryos are subjected to during assisted reproduction, it is staggering to consider that we have not already encountered greater developmental problems in human infants. It is also difficult to reconcile the contrasting experiences of human ART with those of rodents and farm animals, particularly as the majority of human ART patients are subfertile and the practice of autotransplantation within days of oocyte retrieval is common. It begs the question whether there is something fundamentally different about human reproductive biology that renders human gametes and pre-implantation embryos less susceptible to environmental insults and epigenetic modifications, or can the contrasting experiences between human ART and assisted reproduction in animals be attributed to procedural differences or even luck? The fortuitously slow clinical uptake of procedures such as IVM and blastocyst culture may, to some extent, account for these observations, and the formulation of modern-sequential media may in the future lessen these risks. More transparency, however, is required with regard to the formulation of commercial culture media and more basic research is needed into each of the separate risk factors identified in the preceding section.

Recent advances in gamete and embryo manipulation are transforming mammalian reproduction and scientists and clinicians are privileged to both witness and contribute to these developments. Our responsibility, however, is to safeguard normal development and so it is beholden on all those involved with ART to closely monitor the consequences of new developments and, wherever possible, to ensure that adequate investigations have been conducted *in vitro* and in appropriate animal models prior to their adoption into clinical practice.

Acknowledgements

Original work in the authors' laboratory is currently supported by grants from the National Institutes of Health (NICHD, USA) and the Biotechnology and Biological Sciences Research Council (BBSRC, UK).

References

1. Seamark RF, Robinson JS. Potential health problems stemming from assisted reproduction programmes. *Hum Reprod* 1995;10:1321–2.
2. te Velde ER, van Baar AL, van Kooij RJ. Concerns about assisted reproduction. *Lancet* 1998;351:1524–5.
3. Winston RM, Hardy K. Are we ignoring potential dangers of *in vitro* fertilization and related

treatments? *Nat Med* 2002;8 Suppl: S14–18.

4. Young LE, Sinclair KD, Wilmut I. Large offspring syndrome in cattle and sheep. *Rev Reprod* 1998;3:155–63.

5. Sinclair KD, Young LE, Wilmut I, McEvoy TG. In-utero overgrowth in ruminants following embryo culture: lessons from mice and a warning to men. *Hum Reprod* 2000;15 Suppl 5:68–86.

6. Young LE, Fernandes K, McEvoy TG, Butterwith SC, Gutierrez CG, Carolan C, *et al*. Epigenetic change in IGF2R is associated with fetal overgrowth after sheep embryo culture. *Nat Genet* 2001;27:153–4.

7. Edwards RG, Ludwig M. Are major defects in children conceived *in vitro* due to innate problems in patients or to induced genetic damage? *Reprod Biomed Online* 2003;7:131–8.

8. Niemitz EL, Feinberg AP. Epigenetics and assisted reproductive technology: a call for investigation. *Am J Hum Genet* 2004;74:599–609.

9. Westergaard HB, Johansen AM, Erb K, Andersen AN. Danish National In-Vitro Fertilization Registry 1994 and 1995: a controlled study of births, malformations and cytogenetic findings. *Hum Reprod* 1999;14:1896–902.

10. Schieve LA, Meikle SF, Ferre C, Peterson HB, Jeng G, Wilcox LS. Low and very low birth weight in infants conceived with use of assisted reproductive technology. *N Engl J Med* 2002;346:731–7.

11. Koivurova S, Hartikainen AL, Gissler M, Hemminki E, Sovio U, Jarvelin MR. Neonatal outcome and congenital malformations in children born after in-vitro fertilization. *Hum Reprod* 2002;17:1391–8.

12. Hansen M, Kurinczuk JJ, Bower C, Webb S. The risk of major birth defects after intracytoplasmic sperm injection and *in vitro* fertilization. *N Engl J Med* 2002;346:725–30.

13. Stromberg B, Dahlquist G, Ericson A, Finnstrom O, Koster M, Stjernqvist K. Neurological sequelae in children born after in-vitro fertilisation: a population-based study. *Lancet* 2002;359:461–5.

14. Olivennes F, Fanchin R, Ledee N, Righini C, Kadoch IJ, Frydman R. Perinatal outcome and developmental studies on children born after IVF. *Hum Reprod Update* 2002;8:117–28.

15. Retzloff MG, Hornstein MD. Is intracytoplasmic sperm injection safe? *Fertil Steril* 2003;80:851–9.

16. Kurinczuk JJ. Safety issues in assisted reproduction technology. From theory to reality – just what are the data telling us about ICSI offspring health and future fertility and should we be concerned? *Hum Reprod* 2003;18:925–31.

17. Sauer MV. The impact of age on reproductive potential: lessons learned from oocyte donation. *Maturitas* 1998;30:221–5.

18. Hassold T, Hunt P. To err (meiotically) is human: the genesis of human aneuploidy. *Nat Rev Genet* 2001;2:280–91.

19. Hassold T, Chiu D. Maternal age-specific rates of numerical chromosome abnormalities with special reference to trisomy. *Hum Genet* 1985;70:11–17.

20. Lamb NE, Freeman SB, Savage-Austin A, Pettay D, Taft L, Hersey J, *et al*. Susceptible chiasmate configurations of chromosome 21 predispose to non-disjunction in both maternal meiosis I and meiosis II. *Nat Genet* 1996;14:400–5.

21. Simon C, Rubio C, Vidal F, Gimenez C, Moreno C, Parrilla JJ, *et al*. Increased chromosome abnormalities in human preimplantation embryos in in-vitro fertilization in patients with recurrent miscarriage. *Reprod Fertil Dev* 1998;10:87–92.

22. Ruangvutilert P, Delhanty JD, Serhal P, Simopoulou M, Rodeck CH, Harper JC. FISH analysis on day 5 post-insemination of human arrested and blastocyst stage embryos. *Prenat Diagn* 2000;20:552–60.

23. Bean CJ, Hunt PA, Millie EA, Hassold TJ. Analysis of a malsegregating mouse Y chromosome: evidence that the earliest cleavage divisions of the mammalian embryo are non-disjunction-prone. *Hum Mol Genet* 2001;10:963–72.

24. Viuff D, Hendriksen PJ, Vos PL, Dieleman SJ, Bibby BM, Greve T, *et al*. Chromosomal abnormalities and developmental kinetics in *in vivo*-developed cattle embryos at days 2 to 5 after ovulation. *Biol Reprod* 2001;65:204–8.

25. Bean CJ, Hassold TJ, Judis L, Hunt PA. Fertilization *in vitro* increases non-disjunction during early cleavage divisions in a mouse model system. *Hum Reprod* 2002;17:2362–7.

26. Draper ES, Kurinczuk JJ, Abrams KR, Clarke M. Assessment of separate contributions to perinatal mortality of infertility history and treatment: a case–control analysis. *Lancet* 1999;353:1746–9.

27. Gaudoin M, Dobbie R, Finlayson A, Chalmers J, Cameron IT, Fleming R. Ovulation induction/intrauterine insemination in infertile couples is associated with low-birth-weight infants. *Am J Obstet Gynecol* 2003;188:611–16.

28. Pandian Z, Bhattacharya S, Templeton A. Review of unexplained infertility and obstetric outcome: a 10 year review. *Hum Reprod* 2001;16:2593–7.

29. Serafini P. Outcome and follow-up of children born after IVF-surrogacy. *Hum Reprod Update* 2001;7:23–7.
30. Olivennes F, Rufat P, Andre B, Pourade A, Quiros MC, Frydman R. The increased risk of complication observed in singleton pregnancies resulting from in-vitro fertilization (IVF) does not seem to be related to the IVF method itself. *Hum Reprod* 1993;8:1297–300.
31. Brinton LA, Scoccia B, Moghissi KS, Westhoff CL, Althuis MD, Mabie JE, *et al*. Breast cancer risk associated with ovulation-stimulating drugs. *Hum Reprod* 2004;19:2005–13.
32. Oktay K, Berkowitz P, Berkus M, Schenken RS, Brzyski RG. The re-incarnation of an old question – clomid effect on oocyte and embryo? *Fertil Steril* 2000;74:422–3.
33. London SN, Young D, Caldito G, Mailhes JB. Clomiphene citrate-induced perturbations during meiotic maturation and cytogenetic abnormalities in mouse oocytes *in vivo* and *in vitro*. *Fertil Steril* 2000;73:620–6.
34. Van der Auwera I, Pijnenborg R, Koninckx PR. The influence of in-vitro culture versus stimulated and untreated oviductal environment on mouse embryo development and implantation. *Hum Reprod* 1999;14:2570–4.
35. Van der Auwera I, D'Hooghe T.. Superovulation of female mice delays embryonic and fetal development. *Hum Reprod* 2001;16:1237–43.
36. Ertzeid G, Storeng R. The impact of ovarian stimulation on implantation and fetal development in mice. *Hum Reprod* 2001;16:221–5.
37. Picton HM. Oocyte maturation *in vitro*. *Curr Opin Obstet Gynecol* 2002;14:295–302.
38. Trounson A, Anderiesz C, Jones G. Maturation of human oocytes *in vitro* and their developmental competence. *Reproduction* 2001;121:51–75.
39. Bjercke S, Dale PO, Tanbo T, Storeng R, Ertzeid G, Abyholm T. Impact of insulin resistance on pregnancy complications and outcome in women with polycystic ovary syndrome. *Gynecol Obstet Invest* 2002;54:94–8.
40. Hardy K, Wright CS, Franks S, Winston RM. *In vitro* maturation of oocytes. *Br Med Bull* 2000;56:588–602.
41. Merton JS, de Roos AP, Mullaart E, de Ruigh L, Kaal L, Vos PL, *et al*. Factors affecting oocyte quality and quantity in commercial application of embryo technologies in the cattle breeding industry. *Theriogenology* 2003;59:651–74.
42. Teixeira Filho FL, Baracat EC, Lee TH, Suh CS, Matsui M, *et al*. Aberrant expression of growth differentiation factor-9 in oocytes of women with polycystic ovary syndrome. *J Clin Endocrinol Metab* 2002;87:1337–44.
43. Dumesic DA, Schramm RD, Peterson E, Paprocki AM, Zhou R, Abbott DH. Impaired developmental competence of oocytes in adult prenatally androgenized female rhesus monkeys undergoing gonadotropin stimulation for *in vitro* fertilization. *J Clin Endocrinol Metab* 2002;87:1111–19.
44. Wallace DC. Mitochondrial diseases in man and mouse. *Science* 1999;283:1482–8.
45. Keefe DL, Niven-Fairchild T, Buradagunta S. Mitochondrial deoxyribonucleic acid deletions in oocytes and reproductive ageing in women. *Fertil Steril* 1995;64:577–83.
46. Barritt JA, Willadsen S, Brenner C, Cohen J. Cytoplasmic transfer in assisted reproduction. *Hum Reprod Update* 2001;7:428–35.
47. St John JC. The need to investigate the transmission of mitochondrial DNA following cytoplasmic transfer. *Hum Reprod* 2002;17:1954–8.
48. Yanagimachi R. Gamete manipulation for development: new methods for conception. *Reprod Fertil Dev* 2001;13:3–14.
49. Hewitson L, Takahashi D, Dominko T, Simerly C, Schatten G. Fertilization and embryo development to blastocysts after intracytoplasmic sperm injection in the rhesus monkey. *Hum Reprod* 1998;13:3449–55.
50. Ramalho-Santos J, Sutovsky P, Simerly C, Oko R, Wessel GM, Hewitson L, *et al*. ICSI choreography: fate of sperm structures after monospermic rhesus ICSI and first cell cycle implications. *Hum Reprod* 2000;15:2610–20.
51. Wall RJ. New gene transfer methods. *Theriogenology* 2002;57:189–201.
52. Bonduelle M, Liebaers I, Deketelaere V, Derde MP, Camus M, Devroey P, *et al*. Neonatal data on a cohort of 2889 infants born after ICSI (1991–1999) and of 2995 infants born after IVF (1983–1999). *Hum Reprod* 2002;17:671–94.
53. Egozcue S, Blanco J, Vendrell JM, Garcia F, Veiga A, Aran B, *et al*. Human male infertility: chromosome anomalies, meiotic disorders, abnormal spermatozoa and recurrent abortion. *Hum Reprod Update* 2000;6:93–105.
54. Rubio C, Gil-Salom M, Simon C, Vidal F, Rodrigo L, Minguez Y, *et al*. Incidence of sperm

chromosomal abnormalities in a risk population: relationship with sperm quality and ICSI outcome. *Hum Reprod* 2001;16:2084–92.

55. Vendrell JM, Aran B, Veiga A, Garcia F, Coroleu B, Egozcue S, et al. Spermatogenic patterns and early embryo development after intracytoplasmic sperm injection in severe oligoasthenozoospermia. *J Assist Reprod Genet* 2003;20:106–12.

56. Menezo YJ, Hamamah S, Hazout A, Dale B. Time to switch from co-culture to sequential defined media for transfer at the blastocyst stage. *Hum Reprod* 1998;13:2043–4.

57. Quinn P. The development and impact of culture media for assisted reproductive technologies. *Fertil Steril* 2004;81:27–9.

58. Khosla S, Dean W, Brown D, Reik W, Feil R. Culture of preimplantation mouse embryos affects fetal development and the expression of imprinted genes. *Biol Reprod* 2001;64:918–26.

59. Fernandez-Gonzalez R, Moreira P, Bilbao A, Jimenez A, Perez-Crespo M, Ramirez MA, et al. Long-term effect of *in vitro* culture of mouse embryos with serum on mRNA expression of imprinting genes, development, and behavior. *Proc Natl Acad Sci U S A* 2004;101:5880–5.

60. Sinclair KD, McEvoy TG, Ashworth CJ, Rooke JA, Young LE, Wilmut I, et al. Effects of timing of serum exposure during embryo culture on ovine fetal development. *Reproduction Abstract Series* 2002;28:15.

61. Sinclair KD, Powell KA, McEvoy TG, Ashworth CJ, Rooke JA, Young LE, et al. Zygote donor nutrition affects ovine fetal development following *in vitro* embryo culture. *Reprod Abstr Ser* 2003;30:55–6.

62. Lazzari L, Lucchi S, Montemurro T, Porretti L, Lopa R, Rebulla P, et al. Evaluation of the effect of cryopreservation on *ex vivo* expansion of hematopoietic progenitors from cord blood. *Bone Marrow Transplant* 2001;28:693–8.

63. Lane M, Gardner DK. Increase in postimplantation development of cultured mouse embryos by amino acids and induction of fetal retardation and exencephaly by ammonium ions. *J Reprod Fertil* 1994;102:305–12.

64. Doherty AS, Mann MR, Tremblay KD, Bartolomei MS, Schultz RM. Differential effects of culture on imprinted H19 expression in the preimplantation mouse embryo. *Biol Reprod* 2000;62:1526–35.

65. Lane M, Gardner DK. Ammonium induces aberrant blastocyst differentiation, metabolism, pH regulation, gene expression and subsequently alters fetal development in the mouse. *Biol Reprod* 2003;69:1109–17.

66. Sinawat S, Hsaio WC, Flockhart JH, Kaufman MH, Keith J, West JD. Fetal abnormalities produced after preimplantation exposure of mouse embryos to ammonium chloride. *Hum Reprod* 2003;18:2157–65.

67. Sills ES, Tucker MJ, Palermo GD. Assisted reproductive technologies and monozygous twins: implications for future study and clinical practice. *Twin Res* 2000;3:217–23.

68. da Costa AL, Abdelmassih S, de Oliveira FG, Abdelmassih V, Abdelmassih R, Nagy ZP, et al. Monozygotic twins and transfer at the blastocyst stage after ICSI. *Hum Reprod* 2001;16:333–6.

69. Milki AA, Jun SH, Hinckley MD, Behr B, Giudice LC, Westphal LM. Incidence of monozygotic twinning with blastocyst transfer compared to cleavage-stage transfer. *Fertil Steril* 2003;79:503–6.

70. Tarlatzis BC, Qublan HS, Sanopoulou T, Zepiridis L, Grimbizis G, Bontis J. Increase in the monozygotic twinning rate after intracytoplasmic sperm injection and blastocyst stage embryo transfer. *Fertil Steril* 2002;77:196–8.

71. Hershlag A, Paine T, Cooper GW, Scholl GM, Rawlinson K, Kvapil G. Monozygotic twinning associated with mechanical assisted hatching. *Fertil Steril* 1999;71:144–6.

72. Gardner DK, Surrey E, Minjarez D, Leitz A, Stevens J, Schoolcraft WB. Single blastocyst transfer: a prospective randomized trial. *Fertil Steril* 2004;81:551–5.

73. Jain JK, Boostanfar R, Slater CC, Francis MM, Paulson RJ. Monozygotic twins and triplets in association with blastocyst transfer. *J Assist Reprod Genet* 2004;21:103–7.

74. Botchan A, Hauser R, Gamzu R, Yogev L, Paz G, Yavetz H. Results of 6139 artificial insemination cycles with donor spermatozoa. *Hum Reprod* 2001;16:2298–304.

75. Gorrill MJ, Burry KA, Patton PE. Pregnancy outcomes using donor sperm insemination after failed *in vitro* fertilization with intracytoplasmic sperm injection cycles in couples with complex infertility disorders. *Fertil Steril* 2003;80:936–8.

76. Lansac J, Royere D. Follow-up studies of children born after frozen sperm donation. *Hum Reprod Update* 2001;7:33–7.

77. Holt WV, Watson PF. Role of new and current methods in semen technology for genetic resource conservation. In: *Farm Animal Genetic Resources*, BSAS Publication No. 30. Simm G, Villanueva B, Sinclair KD, Townsend S, editors. Nottingham: Nottingham University Press; 2004. p. 191–205.

78. Morris GJ. A new development in the cryopreservation of sperm. *Hum Fertil (Camb)* 2002;5:23–9.

79. Seli E, Gardner DK, Schoolcraft WB, Moffatt O, Sakkas D. Extent of nuclear DNA damage in ejaculated spermatozoa impacts on blastocyst development after *in vitro* fertilization. *Fertil Steril* 2004;82:378–83.

80. Thompson-Cree ME, McClure N, Donnelly ET, Steele KE, Lewis SE. Effects of cryopreservation on testicular sperm nuclear DNA fragmentation and its relationship with assisted conception outcome following ICSI with testicular spermatozoa. *Reprod Biomed Online* 2003;7:449–55.

81. Park YS, Lee SH, Song SJ, Jun JH, Koong MK, Seo JT. Influence of motility on the outcome of *in vitro* fertilization/intracytoplasmic sperm injection with fresh vs. frozen testicular sperm from men with obstructive azoospermia. *Fertil Steril* 2003;80:526–30.

82. Ramos L, De Boer P, Meuleman EJ, Braat DD, Wetzels AM. Evaluation of ICSI-selected epididymal sperm samples of obstructive azoospermic males by the CKIA system. *J Androl* 2004;25:406–11.

83. Wennerholm UB, Bergh C, Hamberger L, Westlander G, Wikland M, Wood M. Obstetric outcome of pregnancies following ICSI, classified according to sperm origin and quality. *Hum Reprod* 2000;15:1189–94.

84. Kolibianakis EM, Zikopoulos K, Devroey P. Implantation potential and clinical impact of cryopreservation – a review. *Placenta* 2003;24 Suppl B:S27–33.

85. Winston RM, Hardy K. Are we ignoring potential dangers of *in vitro* fertilization and related treatments? *Nat Cell Biol* 2002;4 Suppl:S14–18.

86. Paynter SJ. Current status of the cryopreservation of human unfertilized oocytes. *Hum Reprod Update* 2000;6:449–56.

87. Mandelbaum J, Anastasiou O, Levy R, Guerin JF, de Larouzier V, Antoine JM. Effects of cryopreservation on the meiotic spindle of human oocytes. *Eur J Obstet Gynecol Reprod Biol* 2004;113 Suppl 1:S17–23.

88. Jones A, Van Blerkom J, Davis P, Toledo AA. Cryopreservation of metaphase II human oocytes effects mitochondrial membrane potential: implications for developmental competence. *Hum Reprod* 2004;19:1861–6.

89. Coticchio G, Bonu MA, Borini A, Flamigni C. Oocyte cryopreservation: a biological perspective. *Eur J Obstet Gynecol Reprod Biol* 2004;115 Suppl 1:S2–7.

90. Mavrides A, Morroll D. Cryopreservation of bovine oocytes: is cryoloop vitrification the future to preserving the female gamete? *Reprod Nutr Dev* 2002;42:73–80.

91. Liebermann J, Tucker MJ, Sills ES. Cryoloop vitrification in assisted reproduction: analysis of survival rates in > 1000 human oocytes after ultra-rapid cooling with polymer augmented cryoprotectants. *Clin Exp Obstet Gynecol* 2003;30:125–9.

92. Auroux M. Long-term effects in progeny of paternal environment and of gamete/embryo cryopreservation. *Hum Reprod Update* 2000;6:550–63.

93. Humpherys D, Eggan K, Akutsu H, Hochedlinger K, Rideout WM 3rd, Biniszkiewicz D, *et al.* Epigenetic instability in ES cells and cloned mice. *Science* 2001;293:95–7.

94. Young LE, Schnieke AE, McCreath KJ, Wieckowski S, Konfortova G, Fernandes K, *et al.* Conservation of IGF2-H19 and IGF2R imprinting in sheep: effects of somatic cell nuclear transfer. *Mech Dev* 2003;120:1433–42.

95. Beaujean N, Hartshorne G, Cavilla J, Taylor J, Gardner J, Wilmut I, *et al.* Non-conservation of mammalian preimplantation methylation dynamics. *Curr Biol* 2004;14:R266–7.

96. Sinclair KD, McEvoy TG, Maxfield EK, Maltin CA, Young LE, Wilmut I, *et al.* Aberrant fetal growth and development after *in vitro* culture of sheep zygotes. *J Reprod Fertil* 1999;116:177–86.

97. Dean W, Bowden L, Aitchison A, Klose J, Moore T, Meneses JJ, *et al.* Altered imprinted gene methylation and expression in completely ES cell-derived mouse fetuses: association with aberrant phenotypes. *Development* 1998;125:2273–82.

98. Lucifero D, Mann MRW, Bartolomei MS, Trasler JM. Gene-specific timing and epigenetic memory in oocyte imprinting. *Hum Mol Genet* 2004;13:839–49.

99. Shi W, Haaf T. Aberrant methylation patterns at the two-cell stage as an indicator of early developmental failure. *Mol Reprod Dev* 2002;63:329–34.

100. Cox GF, Burger J, Lip V, Mau UA, Sperling K, Wu BL, *et al.* Intracytoplasmic sperm injection may increase the risk of imprinting defects. *Am J Hum Genet* 2002;71:162–4.

101. Orstavik KH, Eiklid K, van der Hagen CB, Spetalen S, Kierulf K, Skjeldal O, *et al.* Another case of imprinting defect in a girl with Angelman syndrome who was conceived by intracytoplasmic semen injection. *Am J Hum Genet* 2003;72:218–19.

102. DeBaun MR, Niemitz EL, Feinberg AP. Association of *in vitro* fertilization with Beckwith–Wiedemann syndrome and epigenetic alterations of LIT1 and H19. *Am J Hum Genet* 2003;72:156–60.

103. Gicquel C, Gaston V, Mandelbaum J, Siffroi JP, Flahault A, Le Bouc Y. *In vitro* fertilization may

increase the risk of Beckwith–Wiedemann syndrome related to the abnormal imprinting of the KCN1OT gene. *Am J Hum Genet* 2003;72:1338–41.

104. Maher ER, Brueton LA, Bowdin SC, Luharia A, Cooper W, Cole TR, *et al*. Beckwith–Wiedemann syndrome and assisted reproduction technology (ART). *J Med Genet* 2003;40:62–4.

105. Maher ER, Afnan M, Barratt CL. Epigenetic risks related to assisted reproductive technologies: epigenetics, imprinting, ART and icebergs? *Hum Reprod* 2003;18:2508–11.

106. Wutz A, Theussl HC, Dausman J, Jaenisch R, Barlow DP, Wagner EF. Non-imprinted Igf2r expression decreases growth and rescues the Tme mutation in mice. *Development* 2001;128:1881–7.

107. Killian JK, Nolan CM, Stewart N, Munday BL, Andersen NA, Nicol S, *et al*. Monotreme IGF2 expression and ancestral origin of genomic imprinting. *J Exp Zool* 2001;291:205–12.

108. Gicquel C, Weiss J, Amiel J, Gaston V, Le Bouc Y, Scott CD. Epigenetic abnormalities of the mannose-6-phosphate/IGF2 receptor gene are uncommon in human overgrowth syndromes. *J Med Genet* 2004;41:e4.

Chapter 14
Pre-implantation genetic testing

Peter Braude, Jan Grace and Tarek El Toukhy

Introduction

Since its first clinical use, pre-implantation genetic testing (PGT) has become increasingly available as a method of detecting genetic disorders before pregnancy is established. Based on a difference of purpose, PGT can be classified as either pre-implantation genetic diagnosis (PGD) or pre-implantation genetic screening (PGS). PGD was established in the early 1990s as an alternative to prenatal diagnosis (PND) and termination of pregnancy.[1] PGD describes the testing of oocytes or embryos from patients who have a significant risk of conceiving a pregnancy affected by a known recurrent genetic disorder, in order to preselect for transfer only those embryos found not to carry the disorder. PGS, on the other hand, aims to improve the outcome of assisted reproductive technology (ART) treatment for the subfertile by testing for a number of the more frequent chromosome aneuploidies in an attempt to improve implantation and reduce the incidence of miscarriage. It is estimated that worldwide, more than 1000 children have been born following PGT.[2] The clinical application of PGT is expanding into new areas, creating novel ethical and practical dilemmas.

In order for a pre-implantation genetic test to be performed, a representative sample of the embryo is required. A single cell can be removed from a late cleavage stage embryo (8–16 cells), or a few cells may be taken from the trophectoderm of a blastocyst, or one or both of the polar bodies can be removed from the unfertilised egg or early zygote. First polar body biopsy has advantages in that the test is effectively done pre-fertilisation, and it samples extra-embryonic tissue and thus may be less likely to affect cleavage of the embryo.[3] However, only information about the maternal genotype can be gathered and, since the diagnosis in the oocyte is inferred, cross-over during meiosis may render the result less reliable. For these reasons a complementary cleavage stage biopsy may be required. Cleavage stage biopsy is the most commonly used technique, where embryos are grown until they reach the 6- to 8-cell stage on day 3 after insemination, and one or two blastomeres are then removed (Figure 14.1). Blastocyst biopsy overcomes some of the technical difficulties of molecular diagnosis as more cells are available to be removed from extra-embryonic tissues. However, culturing embryos to the blastocyst stage may reduce the

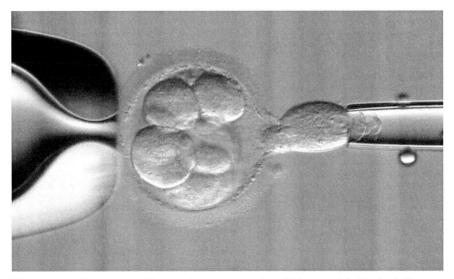

Figure 14.1. Cleavage stage biopsy: a cleavage stage embryo 72 hours post-fertilisation held stationary on a glass micropipette (left) by gentle suction; the zona pellucida has been breached by acid Tyrode's solution; a single nucleated blastomere has been removed using a suction pipette (right); note the clear single nucleus in the blastomere

cohort for biopsy as only 36% of embryos mature this far, and the time available for diagnosis is limited by the need for transfer on the same day as biopsy.[4]

Pre-implantation genetic diagnosis (PGD)

The first successful clinical application of PGD, to avoid the X-linked condition adrenoleukodystrophy, used polymerase chain reaction (PCR) to amplify a specific repeat on the Y chromosome in order to sex embryos.[5] Proof of principle had been demonstrated in 1968 when rabbit embryos were sexed using sex-specific chromatin following blastocyst biopsies.[6]

Before the advent of PGD there were few reproductive options for couples at high risk of transmission of a serious genetic disorder. These included accepting the risks of the condition and hoping for favourable odds; opting for PND (amniocentesis or chorionic villus sampling) and then being prepared to terminate an affected pregnancy – an option not taken lightly as it is often performed in the second trimester with considerable physical and psychological morbidity; or the use of gametes from donors who are not carriers of the disorder. For X-linked conditions, there is also now the possibility of using fluorescence-activated cell sorting (FACS) to sort semen into separate X- and Y-bearing spermatozoa. Although this process is not totally reliable, it may be used to skew the result in favour of an unaffected pregnancy.[7] Couples may otherwise chose adoption or decide to remain childless.

Patients choose PGD for a variety of reasons. They may already have an affected child, or they may have lost affected children as a result of the genetic condition and wish to avoid further risk. They may have had several terminations of affected pregnancies and wish for another method to eliminate or minimise that outcome, or they may have personal, including religious, objections to termination of pregnancy. Some may carry a dominant disorder and, as such, either are or will become affected by that condition, and wish to avoid having a child affected as they are, and also wish to eliminate the condition from their bloodline. They may have seen the genetic condition affect their family and wish to avoid the risk before attempting pregnancy themselves. They may have suffered multiple miscarriages as a result of a chromosome rearrangement and see PGD as an option to reduce the risk of further miscarriage.

Clinical considerations

In order to offer a safe and effective service, a multidisciplinary team should be established. This should include genetic and infertility counsellors, clinical geneticists, cytogeneticists, molecular biologists, embryologists and reproductive specialists. Those performing embryo biopsy must be approved and licensed by the Human Fertilisation and Embryology Authority (HFEA) after inspection. Twelve clinics are currently licensed for biopsy in the UK and fewer than that for full processing of biopsy samples for diagnosis. Laboratories should participate in external quality assessment and in the UK are expected to have received clinical pathology (CPA) accreditation, or to be working towards accreditation.[8]

A couple considering PGD must receive genetic counselling to confirm that they understand the nature of their particular condition and how it may affect their offspring, and that they are aware of alternative reproductive options. If one of the couple carries a lethal or debilitating progressive disorder they need to consider the welfare of, and make arrangements for, the care of any child born. The need to take account of the welfare of the child and any existing children is a statutory requirement of the Human Fertilisation and Embryology Act.[8] Couples need to understand fully the processes involved in PGD in terms of stimulation and collection of oocytes, fertilisation, development of embryos and the biopsy process, and the risks of superovulation, including hyperstimulation syndrome and multiple pregnancy. Couples should be aware of the large attrition in numbers of embryos that may be available from beginning a cycle to those that may be suitable for replacement after PGD, the predominant factor in the likely success in terms of pregnancy. They also should be aware of the risk of misdiagnosis after PGD and should consider whether they would accept confirmatory PND.

PGD is a major undertaking for any couple, and the psychological, medical and financial costs are considerable. A single cycle might cost anything from £4000 to £7000, with a likely 'take-home baby' rate not much above 20% wherever this is undertaken.[9] In our practice, approximately half of UK patients are likely to obtain NHS funding for at least one cycle. Funding of PGD is not one of the issues considered in the 2004 National Institute for Clinical Excellence (NICE) fertility guideline as this service appropriately falls within the consideration and funding of genetic services.[10] In some areas specialist local consortia are being established to advise primary care trusts about the appropriateness of cases for NHS funding (*Pre-implantation Genetic Diagnosis (PGD) – Guiding Principles for Commissioners of NHS Services* [www.dh.gov.uk/PolicyAndGuidance/HealthAndSocialCareTopics/Genetics/

GeneticsGeneralInformation/GeneticsGeneralArticle/fs/en?CONTENT_ID=4072 467&chk=hX18v9]).

Of 275 cycles performed for 149 couples in our unit, the cumulative clinical pregnancy rate per couple treated was 36% (live birth rate 20% per cycle started). On average, the time interval from referral to consultation is six months. Auditing over a 19 month period revealed that of 158 couples referred only one-third started treatment, most dropped out having established what PGD entailed. Thus fewer than 10% of those referred originally went on with treatment and achieved a clinical pregnancy.[11]

Clinical procedures and embryology

Although patients seeking PGD are generally fertile, ART techniques are required to access the embryo *in vitro* for testing. Ovarian stimulation, monitoring and egg collection are identical to those used for ART for alleviating subfertility, but since the number of eggs (and hence embryos) available is critical to success, regimens tend to be more aggressive. Oocytes may be fertilised using *in vitro* fertilisation (IVF) where the sperm quality is deemed adequate. Intracytoplasmic sperm injection (ICSI) is essential when the diagnostic test requires the use of PCR, as the presence of additional sperm buried in the zona pellucida may lead to contamination of the PCR reactions with paternal DNA, thus risking misdiagnosis.

For whom may PGD be suitable?

Once a biopsy is performed the type of test applied to the cell depends on the genetic condition being tested. PGD is offered for three main categories of disease (Table 14.1):

1. to determine the sex of an embryo for an X-linked condition whose specific gene defect at a molecular level is unknown, highly variable or unsuitable for testing on single cells
2. to detect a variety of chromosomal rearrangements such as translocations, inversions, deletions or insertions on interphase nuclei using fluorescence *in situ* hybridisation (FISH)
3. to identify single-gene disorders, which may be recessive or dominant, where the molecular abnormality is tested following amplification by PCR of DNA extracted from single cells.

X-linked disorders

Where a specific test at the single-cell level is not available, couples may opt to have sex selection of the embryos using FISH with the intention of replacing female embryos in order to prevent transmission of the condition.[12] This does not eliminate the disease from the family in the future, as half of these female embryos will be carriers. It is often assumed that since on average half the embryos will be of either sex, the use of sex selection gives a 50:50 chance of being able to select an unaffected embryo from the cohort. In practice the odds are worse than this, since some embryos may be unsuitable for replacement because the test has revealed aneuploidy, or an uncertain diagnosis owing to FISH failure.[13] Also, the fact that half the non-

Table 14.1. Common indications for PGD arranged by mode of inheritance

Disorder	Condition
Single-gene disorders	
Autosomal recessive	Huntington disease
	Myotonic dystrophy
	Neurofibromatosis
	Charcot–Marie–Tooth 1a and 2a
	Osteogenesis imperfecta I and IV
	Stickler syndrome
	Tuberous sclerosis
	Marfan syndrome
Autosomal dominant	Cystic fibrosis
	Beta-thalassaemia
	Spinal muscular atrophy
	Sickle cell disease
	Epidermolysis bullosa
	Gaucher disease
	Tay–Sachs disease
Sex-linked dominant	Fragile X syndrome
	Oral-facial-digital syndrome type I
Sex-linked recessive	Duchenne muscular dystrophy
	Spinal and bulbar atrophy
	Agammaglobulinaemia
	Hunter syndrome
Chromosomal disorders	
Structural aberrations	Reciprocal translocation
	Robertsonian translocation
	Inversion
	Deletion
Numerical aberrations	47 XXY (Klinefelter syndrome)
	47 XYY
	Sex chromosomal mosaicism
	Male meiotic abnormalities

transferred male embryos could be normal may raise ethical objections. As mentioned, FACS may be used to increase the number of X-bearing spermatozoa before IVF so as to increase the number of unaffected embryos available.[7] In general, this FISH for sex determination is robust, as misdiagnosis would have to involve two errors; loss of a Y signal and gain of an X. Despite this, one FISH misdiagnosis for sexing has been reported.[9]

Chromosomal rearrangements

Chromosomal rearrangements are a well-recognised cause of reproductive failure.[14] Reciprocal translocations (where there is an exchange of terminal segments from two different chromosomes), occur in about 1 in every 500 of the general population. They are more common in infertile couples (0.6%), men with oligoastheno-teratospermia (3%), and in couples with repeated IVF failures (3.2%).[15,16] In fertile couples with three or more consecutive first-trimester miscarriages they may be present in almost 10% of cases. A carrier of a balanced reciprocal translocation is phenotypically normal but, owing to abnormal segregation at meiosis, 50–70% of their gametes are likely to be unbalanced. Since each translocation is unique, and there are 32 possible segregation products, only two of which are phenotypically normal (balanced and normal), the significant effects of the translocation, such as miscarriage, affected liveborn risk and reproductive failure, will be particular to the specific chromosomes involved and their breakpoints.[17]

In order to perform PGD for reciprocal translocations, fluorescent probes specific for the subtelomeric regions of the translocated segments and the centromere regions of centric segments are hybridised to the interphase nucleus of the biopsied cell. For Robertsonian translocations (where two acrocentric chromosomes fuse to give one derivative chromosome), chromosome enumerator probes, which can be chosen to bind at any point on the long arm of the chromosome that is involved in the translocation, are used to count the chromosomes in the nuclei of the cells.[18]

The most common indication for PGD for translocations is to prevent repeated miscarriage. Other causes of miscarriage such as antiphospholipid syndrome or intrauterine abnormalities must first be excluded as they cannot be prevented using PGD but may be present in addition to the chromosome rearrangement. The chance of a live birth following spontaneous conception in the next pregnancy even after three first-trimester losses is in excess of 65% and still 62% after four losses.[19] So the decision to use PGD, where the liveborn chance is only of the order of 20%,[9] is debatable and needs to take account of other factors such as the psychological consequences of loss and subfertility.

Single-gene disorders

As the amount of DNA available for diagnosis in a single-cell biopsy is tiny, a direct test cannot be performed without amplification of the DNA using PCR to an amount where the specific mutation can be detected.[1] At this level, PCR may not be wholly reliable such that, occasionally, sequences may fail to amplify. This can result in a heterozygous embryo being typed as a homozygous affected, and thus excluded from the cohort of embryos available for transfer – a false positive.[20,21] Equally, the classification of a heterozygote as homozygous normal owing to absence of the affected allele (false negative) may still be safe in autosomal recessive disorders since there are no adverse phenotypes in carriers (Figure 14.2), but in autosomal dominant conditions where heterozygotes are affected, problems of undetected allele drop-out (ADO) or amplification failure make the possibility of misdiagnosis too great for a simple test to be acceptable.[22] In addition, the sample could become contaminated with extraneous non-embryonic DNA, leading to misdiagnosis. The accuracy of the test can be improved and the possibility of misdiagnosis (around 4–7%) decreased by the use of multiplex fluorescent PCR.[23,24] Here, simultaneous amplification of two or

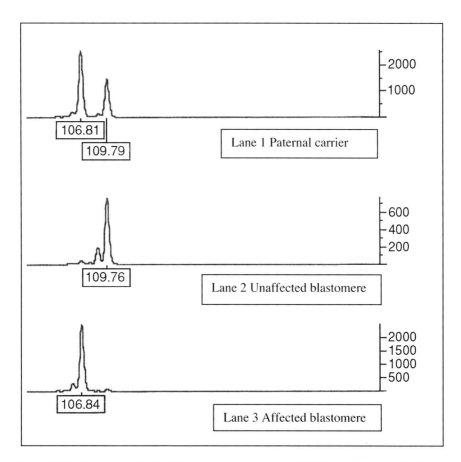

Figure 14.2. Fluorescent-labelled PCR product analysed on an ABI 3100 genetic analyser for the presence or absence of the cystic fibrosis ΔF508 mutation: Lane 1 shows heterozygous paternal carrier buccal cell, where the normal allele and the affected allele are represented by the 109 base pair (bp) and 106 bp peaks, respectively; Lane 2 shows the result from a blastomere taken from a normal embryo with only the normal allele (109 bp) present; Lane 3 shows the result from a blastomere taken from an affected embryo with only the affected allele (106 bp) present (courtesy of Cheryl Black)

more loci, one containing the mutation and one or more containing informative polymorphic markers in close proximity to the mutation (acting as a mini-fingerprint), confirms the embryonic origin of the DNA. The enhanced sensitivity of fluorescence PCR makes ADO less frequent and, since contamination by rogue DNA can be detected as it can be distinguished from DNA of embryonic origin, the risk of misdiagnosis is reduced significantly (< 1%).

Regulation of PGD

There are substantial international differences in the regulation of PGD. In the UK, all assisted reproduction techniques, including PGD, are regulated by the HFEA under the terms of the Human Fertilisation and Embryology Act (1990). According to the Act and the HFEA's *Code of Practice* (6th edition, 2003), an embryo may only be used for PGD or for research to develop diagnostic methods under licence from the HFEA.[8] The HFEA provides reassurance to the public that PGD is being undertaken only for serious genetic conditions and not simply for social reasons. PGD has only recently been allowed in France in three specified centres. It is disallowed in several countries, including Austria, Germany and Switzerland. Recent restrictive legislation in Italy has caused consternation, as it essentially outlaws all pre-implantation procedures on embryos. There is no federal regulation of PGD in the USA.

There are understandable concerns regarding the safety of PGD. The long-term effects of removal of one or more cells at cleavage stage, which will decrease the cellular mass of the embryo, are unknown. Although animal experiments suggest that this does not adversely affect *in vitro* and *in vivo* development, there are few good follow-up studies of embryo biopsy in humans. In one small study of 123 deliveries, the complications of pregnancy, birthweight and length of pregnancy were found to be similar to ICSI. Of 109 infants born following polar body biopsy, six birth defects – two major (an amniotic band and neonatal seizures) and four minor – were reported.[25] An increased multiple monozygotic pregnancy rate has also been reported (27–31%), and triplets have occurred following double-embryo transfer (DET), although whether this is increased significantly is still under investigation. Success of PGD seems to be universally similar, with quoted rates of clinical pregnancy of 19% per oocyte retrieval and 23% per embryo transfer. So far, the reported misdiagnosis rate is higher in the PCR group (3.4%) than in the FISH group (0.9%).[9] In Europe, the European Society of Human Reproduction and Embryology (ESHRE) PGD Consortium was formed in 1997 to undertake a long-term study of the efficacy, safety and clinical outcome of PGD. It reports its findings annually at the ESHRE meeting (www.eshre.com). In 2002 an international society, the Pre-implantation Genetic Diagnosis International Society (PGDIS) was formed to encourage and coordinate research, education and training in PGD on a more international basis.

Advances in pre-implantation genetic testing (PGT)

Pre-implantation genetic screening (PGS)

The use of PGD for the prevention of transmission of serious genetic disease has largely been overtaken in volume by use of embryo biopsy to improve IVF outcome for subfertile couples.[26] The application of FISH as well as other more sophisticated techniques has been extended to detect embryos that contain major sporadic chromosomal or age-related aneuploidies that may result in failure of implantation or spontaneous miscarriage, and to remove them from the cohort available for transfer. This technique is variously called pre-implantation genetic screening (PGS) by the HFEA in the UK, or aneuploidy screening (PGD-AS) in other parts of Europe and by the ESHRE Consortium. In the USA it tends to be included under the overall banner of PGD, which inflates the number of PGD cycles that have been reported from there.

During PGS, individual embryos are biopsied and single blastomeres are examined using between 5 and 14 FISH probes (most commonly X,Y, 13, 15, 16, 17, 18, 21 and 22).[27] The technique has so far been advocated for three main groups, recurrent miscarriage, poor-prognosis IVF patients and severe male-factor infertility, as discussed below.

Recurrent miscarriage

Recurrent miscarriage affects about 1% of couples of reproductive age.[28] Although chromosomal abnormalities are implicated in up to 60% of first-trimester miscarriages, fewer than 5% of couples with two or more miscarriages carry a balanced chromosomal rearrangement.[29] *De novo* numerical abnormalities (in particular monosomy X and autosomal trisomies involving chromosomes 16, 21 and 22 and to a lesser extent chromosomes 13 and 18) account for the vast majority of spontaneous miscarriages caused by chromosomal aberrations. Thus, screening embryos with FISH analysis using probes specific for these chromosomes could detect approximately 70% of the chromosomal abnormalities found in spontaneous miscarriages and provide a means of improving reproductive outcome in affected couples.

Poor-prognosis IVF patients

Advanced maternal age and recurrent implantation failures (defined as three or more failed IVF attempts) are poor prognostic factors for successful IVF treatment.[30] Studies of pre-implantation embryos in women of advanced maternal age suggest that more than half have aneuploidies that would be detectable by FISH, including trisomies involving chromosomes 16 and 21. Likewise, up to 75% of embryos from patients with repeated IVF failures may be chromosomally abnormal, the most common abnormalities encountered being aneuploidies of chromosomes 13, 16, 21 and 22.[31] Since good morphology and developmental stage cannot reliably predict chromosomal normality of early human embryos, the use of FISH to exclude chromosomally abnormal embryos has been advocated to improve the success rate of IVF in these poor-prognosis patients, particularly in light of the current tendency to limit the number of transferred embryos to avoid multiple pregnancies.

Severe male-factor infertility

Although ICSI has dramatically changed the outlook for conception in couples with severe male-factor infertility, it appears that among these patients there are various underlying genetic abnormalities that may be involved in the aetiology of their infertility. For example, patients with non-obstructive azoospermia or severe oligospermia may have microdeletions in the long arm of the Y chromosomes.[32] In addition, ICSI cycles aimed at the treatment of severe male-factor infertility are associated with an increased risk of *de novo* chromosomal aberrations, especially aneuplodies involving the sex chromosomes.[33] These may be secondary to increased aneuploidy rates in the sperm used.[34] Hence, applying the appropriate FISH probes to those ICSI-generated embryos may reduce transfer of such embryos.

Limitations and drawbacks of PGS

Despite a decade of experience, over 3000 treatment cycles of PGS reported and over 500 babies born, data from randomised controlled trials demonstrating the efficacy of the technique over less-invasive alternative therapies are lacking. Furthermore, there are no studies clearly showing improvement in live birth rates per stimulated cycle with the use of PGS, particularly when taking into account the advantage that additional frozen embryos may confer. To date, most studies have reported their results in terms of implantation and clinical pregnancy rates per transfer, falsely inflating the reported success rate by excluding cycles where embryo transfer was not performed because no normal embryos were available for transfer (usually in the range 20–65% of cycles). Only one recent multicentre study of PGS showed a significant two-fold increase of implantation from 10.2% to 22.5% based on clinical pregnancy, and a decrease in the miscarriage rate from 27.5% per patient in the control group to 14.3% in the group undergoing PGD-AS testing. Although clinically impressive, this difference was not yet statistically significant.[35,36]

False-positive and false-negative FISH results (due to hybridisation failure, weak or overlapping signals and cross-hybridisation), estimated in various studies to be between 5% and 12%, can lead to chromosomally normal embryos being excluded from the cohort suitable for transfer. In addition, the fact that mosaicism is a natural event in early human embryos, even in morphologically normal good-quality embryos, undermines the accuracy of PGS as a screening test for embryo karyotype normality since the cell removed and tested may not be representative of the entire embryo.[37] The overall outcome of these pitfalls is that 12–20% of normal embryos may be excluded from transfer, placing women with a low embryo yield at a significant risk of not having embryos transferred at all. Finally, even if a good number of biopsied embryos have been found 'normal', women failing to conceive after the fresh transfer are disadvantaged since the surplus 'normal' embryos do not have the same potential for survival after cryopreservation and thawing compared with intact embryos without a zona breach.

There is a clear need for randomised controlled trials examining the outcome of PGS in terms of live birth per cycle started in order to define the groups for whom this technique may be beneficial over conventional IVF. This is an expensive, and yet unproven, test that is taken up by women desperate to gain a pregnancy when, for some, it might actually decrease their chances of pregnancy by reducing the cohort of normal embryos available for transfer.

Social sex selection

The use of PGD for sex selection to prevent X-linked disorders has been extended to the selection of a child of a particular gender. This may be either by preference where selection is predominantly for one sex when only one child is allowed, or where male offspring are favoured over female for cultural or economic reasons. Alternatively, it may be performed for 'family balancing' where there is already one or more child of a particular sex in the family and there is a desire for a child of the other sex. In the UK, after a second public consultation, the HFEA has reaffirmed its original position in opposing any form of sex selection for non-medical reasons.[38]

This is not the case in many other countries in the world where sex selection is viewed as acceptable and sex selection by FISH is permitted as an alternative to PND, with a predictable bias towards male children.[39] However, as it is still an expensive technique that requires substantial expertise and equipment, it is not widely available and thus has little chance of altering the sex ratio compared with abortion or feticide, which is still practised in a number of countries even where it is outlawed.

Pre-implantation HLA typing

Pre-implantation human leukocyte antigen (HLA) matching has been used to ensure that an embryo to be replaced after IVF and PGD will be a suitable tissue match for an affected sibling, where it is intended that cord blood will be harvested at birth for use in bone marrow cell therapy.[40] The first such case was Adam Nash, born following PGD not only to exclude his being affected by Fanconi anaemia, but also so that he would be a suitable match for his sister Molly who suffered from the condition and required a bone marrow transplant.[41] In these situations, a large number of embryos are likely to be discarded as only 3 in 16 embryos will both be unaffected by the recessive disorder and be a full HLA match. Coupled with this is a 20–25% success rate of pregnancy, which may be worse depending on the woman's age. Several PGD cycles might have to be performed to achieve a match, let alone a successful pregnancy. Pre-implantation HLA genotyping in combination with PGD for causative genes has also been performed for thalassaemia, hyperimmunoglobulin M syndrome, X-linked adrenoleukodystrophy and Wiskott–Aldrich syndrome.[2] HLA typing without PGD in the absence of a high-risk genetic transmissible disease is even more controversial. Here, there may be no pre-existing genetic condition to be avoided, but the PGD performed with the sole objective of pre-selecting HLA-matched progeny for cell therapy treatment of siblings. Although the likelihood of match is higher, (one in four embryos is likely to be a suitable match), the fact that 75% of the created essentially normal embryos will be unsuitable and discarded leads to substantial ethical disquiet as the embryos are being typed and conceived for no other reason than to be a match for an affected brother or sister.[42] Issues of consent and protection of the children's autonomy are raised, especially should the cord blood fail to yield sufficient stem cells or if the cell therapy should fail.

Future developments

Rapid and efficient analysis of all 46 chromosomes is the ideal as some embryos diagnosed as normal can still be abnormal for other aneuploidies not currently analysed. So far the most promising method is comparative genomic hybridisation (CGH), where molecular techniques are used to perform a quantitative analysis of the whole genome, although polyploidy and balanced translocations cannot be detected.[43] This technique currently requires two or three days for diagnosis and is therefore not yet suitable for routine use on cleavage stage embryos or blastocysts, which need to be cryopreserved until the diagnosis has been made. Several continuing pregnancies and the birth of one healthy child have been reported, but at present the delay in diagnosis and damage caused by the freezing and thawing of biopsied embryos probably outweigh the benefits of CGH.

Faster and more robust techniques such as DNA microarrays may obviate the need for embryo freezing. This is a method of molecular analysis primarily used for gene expression analysis. However, it could also be applied to routine PGD to screen for mutations in any one gene, or for screening several genes for several mutations.[44] Microarrays might also be useful in PGD of specific conditions that are genetically heterogeneous and for which there are few common mutations, such as Duchenne muscular dystrophy, where it could provide a generic testing procedure applicable to all patients carrying the gene. The ability to screen mutations in one gene or several mutations for several genes would allow embryos to be screened for serious susceptibility traits loci, such as the breast cancer gene *BRCA1* or that for familial adenomatous polyposis coli. Finally, appropriately constructed microarrays might replace the need for metaphase spreads now used to assess chromosome imbalance during CGH.

Conclusion

PGD combines the technology of assisted reproduction and molecular and cytogenetics in order to perform a very early form of PND. Preliminary information and results so far suggest that it is probably safe and reliable. Although there is little evidence of impairment of embryonic development, there is also no good evidence for estimating its long-term safety, and there is still a small but significant risk of misdiagnosis. Thus quality standards should be as rigorous as for other forms of prenatal testing. Rapid advances in molecular genetics will allow efficient examination of the entire chromosomes of the embryo. More couples are likely to seek using the technology in order to improve their chances of successful IVF. Thus it is important that the use of PGD is strictly regulated for medical purposes and prohibited for social eugenic selection, and that the place of PGS to enhance IVF success is fully evaluated.

Acknowledgement

This chapter was modified from an article that appeared in *BJOG* in November 2004.[45]

References

1. Handyside AH, Lesko JG, Tarin JJ, Winston RM, Hughes MR. Birth of a normal girl after *in vitro* fertilization and preimplantation diagnostic testing for cystic fibrosis. *N Engl J Med* 1992;327:905–9.
2. Kuliev A, Verlinsky Y. Thirteen years' experience of preimplantation diagnosis: report of the Fifth International Symposium on Preimplantation Genetics. *Reprod Biomed Online* 2004;8:229–35.
3. Verlinsky Y, Ginsberg N, Lifchez A, Valle J, Moise J, Strom CM. Analysis of the first polar body: preconception genetic diagnosis. *Hum Reprod* 1990;5:826–9.
4. Magli MC, Gianaroli L, Fortini D, Ferraretti AP, Munne S. Impact of blastomere biopsy and cryopreservation techniques on human embryo viability. *Hum Reprod* 1999;14:770–3.
5. Handyside AH, Kontogianni EH, Hardy K, Winston RM. Pregnancies from biopsied human preimplantation embryos sexed by Y-specific DNA amplification. *Nature* 1990;344:768–70.
6. Gardner RL, Edwards RG. Control of the sex ratio at full term in the rabbit by transferring sexed blastocysts. *Nature* 1968;218:346–9.
7. Vidal F, Fugger EF, Blanco J, Keyvanfar K, Catala V, Norton M, *et al*. Efficiency of MicroSort flow cytometry for producing sperm populations enriched in X- or Y-chromosome haplotypes: a blind trial assessed by double and triple colour fluorescent in-situ hybridization. *Hum Reprod* 1998;13:308–12.
8. Human Fertilisation and Embryology Authority (HFEA). *Code of Practice*. 6th ed. London: HFEA; 2003.
9. ESHRE PGD Consortium Steering Committee.. ESHRE Preimplantation Genetic Diagnosis Consortium: data collection III (May 2001). *Hum Reprod* 2002;17:233–46.
10. National Institute for Clinical Excellence (NICE). *Fertility Assessment and Treatment for People with Fertility Problems*. London: National Collaborating Centre For Women and Children's Health; 2004 [www.nice.org.uk/CG011].
11. Caller J, Watson S. All work no go. Audit of PGD Referrals. Abstract presented at the British Society for Human Genetics, September 2004.
12. Griffin DK, Wilton LJ, Handyside AH, Atkinson GH, Winston RM, Delhanty JD. Diagnosis of sex

in preimplantation embryos by fluorescent *in situ* hybridisation. *BMJ* 1993;306:1382.

13. Munne S, Dailey T, Finkelstein M, Weier HU. Reduction in signal overlap results in increased FISH efficiency: implications for preimplantation genetic diagnosis. *J Assist Reprod Genet* 1996;13:149–56.

14. Gardner RGS. *Chromosome Abnormalities and Genetic Counselling*. 2nd ed. Oxford: Oxford University Press; 1996.

15. Zuffardi O, Tiepolo L. Frequencies and types of chromosome abnormalities associated with male infertility. In: Croigani P, Rubin B, editors. *Genetic Control of Gamete Production and Function*. London: Academic; 1982. p. 261–73.

16. Hook E. Chromosome abnormalities: prevalence, risks and recurrence. In: Broch D, Rodeck C, Ferguson-Smith M, editors. *Prenatal Diagnosis and Screening*. Edinburgh: Churchill Livingstone; 1992. p. 351–92.

17. Scriven PN, Flinter FA, Braude PR, Ogilvie CM. Robertsonian translocations – reproductive risks and indications for preimplantation genetic diagnosis. *Hum Reprod* 2001;16:2267–73.

18. Scriven PN, Handyside AH, Ogilvie CM. Chromosome translocations: segregation modes and strategies for preimplantation genetic diagnosis. *Prenat Diagn* 1998;18:1437–49.

19. Rai R, Backos M, El Gaddal S, Regan L. Recurrent miscarriage and parental karyotype abnormalities – prospective pregnancy outcome of spontaneously conceived pregnancies. In: *The Society for Gynecological Investigation Annual Meeting, 2004 March 24–27*. Houston, TX; 2004.

20. Ray PF, Ao A, Taylor DM, Winston RM, Handyside AH. Assessment of the reliability of single blastomere analysis for preimplantation diagnosis of the delta F508 deletion causing cystic fibrosis in clinical practice. *Prenat Diagn* 1998;18:1402–12.

21. Thornhill AR, McGrath JA, Eady RA, Braude PR, Handyside AH. A comparison of different lysis buffers to assess allele dropout from single cells for preimplantation genetic diagnosis. *Prenat Diagn* 2001;21:490–7.

22. Moutou C, Rongieres C, Bettahar-Lebugle K, Gardes N, Philippe C, Viville S. Preimplantation genetic diagnosis for achondroplasia: genetics and gynaecological limits and difficulties. *Hum Reprod* 2003;18:509–14.

23. Sermon K, De Vos A, Van de Velde H, Seneca S, Lissens W, Joris H, *et al.* Fluorescent PCR and automated fragment analysis for the clinical application of preimplantation genetic diagnosis of myotonic dystrophy (Steinert's disease). *Mol Hum Reprod* 1998;4:791–6.

24. Findlay I, Quirke P, Hall J, Rutherford A. Fluorescent PCR: a new technique for PGD of sex and single-gene defects. *J Assist Reprod Genet* 1996;13:96–103.

25. Strom CM, Levin R, Strom S, Masciangelo C, Kuliev A, Verlinsky Y. Neonatal outcome of preimplantation genetic diagnosis by polar body removal: the first 109 infants. *Pediatrics* 2000;106:650–3.

26. Kuliev A, Cieslak J, Ilkevitch Y, Verlinsky Y. Chromosomal abnormalities in a series of 6,733 human oocytes in preimplantation diagnosis for age-related aneuploidies. *Reprod Biomed Online* 2003;6:54–9.

27. Munne S, Magli C, Bahce M, Fung J, Legator M, Morrison L, *et al.* Preimplantation diagnosis of the aneuploidies most commonly found in spontaneous abortions and live births: XY, 13, 14, 15, 16, 18, 21, 22. *Prenat Diagn* 1998;18:1459–66.

28. Cramer DW, Wise LA. The epidemiology of recurrent pregnancy loss. *Semin Reprod Med* 2000;18:331–9.

29. De Braekeleer M, Dao TN. Cytogenetic studies in couples experiencing repeated pregnancy losses. *Hum Reprod* 1990;5:519–28.

30. Spandorfer SD, Chung PH, Kligman I, Liu HC, Davis OK, Rosenwaks Z. An analysis of the effect of age on implantation rates. *J Assist Reprod Genet* 2000;17:303–6.

31. Pehlivan T, Rubio C, Rodrigo L, Remohi J, Pellicer A, Simon C. Preimplantation genetic diagnosis by fluorescence *in situ* hybridization: clinical possibilities and pitfalls. *J Soc Gynecol Investig* 2003;10:315–22.

32. Kent-First MG, Kol S, Muallem A, Ofir R, Manor D, Blazer S, *et al.* The incidence and possible relevance of Y-linked microdeletions in babies born after intracytoplasmic sperm injection and their infertile fathers. *Mol Hum Reprod* 1996;2:943–50.

33. Bonduelle M, Van Assche E, Joris H, Keymolen K, Devroey P, Van Steirteghem A, *et al.* Prenatal testing in ICSI pregnancies: incidence of chromosomal anomalies in 1586 karyotypes and relation to sperm parameters. *Hum Reprod* 2002;17:2600–14.

34. Levron J, Aviram-Goldring A, Madgar I, Raviv G, Barkai G, Dor J. Studies on sperm chromosomes in patients with severe male factor infertility undergoing assisted reproductive technology treatment. *Mol Cell Endocrinol* 2001;183 Suppl 1:S23–8.

35. Munne S, Magli C, Cohen J, Morton P, Sadowy S, Gianaroli L, *et al.* Positive outcome after

preimplantation diagnosis of aneuploidy in human embryos. *Hum Reprod* 1999;14:2191–9.

36. Munne S. Preimplantation genetic diagnosis and human implantation – a review. *Placenta* 2003;24 Suppl B:S70–6.

37. Harper JC, Coonen E, Handyside AH, Winston RM, Hopman AH, Delhanty JD. Mosaicism of autosomes and sex chromosomes in morphologically normal, monospermic preimplantation human embryos. *Prenat Diagn* 1995;15:41–9.

38. Human Fertilisation and Embryology Authority (HFEA). *Sex Selection: Options for Regulation.* London: HFEA; 2003.

39. Kilani Z, Haj Hassan L. Sex selection and preimplantation genetic diagnosis at The Farah Hospital. *Reprod Biomed Online* 2002;4:68–70.

40. Verlinsky Y, Rechitsky S, Sharapova T, Morris R, Taranissi M, Kuliev A. Preimplantation HLA testing. *JAMA* 2004;291:2079–85.

41. Verlinsky Y, Rechitsky S, Schoolcraft W, Strom C, Kuliev A. Preimplantation diagnosis for Fanconi anemia combined with HLA matching. *JAMA* 2001;285:3130–3.

42. Boyle RJ, Savulescu J. Ethics of using preimplantation genetic diagnosis to select a stem cell donor for an existing person. *BMJ* 2001;323:1240–3.

43. Wells D, Delhanty JD. Comprehensive chromosomal analysis of human preimplantation embryos using whole genome amplification and single cell comparative genomic hybridization. *Mol Hum Reprod* 2000;6:1055–62.

44. Clarke PA, te Poele R, Wooster R, Workman P. Gene expression microarray analysis in cancer biology, pharmacology, and drug development: progress and potential. *Biochem Pharmacol* 2001;62:1311–36.

45. Grace J, El Toukhy T, Braude P. Pre-implantation genetic testing. *BJOG* 2004;111:1165–73.

SECTION 3

LESSONS FROM ANIMAL MODELS (TRANSGENICS) AND NOVEL TECHNOLOGIES

Chapter 15

To implant or not to implant: the role of leukaemia inhibitory factor

Susan J Kimber, Ali A Fouladi-Nashta, Lisa Mohamet,
Carolyn JP Jones and Gemma Schofield

Introduction

Embryo implantation in the uterus is a unique feature of mammalian reproduction and a tightly regulated process. Changes in ovarian steroids during the pre-implantation period instigate the maturation of the endometrial epithelium and stroma required for implantation to occur in all mammals. In rodents, following priming with pre-ovulatory oestrogen, increased ovarian progesterone produces a sensitised uterus, which becomes receptive to interaction with the blastocyst after a subsequent small transient increase in oestrogen.[1] Implantation is restricted to a short period of the reproductive cycle, the receptive period, which is about 18–24 h in rodents and probably several days in the human.[2] Experimentally, the amount of oestrogen given can influence the duration of the receptive phase.[3] The endometrial response involves differentiation of the endometrial epithelium and stroma to facilitate implantation and allow interaction with the blastocyst trophectoderm. It is the luminal epithelium (LE) with which the trophectoderm of the activated blastocyst first interacts and the epithelial changes are essential for the initiation of implantation.[4,5]

For successful completion of implantation and placenta formation, the steroid-prepared stroma must undergo a process of further differentiation, known as decidualisation, triggered by blastocyst signals. This requires an embryonic signal (or artificial mimic) and is induced in stroma around the implantation site from late day 4 of pregnancy in mice. In women, decidualisation can occur in the absence of an embryo. Decidualisation involves changes in expression of a large number of genes[6,7] and is marked by a rapid increase in vascular permeability with resulting oedema in the stroma around the implantation site.[8] Furthermore, in mice it has been shown to occur in the absence of a functional oestrogen receptor (ERα)[9–11] in spite of the well-established requirement for oestrogen priming before blastocyst signals can establish a decidual response. Following the receptive period, the uterus becomes refractory, no longer allowing implantation of any remaining blastocysts. Thus tightly regulated synchrony between embryonic development and uterine maturation is essential for successful pregnancy.

This synchrony makes it clear that implantation of the mammalian embryo requires a strictly coordinated interaction between the embryo and the uterus. Although it has long been known that ovarian steroids regulate this process, it is only in the past two decades that some of the local factors have been identified. Steroidal regulation of uterine function is mediated to a large extent through the action of a number of growth factors and cytokines and their receptors (reviewed by Saito[12] and Sharkey[13]). One essential cytokine is leukaemia inhibitory factor (LIF), a member of the interleukin 6 (IL6) family. LIF is a highly glycosylated 40–50 kDa glycoprotein with a range of biological functions. It is expressed in various embryonic and adult tissues,[14,15] with particularly high levels in the uterus. At the cell surface, LIF receptor β (LIFRβ) binds the glycoprotein gp130 (the common signalling receptor for IL6 family cytokines) to form a high-affinity receptor through which LIF signalling occurs.[16] In inbred female C57BL mice null for the LIF gene, embryos develop to the blastocyst stage but do not implant[17,18] and their uteri show little evidence of decidualisation.[19] We observed the same phenotype in LIF knockout animals on an outbred, MF1 background[20] using LIF-null animals derived by Dani and colleagues.[21] In spite of the presence of antimesometrially located blastocysts in the uterine lumen, no decidual reaction was evident at the light or electron microscope level, nor was there penetration of the LE by trophoblast even by day 7 of pregnancy (Figure 15.1). LIF-null embryos can implant in the uteri of wild-type female mice and delivery of LIF by microosmotic pump, or by injection, on day 4 restores implantation in homozygous mutant females.[17,19,22] Since LIF-null embryos develop to term in heterozygous dams and can implant after transfer to wild-type females of appropriate endocrine status, it is clear that the major implantation defect is on the maternal side. This is supported by the successful implantation of embryos lacking components of the LIF signalling cascade. For instance, gp130-null embryos die during the second half of gestation,[23] and LIFRβ knockout animals implant normally but have placental defects and motor neuron degeneration and die at birth.[24] However, prevention of gp130 signalling leads to an identical implantation failure to LIF-null mice (see below).[25] Thus the lack of LIF signalling in a pregnant female prevents implantation, showing that the action of LIF in the uterus is essential for this process. However, the precise role of maternal LIF at the molecular level is still not clear in any species.

LIF in humans

LIF is also involved in endometrial function in humans and domestic species.[15,26,27] In the human, LIF mRNA and protein are expressed in the endometrial glands during the luteal phase of the menstrual cycle when implantation would occur,[28,29] and LIFRβ and gp130 are expressed in LE throughout the cycle in women of proven fertility[30] but LIF mRNA is also expressed in stroma.[31] A correlation between LIF and LIFR levels and the formation on LE of bulbous protrusions known as pinopodes or uterodomes (indicative of receptivity) has been suggested.[32] Furthermore, recent evidence indicates that human chorionic gonadotrophin (hCG) as well as transforming growth factor β (TGFβ) and insulin–like growth factors IGF1 and IGF2 can stimulate LIF secretion by isolated endometrial epithelial cells in the human, suggesting a role for the peri-implantation blastocyst in regulating endometrial LIF.[33] TGFβ and interleukin 1β (IL1β) have already been demonstrated to stimulate LIF expression in human uterine stromal cultures.[34] Levels of LIF in uterine flushings were suggested to be lower in women with unexplained infertility,[35] but in another study lower levels of LIF were suggested as predictive of implantation success.[36] Since these levels may not reflect the LIF concentration to which (basal) LE is exposed, and

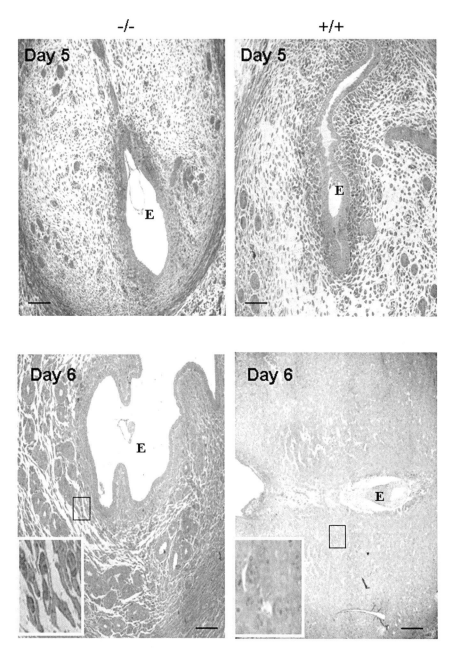

Figure 15.1. Histological features of the uterus in LIF-null and wild-type mice. Semi-thin resin sections from day 5 and 6 of pregnancy were stained with toluidine blue. The insets show high magnification of differentiated polygonal stromal cells in the wild-type and undifferentiated fibroblast-like stroma cells in the LIF-null mice on day 6 of pregnancy. E = embryo; scale bar = 50 μm; reproduced with permission from Fouladi-Nashta et al.[20] (Developmental Biology, © 2005 Elsevier)

in any case the concentration of LIF required for threshold responses of LE *in vivo* is unknown, interpretation of these observations is difficult. No statistically significant difference was found in LIF levels between women with recurrent implantation failure and multiparous women in the control group.[37] Defects in LIF expression are associated with recurrent miscarriage and a subset of conditions of unexplained infertility, suggesting one or more roles in early events in pregnancy.[26,27]

Regulation of LIF

In mice, the highest levels of LIF mRNA are found prior to implantation in glandular epithelium following the nidatory surge of oestrogen on the morning of day 4 of pregnancy.[17,19] The highest levels of LIF protein have also been reported on day 4, mainly in the epithelium but also in the stroma.[38,39] In ovariectomised mice, uterine LIF mRNA increases markedly within 1 h of oestrogen injection and is not affected by progesterone, strongly suggesting oestrogenic control.[19,40,41] LIF mRNA declines to a low level by day 6/7 of pregnancy and the transient nature of the LIF signal may be important to its role in implantation. Recent evidence suggests that, in human endometrial epithelial cells, LIF and LIFR, IL1β, its receptor and receptor antagonist are all regulated by leptin through interaction with its receptor OBR.[42,43] Moreover, IL1β as well as leptin upregulate LIFR and both effects are blocked by inhibition of IL1 receptor type I (IL1R tI). Thus it appears that leptin may be a primary regulator of LIF, at least in human endometrium, and feedback loops may exist between IL1 and LIF in endometrial epithelial cells. It remains to be demonstrated whether IL1 upregulates LIF and its receptor in murine endometrial epithelial cells or whether there is any cycle-dependent specificity in these interactions. Interestingly, progesterone and IL4 both upregulate LIF in Th2 cells[44] and it is notable that the absence of LIF has recently been shown to result in low levels of a number of progesterone-responsive genes in the uterus (see below).[22]

Cellular targets of LIF in the uterus

A key cellular target for LIF appears to be the LE. Here, LIF-receptor mRNA increases from day 3 to 4 of pregnancy, just at the time of implantation. However, both LIFR and gp130 protein can be detected in LE on all of days 3–5 of pregnancy. Expression of gp130 in LE is stimulated by oestrogen together with progesterone.[45,46] LIF signalling in the uterus occurs mainly through the JAK/STAT pathway (rather than the SHP-2/Ras/ERK pathway), via STAT3 which is present in LE throughout early pregnancy but only susceptible to activation (via tyrosine phosphorylation) on day 4, just prior to implantation.[45] This indicates that the temporal response to LIF in LE may partly be regulated at the level of STAT3 phosphorylation. Indeed, mice homozygous for deletion of the gp130 STAT activation site show an identical infertility defect to LIF-null females.[25] Suppressor of cytokine signalling protein 3 (SOCS3) is induced by LIF and inhibits phosphorylation of gp130 and STATs. It has been implicated in regulating uterine LIF signalling. SOCS3 knockout mice are also embryonic lethal.[47] It is therefore likely that LIF acts to facilitate blastocyst-induced decidualisation on days 4–5 of pregnancy by activation of STAT3 signalling in the LE and subsequent gene expression. At the implantation site, the progesterone-primed LE is now able to respond to LIF combined with blastocyst signals which trigger production of local decidualising molecules. In culture, we have shown that LIF induces IL1α secretion by semi-polarised LE, an effect blocked by a competitive inhibitor of LIF.[48] IL1 has previously been shown to induce stromal expression of cyclooxygenase 2 (COX2), a key enzyme in prostaglandin (PG) synthesis, as well as PGE$_2$ synthesis *in vitro*.[49–51] Since PGE$_2$ is a well-established stimulus for vascular oedema, angiogenesis and decidual cell differentiation,[52–54] it is possible that LIF together with a blastocyst signal(s) is transduced by LE which is induced to secrete IL1 that in turn triggers local decidual changes. One problem with this scheme is that, *in vitro,* LIF was found to induce greater apical secretion of IL1 by LE, although it is possible that, under *in vivo* conditions, secretion is directed basally, or that basal secretion is induced by the presence of the blastocyst.

However, LIFR and gp130 are also expressed in decidualising stroma[39,46] and we have shown that LIF has a moderate dose-dependent inhibitory effect on stromal decidualisation *in vitro*.[39] This direct effect may limit decidualisation to the implantation site, thus helping to account for the discrete domain of the decidual reaction and preventing the wasted energy involved in its spread to uterine segments lacking an implanting embryo.

Although the major emphasis has been on the role of LIF at the time of implantation, it is important to realise that LIF may also affect uterine cells in the pre-implantation period since it is transiently expressed after ovulation on day 1 of pregnancy, mainly by the LE. Since LIF appears to be a downstream mediator of oestrogen action in the uterus, one possible role for LIF might be regulation of uterine cell proliferation. During the reproductive cycle, pre-ovulatory oestrogen stimulates luminal and glandular proliferation, which is curtailed by the rise in progesterone on days 2–3 of pregnancy. This inhibits epithelial proliferation and induces changes necessary for stromal proliferation to occur. Following the increase in progesterone, the transient rise in oestrogen early on day 4 of pregnancy stimulates stromal proliferation. It has been reported that LIF has no effect on proliferation in either LE or stroma during the pre-implantation period.[19] However, detailed comparison of different regions of the uterus between LIF–null and wild-type animals after labelling with the nucleotide precursor bromodeoxyuridine (BrdU) has revealed that cell proliferation is indeed altered in the absence of LIF. The overall percentage of proliferative cells was found to be reduced in the LIF–null uterus compared with wild type on days 4 and 5 of pregnancy. Regional differences were evident on days 4 and 5 of pregnancy: there was a significant decrease in proliferation in the outer stroma on day 4 while on day 5 a significant reduction in labelling in stroma adjacent to the LE was observed.[55] The latter may be partly accounted for by the lack of secondary signalling from unstimulated LE of the LIF–null uterus.

Our examination of sections through the LIF–null uterus suggested a greater number of gland profiles in LIF–null compared with wild-type uterus. We therefore carried out a morphometric analysis of uterine sections to quantify this (Figure 15.2).[55] Our results indicate that there are significantly more glandular profiles from day 3 of pregnancy in the absence of LIF. Thus LIF appears to have a cytostatic effect on glandular proliferation or branching morphogenesis. Interestingly, the *Hoxa11* knockout mouse does not express LIF in the uterus and shows a deficit of uterine glands. It is also known that oestrogen exposure at the correct time is critical to regular glandular morphogenesis. Diethylstilboestrol given *in utero* perturbs proper reproductive tract morphogenesis including inhibiting uterine gland development; an effect mimicked by loss of *Wnt7a*.[56,57] *Wnt7a*-null mice are sterile and in the adults uterine cell death is enhanced in response to diethylstilboestrol while proliferation is

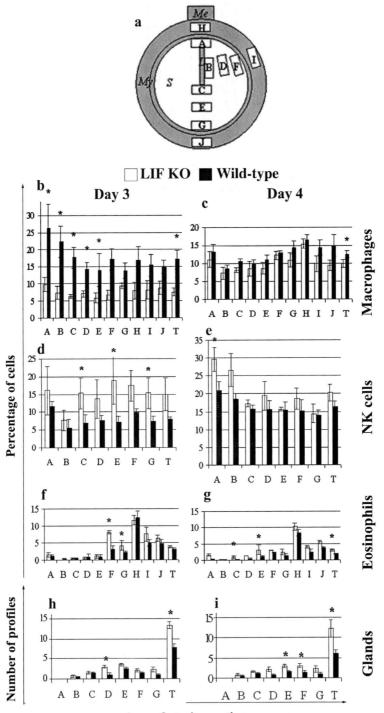

Area of uterine section

Figure 15.2.   The areas (A to J) of transverse uterine sections used for cell counting, shown in (a), were chosen to cover as many different regions of the uterus as possible. The mesometrium (*Me*) was used for orientation and bilateral symmetry was assumed throughout. The dimensions of each area were 100 μm × 200 μm. *L* = lumen; *My* = myometrium; *S* = stroma.

Cell counts for different leukocyte subpopulations in specified areas of the uterus (A to J) were carried out. T shows the total selected cell count for all areas as a % of total cells counted White bars represent LIF knockout mice and black bars wild-type mice. Asterisks indicate significant differences between LIF knockout and wild-type mice. Bar charts (b) and (c) show the percentages of macrophages in the uterus on days 3 and 4 of pregnancy in LIF-null and wild-type uterus. Major differences were seen on day 3 when areas A to E in the stroma as well as the total gave significantly higher percentages of macrophages in the wild-type mice compared with the LIF knockouts. On day 4 differences between the wild-type and the LIF knockout mice were less apparent. Bar charts (d) and (e) show the percentages of natural killer (NK) cells from days 3 and 4 of pregnancy. The biggest differences can be seen on day 3 when areas C, E and G all have significantly higher percentages of NK cells in the LIF knockout mice compared with the wild types. By day 4 only area A adjacent to the lumen shows a higher percentage on NK cells in the LIF knockout uteri. Bar charts (f) and (g) show the percentages of eosinophils on days 3 and 4 of pregnancy. Area H in the mesometrial triangle consistently contained the highest percentage of eosinophils in both wild-type and LIF knockout mice throughout pregnancy. No significant differences were seen between LIF knockout and wild-type mice until day 3 of pregnancy when areas F and G in the outer stroma had a higher proportion of eosinophils in the LIF knockout uteri. On day 4 areas C and E in the inner stroma contained higher percentages of eosinophils in the LIF knockout mice. In (h) and (i) the number of glandular profiles per 20 000 μm^2 areas in wild-type and null uterus are shown. Glandular profiles were increased in LIF-nulls compared with wild-type on days 3 and 4 of pregnancy particularly in mid- and some outer stromal areas. Parts a–g of this figure were originally published in Schofield and Kimber.[61] (*Biology of Reproduction*, © 2005 Elsevier)

unaffected. These animals also show a range of molecular misregulations in the adult uterus.

In addition to epithelial cells and stromal fibroblasts, other cell populations such as leucocytes may be adversely effected in the absence of LIF. Macrophages, natural killer (NK) cells and eosinophils are present in the pregnant uterus and are thought to be beneficial. Alterations in the proportions of NK cells and macrophages can adversely affect pregnancy.[58–60] We used a combination of immunocytochemistry, cell counting and flow cytometry to compare the distributions and dynamics of leucocyte subpopulations in wild-type and LIF knockout mice.[61] It was striking that we found that the percentage of macrophages was reduced by more than half in the LIF knockout mice on day 3 of pregnancy and their distribution was altered (Figure 15.2), suggesting that LIF is a chemokine for these cells. NK cells were detected as early as day 3 of pregnancy in wild-type and LIF-null mice but the LIF-null mice had double the percentage of NK cells compared with wild-type mice at this time, indicating that LIF restricts the migration of NK cells into the uterus. LIF-null mice also had significantly higher percentages of eosinophils in the outer stroma on day 3 and the midstroma on day 4 of pregnancy, so LIF may also restrict eosinophil migration to the uterus. These alterations in the uterine leucocyte subpopulations in LIF-null mice may give rise to a less robust pregnancy and contribute to failure of implantation.

Ultrastructural changes during the peri-implantation period in LIF-null mice

In wild-type animals, luminal epithelial cell polarity becomes less marked in the peri-implantation period when latero-basal markers become detectable in the apical membrane.[62] In LIF-null animals on days 4–5 of pregnancy, the LE cells appear to remain columnar, as for wild-type LE on days 2–3, with a rather domed apical surface. Prior to implantation, LE cells normally become more cuboidal and microvilli are replaced by pinopods,[63–65] which increase in number up to day 5 postcoitus.[66] In rodents these apical modifications of the uterine LE appear to mediate uptake of fluid[67] and macromolecules,[68] although not in humans.[69] In LIF-null mice, pinopods do not develop over the apical cell membranes, which remain microvillous (Figure 15.3) up to day 7 of pregnancy.[20] In humans, equivalent structures, utero-domes, have been associated with receptivity[70] and it has been suggested that they carry potential embryo-adhesion molecules.[71,72] It is likely that the failure of embryos to develop intimate association with the LE of LIF-null mice relates to the lack of apical maturation and pinopod formation by these cells. HOXA10 is also required for pinopod formation: after HOXA10-antisense treatment, pinopods do not appear on the LE at the start of the period of receptivity.[73] Thus both HOXA10 and LIF appear to drive pinopod formation on the murine LE.

Stromal cells at the implantation site show marked signs of differentiation by day 5 of wild-type pregnancy.[8] They enlarge, take on a more epithelial appearance with deposition of glycogen in the cytoplasm and some become binucleate. By day 6, loss of extracellular matrix and close cell–cell apposition is apparent in cells in the primary decidual zone. The LIF-null mice, however, show only features characteristic of the pre-implantation period, with none of the ultrastructural changes in stromal cells indicating decidualisation.

Molecular changes in the luminal epithelium of LIF-null animals

In the LE, a number of molecules are downregulated or disappear at or just after implantation, including the H-type-1 glycan,[4,74] MUC1[75] and desmosomes,[76] while there are also changes in tight junction proteins.[65,77] The mucin MUC1, which has been postulated to form a barrier to embryo attachment and which normally disappears from the LE at implantation, is removed on schedule in the LIF-null uterus.[19,20] However, we detected several molecular defects in the receptive-stage LE. Changes in LE glycosylation occur in the pre-and peri-implantation period[74,78] and the failure to develop uterodomes in LIF-null mice is associated with aberrant retention of glycosyl residues on the surface of the LE. This includes the presence of a more prominent glycocalyx on the luminal epithelial microvilli as seen in the electron microscope (Figure 15.3) as well as the continued expression of H-type-1 antigen to day 6 (Figure 15.4) and increase in fucosylated molecules bound by lectins from *Ulex europaeus* (*Ulex europaeus* lectin 1, UEA1) and *Tetragonolobus purpureus* (*Tetragonolobus purpureus* agglutinin, LTA) over the peri-implantation period.[20] Our

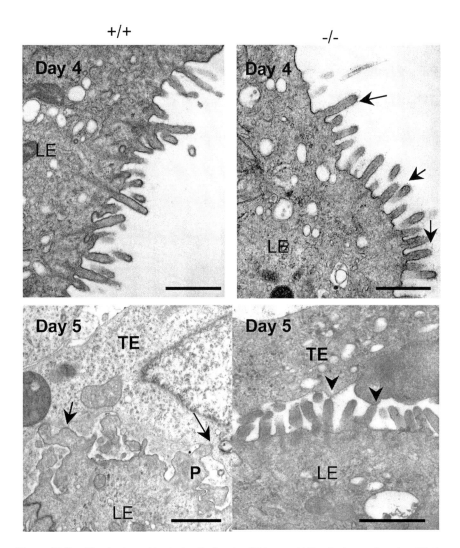

Figure 15.3. Ultrastructure of luminal epithelium in wild-type and LIF-null mice on days 4 and 5 of pregnancy. On day 4, both the wild-type and null mouse have columnar luminal uterine epithelium (LE) bearing microvilli, but the microvilli of the wild-type mouse have less glycocalyx than that of the null animal, which has a prominent filamentous covering over many microvillous processes (arrows). The scale bars represent 0.5 µm except for day 5 +/+ where it represents 1 µm. On the morning of day 5 of pregnancy it can be seen that, in the wild type, pinopods (P) of the LE make close contact, sometimes indenting the surface of the blastocyst (arrows), whereas in the null mouse the blastocyst is only contacted by the tips of untransformed microvilli (arrow heads) and no intimate contact is made. Reproduced with permission from Fouladi-Nashta et al.[20] (*Developmental Biology*, © 2005 Elsevier)

previous data have implicated the H-type-1 antigen in implantation[78–80] and this epitope showed a dramatic enhancement in LE adjacent to the day 5 embryo in the null uterus. Continued presence of H-type-1 on day 6 LE cells may indicate that LIF, either directly, or indirectly in conjunction with embryonic signalling, induces its downregulation as the uterus becomes refractory. A similar misregulation appears to occur for transcripts of the homeodomain protein MSX1.[81] It is absent on day 1 but strongly expressed in LE and glands on the morning of day 4 of pregnancy and then dramatically downregulated by the evening of day 4 in both pregnancy and pseudopregnancy.[81] However, in LIF-null mice this downregulation does not occur.

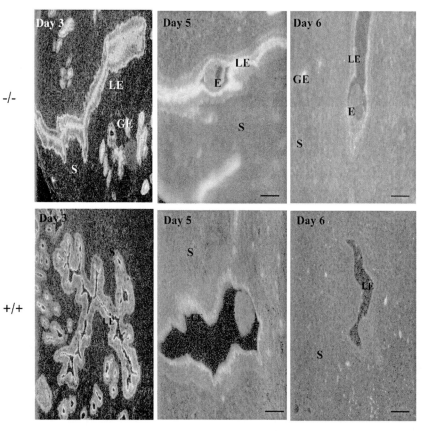

Figure 15.4. Immunofluorescence staining for H-type-1 antigen in LIF-null and wild-type mouse uterus. Frozen sections from days 3, 5 and 6 after mating were stained for H-type-1 using mouse monoclonal 667/9E9, which is expressed in the luminal epithelium. Note the retention of H-type-1 staining on days 5 and 6. E = embryo; GE = glandular epithelium; LE = luminal epithelium; S = stroma. Scale bar = 50 μm. Reproduced with permission from Fouladi-Nashta *et al.*[20] (*Developmental Biology,* © 2005 Elsevier)

Molecular responses to LIF in the stroma

A number of molecules have been suggested to be regulated by LIF during the peri-implantation period but this work has been almost exclusively at the transcript level.[22,81–83] Transcript analysis of expression at the implantation site in LIF-null mice suggests molecular abnormalities associated with the lack of decidualisation. However, it is important to note that many of these aberrations may be secondary effects of the lack of proper signalling between the blastocyst and LE in the absence of the influence of LIF on LE. For example, at the mRNA level there is an absence of expression of stromal COX2 and heparin-binding epidermal growth factor (EGF)-like growth factor (HB-EGF) in the LE at the implantation site.[82] Prostaglandins and prostacyclins, products of COX enzyme activity, have been considered important in initiating decidualisation[50,51,84] (as already mentioned) and local transmembrane HB-EGF on LE is a suggested attachment factor for both murine and human blastocysts.[31,85]

Little is understood about the expression of decidual proteins in LIF-null mice. We therefore examined some of the proteins suggested to be direct or indirect targets of LIF, as well as others with expression patterns fitting that role. We found misexpression of a number of decidual markers such as desmin,[87] bone morphogenetic proteins BMP2 and BMP4[7] and tenascin C, which is located in stroma cells immediately around the implanting embryo.[88] Interestingly, tenascin C has been suggested to be progesterone-regulated through IL1α and prostglandins,[89] both of which are clearly influenced by LIF (see above). COX2 protein, as for the mRNA, is aberrantly expressed: protein is found in the LE adjacent to the embryo but there is extremely limited expression in adjacent stroma (Figure 15.5). Thus misregulation of COX-2 mRNA and protein provides further evidence for the idea that a LIF-mediated signalling cascade involving IL1 induction of PGs is involved in the decidualisation response.

One of the most distinctive aspects of the LIF-null phenotype is the complete absence at the implantation site of expression of oncostatin M (OSM), another member of the IL6 family (Figure 15.5).[20] OSM is a 28kDa protein that binds to a heterodimeric receptor consisting of the OSMRβ and gp130, although human OSM (but not murine) can also signal through the LIFR.[90,91] Signalling leads to activation of STATs (3 and/or 5) and the ERK pathway. While they do have overlapping functions, LIF and OSM have also been shown to have distinct independent functions in the same system.[90] OSM shows exquisitely defined temporal and spatial regulation in the murine uterus, which is quite distinct from the (glandular) expression seen for LIF. OSM is only expressed adjacent to the implanting mouse embryo, first in the LE and then in adjacent stroma at the implantation site (Figure 15.5).[20] The role of OSM has not been investigated before in mouse uterus, but in human it has recently been reported to reduce proliferation and induce differentiation in uterine stroma in the secretory phase.[93,94] In lung carcinoma cells, OSM upregulates the matrix metalloproteinase (MMP) inhibitor TIMP1 and plasminogen activator inhibitor (PAI)[95,96] while in vascular smooth-muscle cells it induces alkaline phosphatase and MMPs.[96] It is of interest that all of these are present in decidualising stroma at the time of implantation and the former two may regulate trophoblast protease activity.

Role of LIF in peri-implantation development of the embryo

As noted above, LIF-null, gp130-null and LIFR-null embryos are all able to progress through the pre-implantation period and implant in the wild-type uterus, suggesting

COX2

Oncostatin M

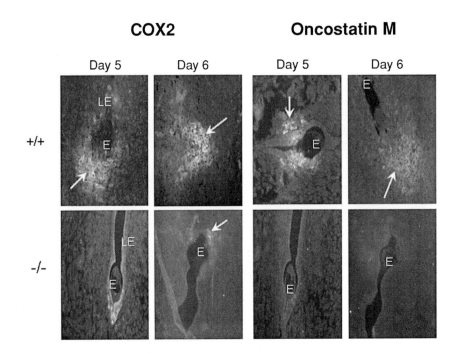

Figure 15.5. Immunofluorescence staining for COX2 and OSM in LIF-null and wild-type mouse uterus on days 5 and 6 of pregnancy. COX2 is strongly expressed in the luminal epithelium (LE) and underlying stromal cells (arrows) at the implantation site on day 5 and expression extended deeper into the stroma by day 6. In LIF-null mice, expression was limited to the LE cells and only a few stromal cells expressed COX2 in the day 6 uterus. The pattern of expression for OSM in wild-type mice was similar to that for COX2. In LIF-null mice, OSM was absent around the embryo on days 5 and 6 of pregnancy. E = embryo. Reproduced with permission from Fouladi-Nashta *et al.*[20] (*Developmental Biology*, © 2005 Elsevier)

that LIF has no function in the embryo during this time. However, gp130 is required for reactivation of the blastocyst to implant after the diapause-like condition induced by experimental delay of implantation.[97] Mammalian blastocysts express LIFR[98–100] and LIF enhances blastocyst development and differentiation *in vitro*.[101,102] Furthermore, it has been reported that the proportion of morulae and/or blastocysts is reduced after microinjection of LIF antisense at the two-cell stage. Blastocyst outgrowths upregulate MMP9 and urokinase-type plasminogen activator in response to LIF,[103] and MMP9 is implicated in trophoblast invasion into the uterus.[104] Moreover, LIF, TGFα and EGF-induced human trophoblast differentiation requires hCG, suggesting hCG is an autocrine or paracrine regulator of syncytiotrophoblast formation.[105] and it has already been mentioned that hCG has been shown to induce endometrial epithelial LIF secretion,[33] completing a possible regulatory cycle.

In our analysis of the progeny of matings involving animals with a deletion of the gene encoding LIF, we found that the number of nulls was 58–68% of that expected for a Mendelian ratio, for both males and females. The lower proportion of LIF-null offspring indicates some embryo loss in the MF1 strain of mouse. It has been reported that on an inbred C57BL6/J background there is no loss of null offspring *in utero* and Mendelian frequencies are obtained.[17] LIF has a variety of effects on different cell types *in vitro*, inhibiting the differentiation of embryonic stem cells and promoting the survival and/or proliferation of neurons, primitive haematopoietic precursors and primordial germ cells.[106] The breadth of influence is reflected in the defects reported in LIFR-null fetuses.[24] LIF-deficient mice derived by gene-targeting techniques have dramatically decreased numbers of stem cells in spleen and bone marrow, while heterozygous animals are intermediate in phenotype, implying that LIF has a dosage effect; defects in stem cell number can be compensated for by the introduction of exogenous LIF.[107]

Our results and those of others are steadily leading to a picture of multiple defects in LIF-null uteri. Working out the sequence of molecular interactions stemming from LIF function that are critical for implantation, rather than merely secondary repercussions of the loss of other primary targets, will require further research. The molecular cascades controlling implantation of the embryo require strict temporal and spatial regulation. A remarkable degree of synchrony is needed between the epithelial and (various) stromal compartments of the uterus together with the developing embryo for successful implantation. This is perhaps most evident in species such as the mouse in which the period during which implantation can occur is so short. Even a short delay in maturation of the uterus will result in asynchrony with the embryo. Although asynchronous embryo transfer studies indicate that the embryo can normally wait while the uterus differentiates to the receptive state,[5] one may speculate that in the absence of LIF even a 24 h asynchrony may be fatal since the embryo can not be reactivated to implant in the absence of LIF. Therefore timeliness of expression, not just expression *per se,* is likely to be particularly important where LIF and its targets in the uterus are concerned.

Acknowledgements

This work was funded by a grant from the BBSRC to SJK, a BBSRC studentship to GS and an MRC studentship to LM. We sincerely thank Nahida Nijjar for technical support.

References

1. Finn CA, Martin L. The role of the oestrogen secreted before oestrus in the preparation of the uterus for implantation in the mouse. *J Endocrinol* 1970;47:431–8.
2. Navot D, Bergh PA, Williams M, Garrisi GJ, Guzman I, Sandler B, et al. An insight into early reproductive processes through the *in vivo* model of ovum donation. *J Clin Endocrinol Metab* 1991;72:408–14.
3. Ma WG, Song H, Das SK, Paria BC, Dey SK. Estrogen is a critical determinant that specifies the duration of the window of uterine receptivity for implantation. *Proc Natl Acad Sci U S A* 2003;100:2963–8.
4. Kimber SJ, Spanswick C. Blastocyst implantation: the adhesion cascade. *Semin Cell Dev Biol* 2000;11:77–92.
5. Aplin JD, Kimber SJ. Trophoblast-uterine interactions at implantation. *Reprod Biol Endocrinol* 2004;2:48.
6. Farrar JD, Carson DD. Differential temporal and spatial expression of mRNA encoding

extracellular matrix components in decidua during the peri-implantation period. *Biol Reprod* 1992;46:1095–108.

7. Paria BC, Ma W, Tan J, Raja S, Das SK, Dey SK, *et al.* Cellular and molecular responses of the uterus to embryo implantation can be elicited by locally applied growth factors. *Proc Natl Acad Sci U S A* 2001;98:1047–52.

8. Abrahamsohn PA, Zorn TM. Implantation and decidualization in rodents. *J Exp Zool* 1993;266:603–28.

9. Curtis SW, Clark J, Myers P, Korach KS. Disruption of estrogen signaling does not prevent progesterone action in the estrogen receptor alpha knockout mouse uterus. *Proc Natl Acad Sci U S A* 1999;96:3646–51.

10. Paria BC, Tan J, Lubahn DB, Dey SK, Das SK. Uterine decidual response occurs in estrogen receptor-alpha-deficient mice. *Endocrinology* 1999;140:2704–10.

11. Curtis Hewitt S, Goulding EH, Eddy EM, Korach KS. Studies using the estrogen receptor alpha knockout uterus demonstrate that implantation but not decidualization-associated signaling is estrogen dependent. *Biol Reprod* 2002;67:1268–77.

12. Saito S. Cytokine cross-talk between mother and the embryo/placenta. *J Reprod Immunol* 2001;52:15–33.

13. Sharkey A. Cytokines and implantation. *Rev Reprod* 1998;3:52–61.

14. Hilton DJ, Gough NM. Leukemia inhibitory factor: a biological perspective. *J Cell Biochem* 1991;46:21–6.

15. Schafer-Somi S. Cytokines during early pregnancy of mammals: a review. *Anim Reprod Sci* 2003;75:73–94.

16. Heinrich PC, Behrmann I, Haan S, Hermanns HM, Muller-Newen G, Schaper F. Principles of interleukin (IL)-6-type cytokine signalling and its regulation. *Biochem J* 2003;374:1–20.

17. Stewart CL, Kaspar P, Brunet LJ, Bhatt H, Gadi I, Kontgen F, *et al.* Blastocyst implantation depends on maternal expression of leukaemia inhibitory factor. *Nature* 1992;359:76–9.

18. Cheng JG, Rodriguez CI, Stewart CL. Control of uterine receptivity and embryo implantation by steroid hormone regulation of LIF production and LIF receptor activity: towards a molecular understanding of "the window of implantation". *Rev Endocr Metab Disord* 2002;3:119–26.

19. Chen JR, Cheng JG, Shatzer T, Sewell L, Hernandez L, Stewart CL. Leukemia inhibitory factor can substitute for nidatory estrogen and is essential to inducing a receptive uterus for implantation but is not essential for subsequent embryogenesis. *Endocrinology* 2000;141:4365–72.

20. Fouladi-Nashta AA, Jones CJ, Nijjar N, Mohamet L, Smith A, Chambers I, *et al.* Characterisation of the uterine phenotype during the peri-implantation period for LIF null, MF1 strain mice. *Dev Biol* 2005 in press online.

21. Dani C, Smith AG, Dessolin S, Leroy P, Staccini L, Villageois P, *et al.* Differentiation of embryonic stem cells into adipocytes *in vitro. J Cell Sci* 1997;110(Pt 11):1279–85.

22. Sherwin JR, Freeman TC, Stephens RJ, Kimber S, Smith AG, Chambers I, *et al.* Identification of genes regulated by leukemia-inhibitory factor in the mouse uterus at the time of implantation. *Mol Endocrinol* 2004;18:2185–95.

23. Yoshida K, Taga T, Saito M, Suematsu S, Kumanogoh A, Tanaka T, *et al.* Targeted disruption of gp130, a common signal transducer for the interleukin 6 family of cytokines, leads to myocardial and hematological disorders. *Proc Natl Acad Sci U S A* 1996;93:407–11.

24. Ware CB, Horowitz MC, Renshaw BR, Hunt JS, Liggitt D, Koblar SA, *et al.* Targeted disruption of the low-affinity leukemia inhibitory factor receptor gene causes placental, skeletal, neural and metabolic defects and results in perinatal death. *Development* 1995;121:1283–99.

25. Ernst M, Inglese M, Waring P, Campbell IK, Bao S, Clay FJ, *et al.* Defective gp130-mediated signal transducer and activator of transcription (STAT) signaling results in degenerative joint disease, gastrointestinal ulceration, and failure of uterine implantation. *J Exp Med* 2001;194:189–203.

26. Lass A, Weiser W, Munafo A, Loumaye E. Leukemia inhibitory factor in human reproduction. *Fertil Steril* 2001;76:1091–6.

27. Hambartsoumian E. Endometrial leukemia inhibitory factor (LIF) as a possible cause of unexplained infertility and multiple failures of implantation. *Am J Reprod Immunol* 1998;39:137–43.

28. Chen DB, Hilsenrath R, Yang ZM, Le SP, Kim SR, Chuong CJ, *et al.* Leukaemia inhibitory factor in human endometrium during the menstrual cycle: cellular origin and action on production of glandular epithelial cell prostaglandin *in vitro. Hum Reprod* 1995;10:911–18.

29. Vogiagis D, Marsh MM, Fry RC, Salamonsen LA. Leukaemia inhibitory factor in human endometrium throughout the menstrual cycle. *J Endocrinol* 1996;148:95–102.

30. Cullinan EB, Abbondanzo SJ, Anderson PS, Pollard JW, Lessey BA, Stewart CL. Leukemia inhibitory factor (LIF) and LIF receptor expression in human endometrium suggests a potential

autocrine/paracrine function in regulating embryo implantation. *Proc Natl Acad Sci U S A* 1996;93:3115–20.

31. Kojima K, Kanzaki H, Iwai M, Hatayama H, Fujimoto M, Inoue T, *et al.* Expression of leukemia inhibitory factor in human endometrium and placenta. *Biol Reprod* 1994;50:882–7.

32. Aghajanova L, Stavreus-Evers A, Nikas Y, Hovatta O, Landgren BM. Coexpression of pinopodes and leukemia inhibitory factor, as well as its receptor, in human endometrium. *Fertil Steril* 2003;79 Suppl 1:808–14.

33. Perrier d'Hauterive S, Charlet-Renard C, Berndt S, Dubois M, Munaut C, Goffin F, *et al.* Human chorionic gonadotrophin and growth factors at the embryonic–endometrial interface control leukemia inhibitory factor (LIF) and interleukin 6 (IL-6) secretion by human endometrial epithelium. *Hum Reprod* 2004;19:2633–43.

34. Arici A, Engin O, Attar E, Olive DL. Modulation of leukaemia inhibitory factor gene expression and protein biosynthesis in human endometrium. *J Clin Endocrinol Metab* 1995;80:1908–15.

35. Laird SM, Tuckerman EM, Dalton CF, Dunphy BC, Li TC, Zhang X. The production of leukaemia inhibitory factor by human endometrium: presence in uterine flushings and production by cells in culture. *Hum Reprod* 1997;12:569–74.

36. Ledee-Bataille N, Lapree-Delage G, Taupin JL, Dubanchet S, Frydman R, Chaouat G. Concentration of leukaemia inhibitory factor (LIF) in uterine flushing fluid is highly predictive of embryo implantation. *Hum Reprod* 2002;17:213–18.

37. Inagaki N, Stern C, McBain J, Lopata A, Kornman L, Wilkinson D. Analysis of intra-uterine cytokine concentration and matrix-metalloproteinase activity in women with recurrent failed embryo transfer. *Hum Reprod* 2003;18:608–15.

38. Yang ZM, Le SP, Chen DB, Cota J, Siero V, Yasukawa K, *et al.* Leukemia inhibitory factor, LIF receptor, and gp130 in the mouse uterus during early pregnancy. *Mol Reprod Dev* 1995;42:407–14.

39. Fouladi Nashta AA, Andreu CV, Nijjar N, Heath JK, Kimber SJ. Role of leukemia inhibitor factor (LIF) in decidualisation of murine uterine stromal cells *in vitro*. *J Endocrinol* 2004;181:477–92.

40. Bhatt H, Brunet LJ, Stewart CL. Uterine expression of leukemia inhibitory factor coincides with the onset of blastocyst implantation. *Proc Natl Acad Sci U S A* 1991;88:11408–12.

41. Stewart CL, Cullinan EB. Preimplantation development of the mammalian embryo and its regulation by growth factors. *Dev Genet* 1997;21:91–101.

42. Gonzalez RR, Leary K, Petrozza JC, Leavis PC. Leptin regulation of the interleukin-1 system in human endometrial cells. *Mol Hum Reprod* 2003;9:151–8.

43. Gonzalez RR, Rueda BR, Ramos MP, Littell RD, Glasser S, Leavis PC. Leptin-induced increase in leukemia inhibitory factor and its receptor by human endometrium is partially mediated by interleukin 1 receptor signaling. *Endocrinology* 2004;145:3850–7.

44. Piccinni MP, Beloni L, Livi C, Maggi E, Scarselli G, Romagnani S. Defective production of both leukemia inhibitory factor and type 2 T-helper cytokines by decidual T cells in unexplained recurrent abortions. *Nat Med* 1998;4:1020–4.

45. Cheng JG, Chen JR, Hernandez L, Alvord WG, Stewart CL. Dual control of LIF expression and LIF receptor function regulate Stat3 activation at the onset of uterine receptivity and embryo implantation. *Proc Natl Acad Sci U S A* 2001;98:8680–5.

46. Ni H, Ding NZ, Harper MJ, Yang ZM. Expression of leukemia inhibitory factor receptor and gp130 in mouse uterus during early pregnancy. *Mol Reprod Dev* 2002;63:143–50.

47. Roberts AW, Robb L, Rakar S, Hartley L, Cluse L, Nicola NA, *et al.* Placental defects and embryonic lethality in mice lacking suppressor of cytokine signaling 3. *Proc Natl Acad Sci U S A* 2001;98:9324–9.

48. Mohamet L, Fouladi-Nashta AA, Nijjar N, Heath JK, Kimber SK. Unpublished data.

49. Jacobs AL, Carson DD. Uterine epithelial cell secretion of interleukin-1 alpha induces prostaglandin E2 (PGE2) and PGF2 alpha secretion by uterine stromal cells *in vitro*. *Endocrinology* 1993;132:300–8.

50. Bany BM, Kennedy TG. Interleukin-1 alpha regulates prostaglandin production and cyclooxygenase activity in sensitized rat endometrial stromal cells *in vitro*. *Biol Reprod* 1995;53:126–32.

51. Jacobs AL, Hwang D, Julian J, Carson DD. Regulated expression of prostaglandin endoperoxide synthase-2 by uterine stroma. *Endocrinology* 1994;135:1807–15.

52. Sananes N, Baulieu EE, Le Goascogne C. Prostaglandin(s) as inductive factor of decidualization in the rat uterus. *Mol Cell Endocrinol* 1976;6:153–8.

53. Kennedy TG, Ross HE. Effect of prostaglandin E2 on rate of decidualization in rats. *Prostaglandins* 1993;46:243–50.

54. Kennedy TG. Evidence for a role for prostaglandins in the initiation of blastocyst implantation in the rat. *Biol Reprod* 1977;16:286–91.

55. Schofield G, Mohamet L, Tickle P, Kimber SK. Unpublished data.

56. Carta L, Sassoon D. Wnt7a is a suppressor of cell death in the female reproductive tract and is required for postnatal and estrogen-mediated growth. *Biol Reprod* 2004;71:444–54.

57. Miller C, Degenhardt K, Sassoon DA. Fetal exposure to DES results in de-regulation of Wnt7a during uterine morphogenesis. *Nat Genet* 1998;20:228–30.

58. Ashkar AA, Croy BA. Interferon-gamma contributes to the normalcy of murine pregnancy. *Biol Reprod* 1999;61:493–502.

59. Guimond MJ, Luross JA, Wang B, Terhorst C, Danial S, Croy BA. Absence of natural killer cells during murine pregnancy is associated with reproductive compromise in TgE26 mice. *Biol Reprod* 1997;56:169–79.

60. Pollard JW, Hunt JS, Wiktor-Jedrzejczak W, Stanley ER. A pregnancy defect in the osteopetrotic (op/op) mouse demonstrates the requirement for CSF-1 in female fertility. *Dev Biol* 1991;148:273–83.

61. Schofield G, Kimber SJ. Leukocyte subpopulations in the uteri of leukemia inhibitory factor knockout mice during early pregnancy. *Biol Reprod* 2004;72:872–8.

62. Thie M, Fuchs P, Denker HW. Epithelial cell polarity and embryo implantation in mammals. *Int J Dev Biol* 1996;40:389–93.

63. Nilsson O. Structural differentiation of luminal membrane in rat uterus during normal and experimental implantations. *Z Anat Entwicklungsgesch* 1966;125:152–9.

64. Kimber SJ. Carbohydrates and implantation of the mammalian embryo. In: Glasser SR, Mulholland J, Psychoyos A, editors. *Endocrinology of Embryo–Endometrium Interactions*. New York: Plenum; 1994. p. 279–96.

65. Murphy CR. Junctional barrier complexes undergo major alterations during the plasma membrane transformation of uterine epithelial cells. *Hum Reprod* 2000;15 Suppl 3:182–8.

66. Bansode FW, Chauhan SC, Makker A, Singh MM. Uterine luminal epithelial alkaline phosphatase activity and pinopod development in relation to endometrial sensitivity in the rat. *Contraception* 1998;58:61–8.

67. Enders AC, Nelson DM. Pinocytotic activity of the uterus of the rat. *Am J Anat* 1973;138:277–99.

68. Parr MB, Parr EL. Uterine luminal epithelium: protrusions mediate endocytosis, not apocrine secretion, in the rat. *Biol Reprod* 1974;11:220–33.

69. Adams SM, Gayer N, Hosie MJ, Murphy CR. Human uterodomes (pinopods) do not display pinocytotic function. *Hum Reprod* 2002;17:1980–6.

70. Nikas G, Drakakis P, Loutradis D, Mara-Skoufari C, Koumantakis E, Michalas S, *et al.* Uterine pinopodes as markers of the 'nidation window' in cycling women receiving exogenous oestradiol and progesterone. *Hum Reprod* 1995;10:1208–13.

71. Bentin-Ley U, Sjogren A, Nilsson L, Hamberger L, Larsen JF, Horn T. Presence of uterine pinopodes at the embryo–endometrial interface during human implantation *in vitro*. *Hum Reprod* 1999;14:515–20.

72. Creus M, Ordi J, Fabregues F, et Creus M, Ordi J, Fabregues F, *et al.* alphavbeta3 integrin expression and pinopod formation in normal and out-of-phase endometria of fertile and infertile women. *Hum Reprod* 2002;17:2279–86.

73. Bagot CN, Kliman HJ, Taylor HS. Maternal Hoxa10 is required for pinopod formation in the development of mouse uterine receptivity to embryo implantation. *Dev Dyn* 2001;222:538–44.

74. Kimber SJ, Lindenberg S, Lundblad A. Distribution of some Gal beta 1-3(4)GlcNAc related carbohydrate antigens on the mouse uterine epithelium in relation to the peri-implantational period. *J Reprod Immunol* 1988;12:297–313.

75. Braga VM, Gendler SJ. Modulation of Muc-1 mucin expression in the mouse uterus during the estrus cycle, early pregnancy and placentation. *J Cell Sci* 1993;105(Pt 2):397–405.

76. Illingworth IM, Kiszka I, Bagley S, Ireland GW, Garrod DR, Kimber SJ. Desmosomes are reduced in the mouse uterine luminal epithelium during the preimplantation period of pregnancy: a mechanism for facilitation of implantation. *Biol Reprod* 2000;63:1764–73.

77. Orchard MD, Murphy CR. Alterations in tight junction molecules of uterine epithelial cells during early pregnancy in the rat. *Acta Histochem* 2002;104:149–55.

78. Kimber SJ, Stones RE, Sidhu SS. Glycosylation changes during differentiation of the murine uterine epithelium. *Biochem Soc Trans* 2001;29:156–62.

79. Lindenberg S, Kimber SJ, Kallin E. Carbohydrate binding properties of mouse embryos. *J Reprod Fertil* 1990;89:431–9.

80. Lindenberg S, Sundberg K, Kimber SJ, Lundblad A. The milk oligosaccharide, lacto-*N*-fucopentaose I, inhibits attachment of mouse blastocysts on endometrial monolayers. *J Reprod Fertil* 1988;83:149–58.

81. Daikoku T, Song H, Guo Y, Riesewijk A, Mosselman S, Das SK, et al. Uterine Msx-1 and Wnt4 signaling becomes aberrant in mice with the loss of leukemia inhibitory factor or Hoxa-10: evidence for a novel cytokine-homeobox-Wnt signaling in implantation. *Mol Endocrinol* 2004;18:1238–50.

82. Song H, Lim H, Das SK, Paria BC, Dey SK. Dysregulation of EGF family of growth factors and COX-2 in the uterus during the preattachment and attachment reactions of the blastocyst with the luminal epithelium correlates with implantation failure in LIF-deficient mice. *Mol Endocrinol* 2000;14:1147–61.

83. Rodriguez CI, Cheng JG, Liu L, Stewart CL. Cochlin, a secreted von Willebrand factor type a domain-containing factor, is regulated by leukemia inhibitory factor in the uterus at the time of embryo implantation. *Endocrinology* 2004;145:1410–18.

84. Lim H, Paria BC, Das SK, Dinchuk JE, Langenbach R, Trzaskos JM, et al. Multiple female reproductive failures in cyclooxygenase 2-deficient mice. *Cell* 1997;91:197–208.

85. Raab G, Kover K, Paria BC, Dey SK, Ezzell RM, Klagsbrun M. Mouse preimplantation blastocysts adhere to cells expressing the transmembrane form of heparin-binding EGF-like growth factor. *Development* 1996;122:637–45.

86. Chobotova K, Spyropoulou I, Carver J, Manek S, Heath JK, Gullick WJ, et al. Heparin-binding epidermal growth factor and its receptor ErbB4 mediate implantation of the human blastocyst. *Mech Dev* 2002;119:137–44.

87. Glasser SR, Lampelo S, Munir MI, Julian J. Expression of desmin, laminin and fibronectin during *in situ* differentiation (decidualization) of rat uterine stromal cells. *Differentiation* 1987;35:132–42.

88. Julian J, Chiquet-Ehrismann R, Erickson HP, Carson DD. Tenascin is induced at implantation sites in the mouse uterus and interferes with epithelial cell adhesion. *Development* 1994;120:661–71.

89. Noda N, Minoura H, Nishiura R, Toyoda N, Imanaka-Yoshida K, Sakakura T, et al. Expression of tenascin-C in stromal cells of the murine uterus during early pregnancy: induction by interleukin-1 alpha, prostaglandin E(2), and prostaglandin F(2 alpha). *Biol Reprod* 2000;63:1713–20.

90. Ichihara M, Hara T, Kim H, Murate T, Miyajima A. Oncostatin M and leukemia inhibitory factor do not use the same functional receptor in mice. *Blood* 1997;90:165–73.

91. Wang Y, Robledo O, Kinzie E, Blanchard F, Richards C, Miyajima A, et al. Receptor subunit-specific action of oncostatin M in hepatic cells and its modulation by leukemia inhibitory factor. *J Biol Chem* 2000;275:25273–85.

92. Hara T, Tamura K, de Miguel MP, Mukouyama Y, Kim H, Kogo H, et al. Distinct roles of oncostatin M and leukemia inhibitory factor in the development of primordial germ cells and sertoli cells in mice. *Dev Biol* 1998;201:144–53.

94. Ogata I, Shimoya K, Moriyama A, Shiki Y, Matsumura Y, Yamanaka K, et al. Oncostatin M is produced during pregnancy by decidual cells and stimulates the release of HCG. *Mol Hum Reprod* 2000;6:750–7.

94. Ohata Y, Harada T, Fujii A, Yoshida S, Iwabe T, Terakawa N. Menstrual cycle-specific inhibition of endometrial stromal cell proliferation by oncostatin M. *Mol Hum Reprod* 2001;7:665–70.

95. Spence MJ, Streiff R, Day D, Ma Y. Oncostatin M induces tissue-type plasminogen activator and plasminogen activator inhibitor-1 in Calu-1 lung carcinoma cells. *Cytokine* 2002;18:26–34.

96. Macfelda K, Weiss TW, Kaun C, Breuss JM, Zorn G, Oberndorfer U, et al. Plasminogen activator inhibitor 1 expression is regulated by the inflammatory mediators interleukin-1alpha, tumor necrosis factor-alpha, transforming growth factor-beta and oncostatin M in human cardiac myocytes. *J Mol Cell Cardiol* 2002;34:1681–91.

97. Nichols J, Chambers I, Taga T, Smith A. Physiological rationale for responsiveness of mouse embryonic stem cells to gp130 cytokines. *Development* 2001;128:2333–9.

98. Charnock-Jones DS, Sharkey AM, Fenwick P, Smith SK. Leukaemia inhibitory factor mRNA concentration peaks in human endometrium at the time of implantation and the blastocyst contains mRNA for the receptor at this time. *J Reprod Fertil* 1994;101:421–6.

99. Nichols J, Davidson D, Taga T, Yoshida K, Chambers I, Smith A. Complementary tissue-specific expression of LIF and LIF-receptor mRNAs in early mouse embryogenesis. *Mech Dev* 1996;57:123–31.

100. Chen HF, Shew JY, Ho HN, Hsu WL, Yang YS. Expression of leukemia inhibitory factor and its receptor in preimplantation embryos. *Fertil Steril* 1999;72:713–19.

101. Dunglison GF, Barlow DH, Sargent IL. Leukaemia inhibitory factor significantly enhances the blastocyst formation rates of human embryos cultured in serum-free medium. *Hum Reprod* 1996;11:191–6.

102. Lavranos TC, Rathjen PD, Seamark RF. Trophic effects of myeloid leukaemia inhibitory factor (LIF) on mouse embryos. *J Reprod Fertil* 1995;105:331–8.

103. Harvey MB, Leco KJ, Arcellana-Panlilio MY, Zhang X, Edwards DR, Schultz GA. Proteinase expression in early mouse embryos is regulated by leukaemia inhibitory factor and epidermal growth factor. *Development* 1995;121:1005–14.
104. Salamonsen LA. Role of proteases in implantation. *Rev Reprod* 1999;4:11–22.
105. Yang M, Lei ZM, Rao ChV. The central role of human chorionic gonadotropin in the formation of human placental syncytium. *Endocrinology* 2003;144:1108–20.
106. Hilton DJ. LIF: lots of interesting functions. *Trends Biochem Sci* 1992;17:72–6.
107. Escary JL, Perreau J, Dumenil D, Ezine S, Brulet P. Leukaemia inhibitory factor is necessary for maintenance of haematopoietic stem cells and thymocyte stimulation. *Nature* 1993;363:361–4.

Chapter 16
Are gene arrays useful for the study of implantation?

Andrew Sharkey, Rob Catalano and Jane Borthwick

Introduction

The recent development of gene expression profiling using DNA microarrays has had a substantial impact on research into endometrial function. This approach allows the abundance of thousands of mRNA transcripts within tissue or isolated cells from endometrium to be measured simultaneously.[1] For the first time, this offers the prospect of understanding the subtle interactions between multiple genes that underlie complex cellular behaviours.

The endometrium is an extremely dynamic tissue that undergoes a series of changes under the influence of steroid hormones during each menstrual cycle. This results in cellular proliferation, maturation and the development of a receptive state, followed by menstruation and endometrial repair. Normal endometrial function therefore involves coordinated interactions between many cell types, including epithelium, stroma, endothelial cells and transient leucocyte populations. Understanding the underlying causes of common endometrial disorders such as menorrhagia, infertility and endometriosis represents a considerable challenge. The traditional approach to the study of such complex systems has been reductionist. Individual pathways and interactions are dissected in isolation in an attempt to explain normal and pathological physiology. Although immensely powerful, this approach has clear limitations. For example, when a cytokine binds to its receptor, several intracellular signalling pathways are activated, including protein phosphorylation, Ca^{2+} mobilisation and activation of transcription factors. Although we can describe in considerable detail each pathway at the molecular level, it is still impossible to predict the overall effect on cellular behaviour.

The use of high-throughput techniques such as microarrays or proteomics methods analysing thousands of genes or proteins simultaneously allows the response of the tissue as a whole integrated system to be determined. This provides a completely new approach to understanding the complex interactions between multiple genes that underlie both healthy and disease states. The responses of endometrium to physiological stimuli such as hormones or to drugs can be studied to define how patterns of gene expression change. In the area of diagnostics, microarrays offer great promise because of their ability to screen all known human transcripts. Their use can also permit more refined classification of diseases that are indistinguishable with current markers. This will allow development of novel therapies for endometrial dysfunction based on targeted drug discovery.

Although microarrays have only been used to study endometrium for a few years, they have significantly advanced our understanding of key areas of endometrial physiology, including infertility, receptivity, endometriosis, decidualisation and endometrial cancer. This article will review how microarray studies to date have advanced our understanding of critical aspects of the biology of implantation and discuss potential applications in the future.

Analysis with microarrays

All gene arrays for expression profiling depend on hybridisation of complementary strands of DNA or RNA. An array consists of the DNA sequences to be probed, attached in an ordered grid on a support of glass or nylon. They come in two main types: oligonucleotide arrays of synthetic DNA sequences between 20 and 80 base pairs long, and cDNA arrays in which portions of cDNA (each of several hundred base pairs) are mechanically spotted in an ordered grid. Small customised arrays targeted at particular pathways are available at low cost, whereas large generic arrays can contain probes complementary to all known transcripts for a particular species. The microarrays are most commonly assayed by hybridisation to the array of fluorescently labelled complex probes prepared from mRNA isolated from the cells or tissue of interest. The signal generated by the hybridisation of each labelled cDNA species to its complementary sequence on the array can then be measured using a confocal laser scanner.

Comparison between two RNA samples can be performed by hybridising each labelled cDNA separately to individual arrays, as occurs in the popular Affymetrix commercial arrays. Alternatively, cDNA from the two sources can be labelled with different fluorophores and hybridised simultaneously to the same array as shown in Figure 16.1. Quantification of the hybridisation of the two different fluorophores allows simultaneous determination of the relative expression levels of all the genes represented in the array between the two samples. A critical point to note is that the hybridisation signal for any one element on the array is not linearly related to abundance of the corresponding cDNA. A hybridisation signal that is two-fold stronger for a particular cDNA in one sample compared with another does not mean the corresponding mRNA is present at twice the level in that sample. Figure 16.2 shows a typical result following two-colour hybridisation to a human cDNA microarray. RNA isolated from endometrial stromal cells treated *in vitro* with 10 pg/ml of interleukin 1β (IL1β) for 24 h was labelled with Cy3 dye (green), and RNA from untreated cells was labelled with Cy5 dye (red). Equal amounts of each labelled cDNA were hybridised to a custom cDNA microarray. The hybridisation signal of the red and green channels from each cDNA spot on the array were quantified and plotted as shown in the figure. Since the majority of genes are equally expressed, these fall along the $y = x$ line with a gradient of 1. Genes that are highly up- or downregulated fall on either side of this line.

A significant challenge with microarray experiments is deciding how to analyse the raw data effectively to identify genes that differ significantly between two samples.[2,3] Many studies express the hybridisation signal obtained for each colour from a particular cDNA as a fold change (i.e. Cy3 signal 350, Cy5 signal 700, so the change

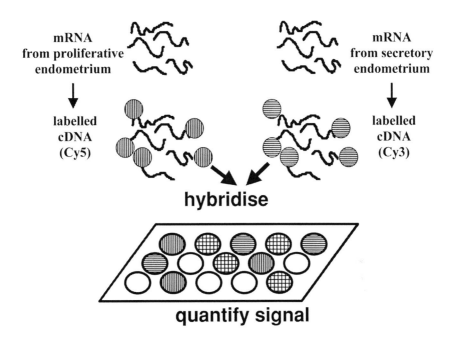

Figure 16.1. Flow diagram of a typical two-colour microarray experiment. In this example, cDNA is synthesised from proliferative endometrium and labelled with the fluorophore Cy5, and cDNA from secretory endometrium is labelled with Cy3. Equal amounts of the two are then hybridised simultaneously to a microarray consisting of amplified cDNA clones spotted in a grid. After hybridisation and washing, the hybridisation signal for each fluorophore is measured on each cDNA spot to determine the relative expression of the corresponding RNA in the two endometrial samples. The majority of RNAs are expressed at the same level in both samples

in levels is two-fold) and accept an arbitrary difference (say two-fold) as significant. This is highly misleading since it ignores the fact that the hybridisation signals obtained for genes expressed at low levels show greater variation than genes expressed at high levels, owing to the influence of background noise. This increase in variation with decreased intensity is apparent in Figure 16.2. A signal that changes from 5000 to 10 000, (a two-fold change) may seem less interesting than a change from 5 to 100 (a twenty-fold change), but the former is more reliable and more likely to be biologically significant.

Use of arrays to identify genes involved in endometrial receptivity

Successful implantation requires the simultaneous development of a competent blastocyst and a receptive endometrium. Embryo-transfer experiments in many species have shown that the uterus becomes receptive to the blastocyst for a relatively short period, known as the implantation window. In mice, the receptive state begins

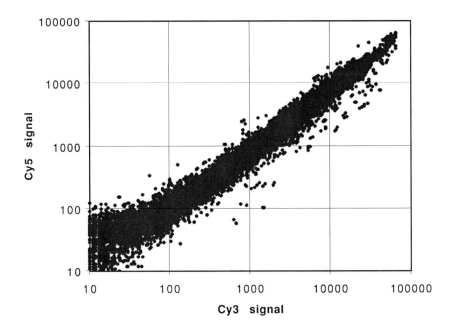

Figure 16.2. Response of endometrial stromal cells to IL1β as assessed by microarrays. Endometrial stromal cells were cultured with or without IL1β for 12 h and total RNA isolated from each paired sample was labelled with Cy3 (untreated) or Cy5 (treated with IL1β). The scatter plot shows the normalised mean signal intensity for the Cy3 and Cy5 signal from each spotted cDNA from a single pair of samples following hybridisation. cDNAs corresponding to RNA species upregulated by IL1β fall above the y = x line (Cy5 signal greater than Cy3 signal), and those downregulated by IL1β fall below the y = x line (Cy5 signal less than Cy3 signal). The majority of genes are equally expressed in both samples and give a Cy5/Cy3 ratio of one

on day 4 of pregnancy and lasts about 20 h.[4] In women, the receptive period is believed to extend from approximately day +5 to day +10 after the luteinising hormone (LH) surge.[5] The receptive state is brought about by the action of progesterone on an oestrogen-primed endometrium. Considerable effort has been devoted to understanding the molecular mechanisms by which the endometrium becomes receptive. Attention has focused primarily on two key questions:

1. the identification of genes whose expression is regulated by progesterone
2. identifying molecular markers that characterise the receptive state.

By 2002, only a handful of genes had been identified in either category in primates and rodents.[6,7] Since then, however, microarray studies have altered this situation dramatically. Hundreds of progesterone-regulated genes have been identified in several landmark studies in mice and humans. Functional analysis has already shown that in mice several of these are essential for normal implantation.

Identification of progesterone-regulated genes in endometrium of mice

To identify progesterone-regulated genes in the mouse uterus during implantation, oligonucleotide microarrays were used to define transcripts whose expression was altered by the progesterone receptor antagonist mifepristone. This drug binds to the progesterone receptor (PR), blocking activation of progesterone-regulated genes. In mice, the action of progesterone is required during the first three days of pregnancy to develop a receptive endometrium.[4] Implantation, which occurs on day 4 of pregnancy, can be prevented by a single injection of mifepristone on day 3, which renders the endometrium nonreceptive. Cheon et al.[8] compared uterine RNA isolated on day 4 of pregnancy from animals treated with mifepristone (nonreceptive) with uterine RNA from normal animals. They used Affymetrix microarrays that contain oligonucleotides corresponding to approximately 6000 known mouse transcripts, and a further 6000 cDNAs of unknown function. A total of 78 known genes were identified as downregulated more than two-fold, and 70 were upregulated by mifepristone. Genes that are downregulated by mifepristone are likely to be upregulated by the PR. Remarkably, only 4 out of 70 of these genes had previously been shown to be upregulated by progesterone. It is also interesting that several genes, such as Hoxa10 and calcitonin, that are present on the array and that are regulated by progesterone were not detected. This is probably because they are expressed at relatively low levels in total RNA from the uterus and are below the detection limit for the microarray.

Although extensive, the gene lists from microarray experiments are never totally comprehensive. Independent verification of ten of these candidate genes by Northern blot confirmed their upregulation following progesterone injection of ovariectomised mice. The effects were completely dependent on the presence of the PR, since no upregulation occurred following progesterone injection of ovariectomised mice lacking PR.

Although PR has long been known to be essential for the preparation of a receptive endometrium, until now relatively little has been known about the molecular pathways regulated by progesterone in the endometrium. Novel targets identified in the Cheon study[8] include transcription factors, peptide hormones, proteases and their inhibitors, metabolic enzymes and molecules involved in immune functions. This is entirely consistent with the known physiological effects of progesterone on endometrium. Among this plethora of genes and pathways must be molecules that are essential for receptivity and implantation – the question is which ones. This illustrates a major challenge with microarrays: how to move from a large candidate list generated by a microarray experiment to then identify the genes with important functions. Mouse knockouts have shown that many genes that are regulated by progesterone in endometrium are nonetheless not essential for implantation.

12/15-lipoxygenase and immune response gene 1 are essential for implantation

In two follow-up papers, Cheon et al. demonstrate the value of such a microarray analysis, by identifying two genes that they show are essential for implantation. One of the novel genes upregulated by progesterone is the lipid-metabolising enzyme leucocyte 12/15-lipoxygenase (Alox15). This generates hydroxy-eicosatetraenoic acids which are known cell differentiation signals. Both epidermal- and leucocyte-

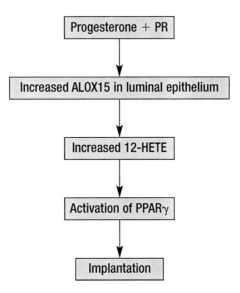

Figure 16.3. Novel signalling pathway identified by microarray analysis of murine endometrium treated with mifepristone. The enzyme ALOX15 is upregulated in luminal epithelium by progesterone, resulting in release of 12-HETE, which in turn activates PPARγ. Inhibition of ALOX15 activity results in implantation failure

specific isoforms are expressed in the luminal epithelium only on the day of implantation, and this is accompanied by a marked increase in their metabolites such as 12-HETE. Blockade of uterine ALOX15 activity by the specific inhibitor AA-861 reduced implantation by more than 80%.[9] Since metabolites such as 12-HETE can function as activating ligands of the peroxisome proliferator-activated receptor gamma (PPARγ), they hypothesised that PPARγ could be a downstream target. Administration of rosiglitazone, a potent PPARγ agonist, restored implantation in animals treated with the ALOX15 inhibitor. Thus the original microarray analysis identified a novel signalling pathway that is critical for implantation (Figure 16.3). Similarly, the mRNA encoding immune response gene 1 (*Irg1*) was shown to be upregulated by progesterone, with expression confined to the luminal epithelium on days 4 and 5 of pregnancy. This closely resembles the expression of the PR in the murine endometrium.[8] *Irg1* was first cloned as a novel lipopolysaccharide-inducible gene in macrophages.[10] The function of IRG1 in implantation was investigated by injection of antisense oligonucleotides to *Irg1* into the uterine lumen on day 3 of pregnancy. The oligonucleotides enter the luminal epithelial cells and were shown to reduce expression levels of IRG1 by more than 90% compared with animals injected with sense oligonucleotides as controls.[11] This treatment reduced the number of implantation sites in each horn from 6.7 ± 1.2 to 1.3 ± 1.2. Although care must be used in interpreting the results of uterine injections of oligonucleotides, because of nonspecific effects, these experiments suggest that IRG1, which is transiently expressed in luminal epithelium through the action of progesterone, is essential for implantation. The molecular function of IRG1 in implantation is unknown.

Receptivity studies in women

In women, the action of the progesterone receptor is also essential for the development of receptivity, which occurs between day LH+5 and day LH+10. Traditionally, this transformation has been assessed histologically according to the criteria of Noyes *et al.*[12] However, more recently, molecular markers have been described that are expressed at different stages of the luteal phase. These provide a novel means to assess whether normal endometrial development is occurring. Their use has revealed that there are subtle differences in the molecular repertoire expressed in the endometrium of patient groups with subfertility such as endometriosis and unexplained infertility compared with fertile women.[13] For example, the frequency of abnormal expression of the integrin $\alpha_v\beta_3$ is increased in the endometrium of subfertile women.[14,15] However, there is substantial overlap in expression levels of these markers between subfertile women and normal controls. Secondly, there is a poor correlation between expression of any one marker and clinical outcome.[16] They are therefore not useful for diagnosis or management of individual women. A major problem is that few prospective controlled studies have been performed and most studies involve small numbers of patients or lack suitable controls. Finally, few genes have been identified that are clearly regulated by progesterone, and only a handful of the total of 30 000 genes in the human genome have been assessed as markers.

Table 16.1. Published microarray studies on human endometrial receptivity using Affymetrix arrays; after Horcajadas *et al.*[36]

Study	Sample type	Number	Analysis	Altered genes
Borthwick *et al.*, 2003[18]	proliferative day 9–11 secretory day LH+(6–8)	5 (pooled) 5 (pooled)	Statistical model	90 up 59 down
Kao *et al.*, 2002[17]	proliferative day 8–10 secretory day LH+(6–8)	4 7	2-fold change	156 up 377 down
Carson *et al.*, 2002[19]	pre-receptive day LH+(2–4) receptive day LH+(7–9)	3 (pooled) 3 (pooled)	2-fold change	323 up 370 down
Riesewijk *et al.*, 2002[20]	pre-receptive day LH+2 receptive day LH+7	5 5	3-fold change	153 up 58 down

The ability of microarrays to analyse thousands of mRNAs simultaneously provides a powerful new approach to the identification of markers of receptivity. Several studies have sought to identify new markers of the receptive state with this technique. These have taken two approaches, and the first has been to compare proliferative and secretory phase endometrium, to identify global gene expression changes between the oestrogen-dominated and progesterone-dominated phases of the cycle. In the second approach, gene expression profiles in normal fertile women at days LH+2 (pre-receptive) and LH+7 (receptive) were analysed. All studies employed the same Affymetrix oligonucleotide arrays, allowing direct comparison of the results. Kao et al.[17] and Borthwick et al.[18] compared gene expression in the late proliferative and mid-secretory endometrium. The latter study pooled RNA from five samples at each time point, whereas Kao et al. hybridised samples individually. Borthwick et al. reported 90 transcripts as significantly upregulated and 59 as significantly downregulated. Using different analysis criteria, Kao et al. reported 156 genes as upregulated and 377 as downregulated (Table 16.1). Approximately 30% of the genes were common to both studies. The concordance between these investigations is striking considering the differences in sample treatment. Furthermore, many of the differences between the lists are likely to be due to the very different methods of analysing the data generated by the same microarray platform. These data represent a molecular signature of the endometrium in the receptive state compared with the proliferative phase. Many of the genes are likely to be upregulated by progesterone directly, but in others this may be due to secondary effects of paracrine mediators. More importantly, new pathways have been found where a function in the endometrium was previously unsuspected. Examples include glutathione peroxidase 3 and manganese superoxide dismutase, which protect cells from reactive oxygen species, and the metallothionein proteins, which may protect the embryo from heavy metal toxicity. Several of the latter are upregulated, indicating coordinated upregulation of the gene family (Table 16.2).

Table 16.2. Metallothionein genes upregulated in secretory-phase endometrium

Genbank accession no.	Gene name	Upregulation fold change[a]	
		Kao et al.[17]	Borthwick et al.[18]
J03910	metallothionein 1G	5.9	25
M10943	metallothionein 1F	3.8	not altered
R93527	metallothionein-like 1H	3.6	6.4
H68340	metallothionein-like 1F	3.5	7.1
K01383	metallothionein 1A	3.0	4.2
M13485	metallothionein 1B	3.5	not altered

[a] The figures show the fold change by which each gene was found to be upregulated in the indicated studies in secretory compared with proliferative endometrium; 'not altered' indicates that the gene was not identified as altered in expression using the analysis criteria

For the comparison of gene expression in pre-receptive (day LH+2) and receptive (day LH+7) endometrium, Carson et al.[19] compared three biopsies from each time point taken from separate women, whereas Riesewijk et al.[20] compared serial biopsies taken from the same woman ($n = 5$) at the two different time points. Carson et al. identified 370 transcripts as downregulated and 323 as upregulated by at least two-fold, whereas Riesewijk et al. identified 153 genes as upregulated and 58 as downregulated by an average of three-fold or more (Table 16.1).

A significant number of the genes identified in these four studies as altering in expression had previously been shown to vary during the menstrual cycle using other methods, such as Northern blotting or immunohistochemistry. This lends support to the microarray approach. More significantly, many new genes were identified as showing regulation, a large number of which had not previously been shown even to be expressed in endometrium. For example, members of the Wnt family of signalling molecules and related inhibitors were identified for the first time in endometrium and may play a role in epithelial/stromal interactions during the receptive phase.[21] Other new genes identified include immune modulators such as chemokines and their receptors that may be involved in regulating the trafficking and function of leucocytes in endometrium.

Difficulties in comparing microarray experiments

Although all four of the above studies tackle a related question, and the gene lists generated display a substantial degree of overlap, they are certainly not identical. This is despite the use of identical commercially available microarrays and hybridisation protocols, and it illustrates a common problem when comparing microarray studies from different laboratories. Some of the differences clearly relate to the study design itself. For example, the Borthwick study[18] pooled endometrial biopsies from five women at each time point prior to hybridisation, whereas Kao et al.[17] hybridised each woman's biopsy separately. In the Riesewijk[20] and Carson[19] studies, there were minor differences in the timing of the biopsies but the substantial differences in the gene lists generated arose instead primarily from differences in the analysis criteria (average change of three-fold or two-fold, respectively, in the two studies). Finally, all these studies involved very small patient groups ($n = 3$ or 5). With such small groups, the natural biological variation between patients due to genotypic and environmental differences may substantially influence the final gene lists. Using genetically identical inbred mice under identical environmental conditions, up to 3.3% of all transcripts showed altered expression in a microarray study of the kidney.[22] This biological variation is natural but, in the context of microarray experiments, 3.3% of 12 000 genes amounts to a substantial number of false positives! This emphasises the need for rigorous and robust experimental design, with especial consideration of the method of analysis to reduce or eliminate false positives.[3] Confirmation of apparent gene expression changes in microarray experiments is therefore essential using an independent method such as Northern blotting or quantitative polymerase chain reaction (PCR). This serves to ensure that the statistical analysis of the microarray data is appropriate and can indicate the true changes in the level of gene expression.

Mifepristone and receptivity in women

Microarray studies in normal endometrium provide the baseline data to define the gene expression 'signature' at defined phases of the menstrual cycle. However, extracting information about which genes are functionally important remains a serious challenge. As countless mouse knockout experiments have shown, just because a gene is present or regulated does not mean that it has a critical function that cannot be compensated by another gene. The next step is to compare the normal gene expression profile with that seen in disorders of endometrium such as implantation-related infertility, endometriosis and menorrhagia and during responses to pharmaceutical agents.

The mifepristone studies in mice described earlier showed how it was possible to identify genes regulated by progesterone and to test which of these are important in implantation. In women, a single dose of mifepristone in the secretory phase rapidly renders the endometrium nonreceptive.[23] The artificial progesterone withdrawal induced by this treatment usually results in endometrial breakdown and menstruation within 48 h.[24] This model provides a system to identify progesterone-regulated genes that may be involved in receptivity or the induction of menstruation in women. We have used microarrays to examine changes in endometrial gene expression following a single dose (200 mg) of mifepristone administered during the implantation window. Pipelle biopsies were taken at 6 h or 24 h after mifepristone administration. At 6 h, six genes were found to be significantly upregulated and 90 were downregulated, compared with controls. Although mifepristone can affect both glucocorticoid and androgen receptor function, the majority of these genes are likely to be directly regulated by progesterone. As in the mouse study, identifying whether these genes are involved in regulating receptivity or blood vessel stability will require localisation of their expression followed by functional studies. However, this clearly shows how microarrays can be used to study drug action on the endometrium *in vivo*.

Microarrays and endometriosis

Endometriosis is characterised by the presence of endometrial tissue at ectopic sites, typically the pelvis and ovary. It is associated with pelvic pain and reduced fertility. Women with endometriosis who undergo *in vitro* fertilisation have reduced implantation rates, thus implicating the endometrium as a cause of the implantation failure.[25] The disease is believed to arise primarily by attachment of fragments of endometrial tissue that enter the pelvis after retrograde menstruation.[26] Although most women have retrograde menstruation, only 10–15% have detectable endometriosis.[27] It is believed that abnormalities in the endometrium of these women trigger a reduced immune response in the pelvis that fails to clear the ectopic tissue. In support of this, several molecules have been shown to exhibit altered expression in endometrium of women with endometriosis during the secretory phase. These include aromatase, endometrial-associated bleeding factor, HOXA10, $\alpha_v\beta_3$ integrin and leukaemia inhibitory factor (LIF) (reviewed in Giudice *et al.*[13]).

A recent microarray study[28] compared the gene expression profile of endometrium obtained at day LH+(8–10) in normal fertile women ($n = 7$) with women with endometriosis ($n = 8$). Ninety-one genes were identified as upregulated and 115 as downregulated by an average of at least two-fold. Functional classification of these altered genes showed that they control functions such as cell adhesion, epithelial secreted proteins, apoptosis and signal transduction. The majority of these had not previously been shown to be dysregulated in endometriosis. They provide new insights into the possible causes of the infertility associated with the disease and the pathogenesis of the condition. For example, the gene *S100E*, which is a member of a family of calcium-binding proteins, is expressed at decreased levels in women with endometriosis. Deletion in mice of a closely related member of the same family, S100A8, results in implantation failure.[29] Downregulation of the calcium-binding protein calbindin d9K using antisense oligonucleotides prevents implantation.[30] Taken together, these results imply a critical role for calcium homeostasis in normal implantation. Dysregulation may contribute to the subfertility associated with endometriosis. These results not only provide new insights into the pathogenesis of endometriosis, but also provide new potential targets for diagnostic screening. Currently, diagnosis requires laparoscopy under general anaesthetic. The identification of a unique gene expression signature that is characteristic of endometriosis may permit routine diagnosis of endometriosis by use of a Pipelle biopsy of eutopic endometrium and gene array profiling rather than more invasive surgical techniques.

Limitations of current microarray studies

The microarray studies performed on endometrium to date have largely used the whole tissue. Although this has been extremely useful in detecting global gene expression changes and may prove satisfactory for diagnostic purposes, it gives little clue as to where the genes are expressed or what they might be doing. Normal endometrial function involves complex interactions among the various cell types, and genes that are expressed at low levels in limited numbers of cells are simply not detected. What is ideally needed are more detailed studies in which the expression profiles of individual cell types are determined at relevant times in the cycle. For example, in seeking to understand embryo attachment, it would be helpful to know the gene expression profile of the luminal epithelium, which is known to differ from the glandular epithelium. One approach has been to isolate the individual cell types and study the responses *in vitro*. Several studies have investigated the responses of isolated endometrial stromal cells to hormones and cytokines such as IL1β.[31–33] However, many relevant cell types are difficult to isolate from endometrium and this ignores the spatial variation in expression that exists, for example in the stromal cells of the functional layer and basal layer. One solution to this problem is the technique of laser capture microdissection (LCM). As a result of improved sensitivity of microarray techniques, individual cell types can now be isolated from tissue sections under the microscope, the RNA isolated and gene expression profiling performed to compare different cell types.[34] This technique will add considerably to our ability to use microarray techniques to understand interactions between different cellular compartments in endometrium.

Although microarray techniques have become extremely powerful tools, it is important to remember that they can only measure RNA levels in tissue or cells. Many cellular functions and responses involve alterations in proteins that are not reflected in steady-state RNA levels. Examples include phosphorylation of signalling intermediaries and control of protein levels through ubiquitination and degradation. The development of high-throughput 'proteomic' techniques is underway and a fuller understanding of endometrial function will require integration of RNA data from microarrays with protein data from other techniques.

Microarrays and the clinic

Microarray studies have provided detailed information about the changes in endometrial gene expression as it goes from a nonreceptive to a receptive state.

Subsets of these genes whose expression during the implantation window is altered in women with unexplained infertility or endometriosis have been identified. These provide new opportunities for targeted drug discovery to develop new treatments for implantation failure. Small, low-cost arrays can now be used to determine whether gene expression profiling can be used to predict uterine receptivity or to tailor-make treatments for individual patients. This approach is already highly successful in cancer diagnostics, where expression profiling of tumours that are apparently identical using conventional histological markers has been able to distinguish between tumours with differing drug sensitivity or prognosis.[35] The diagnostic use of microarrays to distinguish between nonreceptive (day LH+2) and receptive (day LH+7) endometrium has already been demonstrated.[20] This is likely to be extended in future to endometriosis, menorrhagia and endometrial cancer.

Many of the technical difficulties in the use of microarrays, such as sensitivity and reproducibility, have now been overcome. The cost of microarray fabrication and use has fallen dramatically and the entire process of RNA isolation hybridisation and array analysis has been successfully automated. The challenges that remain are primarily in the areas of data analysis and predictive modelling. It is not fanciful to predict that microarray analysis or similar high-throughput proteomics methods will become routine diagnostic tools for the physician treating gynaecological dysfunction in the near future. However, clinical studies are required that will provide the evidence base to assess the practical utility of these techniques in clinical practice.

References

1. DeRisi JL, Iyer VR. Genomics and array technology. *Curr Opin Oncol* 1999;11:76–9.
2. Gaasterland T, Bekiranov S. Making the most of microarray data. *Nat Genet* 2000;24:204–6.
3. Stafford P, Liu P. Microarray technology comparison, statistical analysis and experimental design. In: Hardiman G, editor. *Microarrays Methods and Applications: Nuts & Bolts*. Seattle: DNA Press; 2003. p. 274–324.
4. Psychoyos A. Uterine receptivity for nidation. *Ann N Y Acad Sci* 1986;476:36–42.
5. Navot D, Bergh PA, Williams M, Garrisi GJ, Guzman I, Sandler B, *et al.* An insight into early reproductive processes through the *in vivo* model of ovum donation. *J Clin Endocrinol Metab* 1991;72:408–14.
6. Sharkey AM, Smith SK. The endometrium as a cause of implantation failure. *Best Pract Res Clin Obstet Gynaecol* 2003;17:289–307.
7. Lessey BA. The role of the endometrium during embryo implantation. *Hum Reprod* 2000;15:39–50.
8. Cheon YP, Li Q, Xu X, DeMayo FJ, Bagchi IC, Bagchi MK. A genomic approach to identify novel progesterone receptor regulated pathways in the uterus during implantation. *Mol Endocrinol* 2002;16:2853–71.
9. Li Q, Cheon YP, Kannan A, Shanker S, Bagchi IC, Bagchi MK. A novel pathway involving progesterone receptor, 12/15-lipoxygenase-derived eicosanoids, and peroxisome proliferator-activated receptor gamma regulates implantation in mice. *J Biol Chem* 2004;279:11570–81.
10. Lee CG, Jenkins NA, Gilbert DJ, Copeland NG, O'Brien WE. Cloning and analysis of gene regulation of a novel LPS-inducible cDNA. *Immunogenetics* 1995;41:263–70.
11. Cheon YP, Xu X, Bagchi MK, Bagchi IC. Immune-responsive gene 1 is a novel target of progesterone receptor and plays a critical role during implantation in the mouse. *Endocrinology* 2003;144:5623–30.
12. Noyes RW, Hertig AI, Rock J. Dating the endometrial biopsy. *Fertil Steril* 1950;1:3–25.
13. Giudice LC, Telles TL, Lobo S, Kao LC. The molecular basis for implantation failure in endometriosis: on the road to discovery. *Ann N Y Acad Sci* 2002;955:252–64.
14. Lessey BA, Castelbaum AJ, Sawin SW, Sun J. Integrins as markers of uterine receptivity in women with primary unexplained infertility. *Fertil Steril* 1995;63:535–42.
15. Lessey BA. Implantation defects in infertile women with endometriosis. *Ann N Y Acad Sci* 2002;955:265–80.

16. Damario MA, Lesnick TG, Lessey BA, Kowalik A, Mandelin E, Seppala M, *et al*. Endometrial markers of uterine receptivity utilizing the donor oocyte model. *Hum Reprod* 2001;16:1893–9.
17. Kao LC, Tulac S, Lobo S, Imani B, Yang JP, Germeyer A, *et al*. Global gene profiling in human endometrium during the window of implantation. *Endocrinology* 2002;143:2119–38.
18. Borthwick JM, Charnock-Jones DS, Tom BD, Hull ML, Teirney R, Phillips SC, *et al*. Determination of the transcript profile of human endometrium. *Mol Hum Reprod* 2003;9:19–33.
19. Carson DD, Lagow E, Thathiah A, Al-Shami R, Farach-Carson MC, Vernon M, *et al*. Changes in gene expression during the early to mid-luteal (receptive phase) transition in human endometrium detected by high-density microarray screening. *Mol Hum Reprod* 2002;8:871–9.
20. Riesewijk A, Martin J, van Os R, Horcajadas JA, Polman J, Pellicer A, *et al*. Gene expression profiling of human endometrial receptivity on days LH+2 versus LH+7 by microarray technology. *Mol Hum Reprod* 2003;9:253–64.
21. Tulac S, Nayak NR, Kao LC, Van Waes M, Huang J, Lobo S, *et al*. Identification, characterization, and regulation of the canonical Wnt signaling pathway in human endometrium. *J Clin Endocrinol Metab* 2003;88:3860–6.
22. Pritchard CC, Hsu L, Delrow J, Nelson PS. Project normal: defining normal variance in mouse gene expression. *Proc Natl Acad Sci U S A* 2001;98:13266–71.
23. Danielsson KG, Marions L, Bygdeman M. Effects of mifepristone on endometrial receptivity. *Steroids* 2003;68:1069–75.
24. Hapangama DK, Critchley HO, Henderson TA, Baird DT. Mifepristone-induced vaginal bleeding is associated with increased immunostaining for cyclooxygenase-2 and decrease in prostaglandin dehydrogenase in luteal phase endometrium. *J Clin Endocrinol Metab* 2002;87:5229–34.
25. Barnhart K, Dunsmoor-Su R, Coutifaris C. Effect of endometriosis on *in vitro* fertilization. *Fertil Steril* 2002;77:1148–55.
26. Sampson JA. Peritoneal endometriosis due to the menstrual dissemination of endometrial tissue into the peritoneal cavity. *Am J Obstet Gynecol* 1927;14:422–69.
27. Vigano P, Parazzini F, Somigliana E, Vercellini P. Endometriosis: epidemiology and aetiological factors. *Best Pract Res Clin Gynaecol* 2004;18:177–200.
28. Kao LC, Germeyer A, Tulac S, Lobo S, Yang JP, Taylor RN, *et al*. Expression profiling of endometrium from women with endometriosis reveals candidate genes for disease-based implantation failure and infertility. *Endocrinology* 2003;144:2870–81.
29. Passey RJ, Williams E, Lichanska AM, Wells C, Hu S, Geczy CL, *et al*. A null mutation in the inflammation-associated S100 protein S100A8 causes early resorption of the mouse embryo. *J Immunol* 1999;163:2209–16.
30. Luu KC, Nie GY, Hampton A, Fu GQ, Liu YX, Salamonsen LA. Endometrial expression of calbindin (CaBP)-d28k but not CaBP-d9k in primates implies evolutionary changes and functional redundancy of calbindins at implantation. *Reproduction* 2004;128:433–41.
31. Rossi M, Sharkey AM, Vigano P, Fiore G, Florio P, Furlong R, *et al*. Identification of genes regulated by interleukin-1beta in human endometrial stromal cells. *Reproduction* (in press).
32. Lebovic DI, Baldocchi RA, Mueller MD, Taylor RN. Altered expression of a cell-cycle suppressor gene, Tob-1, in endometriotic cells by cDNA array analyses. *Fertil Steril* 2002;78:849–54.
33. Okada H, Nakajima T, Yoshimura T, Yasuda K, Kanzaki H. Microarray analysis of genes controlled by progesterone in human endometrial stromal cells *in vitro*. *Gynecol Endocrinol* 2003;17:271–80.
34. Matsuzaki S, Canis M, Vaurs-Barriere C, Pouly JL, Boespflug-Tanguy O, Penault-Llorca F, *et al*. DNA microarray analysis of gene expression profiles in deep endometriosis using laser capture microdissection. *Mol Hum Reprod* 2004;10:719–28.
35. Kari L, Loboda A, Nebozhyn M, Rook AH, Vonderheid EC, Nichols C, *et al*. Classification and prediction of survival in patients with the leukemic phase of cutaneous T cell lymphoma. *J Exp Med* 2003;197:1477–88.
36. Horcajadas JA, Riesewijk A, Martin J, Cervero A, Mosselman S, Pellicer A, *et al*. Global gene expression profiling of human endometrial receptivity. *J Reprod Immunol* 2004;63:41–9.

SECTION 4
CLINICAL SEQUELAE

Chapter 17

Sporadic early pregnancy loss: aetiology and management

Siobhan Quenby

Introduction

Sporadic early pregnancy loss occurs in approximately 15% of clinically recognised pregnancies.[1] Despite its high prevalence, a significant amount of confusion exists surrounding the aetiology and management of miscarriage, and this is partly due to the lack of a defined terminology.[2] An optimal terminology would reflect both ultrasound findings and aetiology. At present it is frequently assumed that women with three consecutive miscarriages are losing normal pregnancies but those with only one miscarriage are losing abnormal ones. However, recent data refute this assumption. It is now very important that the diagnosis of miscarriage is refined and women are given more information regarding the aetiology of each pregnancy loss. This requirement can, however, lead to conflicts between treatment modalities and the need for an accurate diagnosis.

Terminology

First-trimester miscarriage

In the past, miscarriage has been referred to as 'blighted ovum' to indicate the absence of an embryo at a very early stage of pregnancy. This is no longer an acceptable term as it implies the mother is at fault.[2] The term 'missed miscarriage' is currently in frequent use to refer to a pregnancy that the uterus does not pass for a prolonged time after fetal demise. However, 'missed miscarriage' implies either the patient or the medical services are at fault for missing the diagnosis and it is an unwieldy and confusing term.

Embryologists define the 'embryonic period' as that of differentiation and formation of major organs that occurs up to 10 weeks of gestation. The 'fetal period' of development is that which occurs after 10 weeks of gestation, when fetal growth predominates.

Clinicians are now beginning to use the terms embryonic and fetal loss to describe miscarriages, but they are using ultrasound-generated information to assign an embryologist's term. This has meant that different authors have assigned different meanings to these terms. In the Liverpool Recurrent Miscarriage Clinic we attempted to simplify the situation by defining embryo losses as those where no fetal heartbeat was ever seen and fetal losses as those where the heart beating was seen prior to the loss.[3,4] However, this definition is only of value in women having serial transvaginal ultrasonography because of a past history of recurrent miscarriage. It is also in conflict with other authors for the cases where a fetal heart is seen beating in a six-week-sized embryo but not in a repeat scan at eight weeks of gestation. The Liverpool system characterises this as a fetal loss but in embryological terms it was an embryonic loss. Another problem surrounds the terminology for the common ultrasound finding of an empty gestation sac, describing this as a 'missed miscarriage' when in fact no fetus developed and this frequently misleads patients and clinicians. There is clearly a need to standardise terms and definitions. The terminology proposed by Nanda and co-workers[2] seems the optimal way to ensure consistency and I suggest that this should be adopted for current use (Table 17.1).

Table 17.1. Terminology of miscarriage; data from Nanda *et al.*[2]

	Definition	Gestation (weeks)	Ultrasound findings
First-trimester miscarriage			
Anembryonic pregnancy	Trophoblast development without the development of an embryo	< 12	Empty gestation sac (diameter > 20 mm, no embryonic pole or yolk sac) or if diameter < 20 mm with no change on rescan 7 days later
Embryonic loss	An early embryo loss before fetal heart activity	< 8	Embryo > 5 mm size but up to 8 weeks size, with no cardiac activity; or crown rump length < 5 mm with no change on rescan 7 days later
Fetal loss	Death of a fetus in the first trimester	8–12	Fetus of 8–12 weeks size with no fetal heart activity
Second-trimester miscarriage			
Late fetal loss	Death of a fetus in the second trimester	12–24	Fetus of 12–24 weeks size with no fetal heart activity
Spontaneous second-trimester loss	Pregnancy loss associated with SROM or cervical dilation	12–24	Fetus of 12–24 weeks size with fetal heart activity

SROM = spontaneous rupture of membranes

Second-trimester miscarriage

There is a significant difference between second-trimester miscarriage identified as a fetal death by ultrasonography compared with one that follows spontaneous rupture of membranes (SROM) or labour. Therefore we have suggested the terms in Table 17.1.[5]

Aetiology

Karyotypical abnormalities

One of the most remarkable, and as yet unexplained, aspects of the first trimester of pregnancy is the fact that the majority (99%) of karyotypically abnormal pregnancies miscarry in the first trimester and the majority (93%) of karyotypically normal pregnancies continue.[6] Hence, miscarriage can be viewed as 'nature's quality control'.[7] It used to be assumed that couples having three or more miscarriages had parental factors contributing to their losses. However, a series of papers has reported an incidence of 29–57% karyotypical abnormality rate in the pregnancies miscarried from women suffering three or more losses.[8–11] Therefore karyotypical abnormality should be excluded before further causes are investigated.

The conventional technique of culture and karyotyping of miscarried tissue has many difficulties. Trophoblasts do not survive in culture long enough to allow conventional karyotyping with G banding; this means that the cytogeneticists, in fact, culture the less common fetal mesenchymal stromal cells and leucocytes. Difficulties in getting miscarried fetal cells to grow means that conventional karyotyping is limited by external contamination, culture failure and selective growth of maternal cells.[12] This problem is illustrated by an audit of 100 consecutive karyotypes of miscarried pregnancies carried out in Liverpool Women's Hospital that had an exceptionally good (96%) successful culture rate owing to highly proficient and motivated staff but a 4:1 female to male sex ratio as against an expected 1:1 ratio. Consequently a result of 46XX has to be considered the result of maternal contamination.

Various options are available to improve the diagnostic accuracy for karyotypical abnormalities. It has been suggested that tissue is collected by chorionic villous sampling immediately prior to the uterine evacuation[13] in order to sample better quality tissue and decrease maternal contamination; however, this is not very practical. Analysis of spontaneous miscarriages by comparative genomic hybridisation (CGH), a technique that detects chromosomal imbalances without the need for culture, has been demonstrated to improve detection rates.[11,14,15] Furthermore, CGH can be used to analyse the cytogenetics of formalin-fixed, paraffin-embedded miscarriage specimens.[16] However, CGH is also susceptible to problems with maternal contamination and is unable to detect mosaicism or balanced structural abnormalities. Mosaicism is a known problem in trophoblastic material. Fluorescence *in situ* hybridisation (FISH) is widely used to detect aneuploidy in samples obtained by amniocentesis, chorioinic villous sampling and pre-gestation diagnosis. FISH had also been used effectively to detect aneuploidy in miscarried tissue where culture fails or maternal contamination occurs.[17] The problem with FISH is that it is too expensive and impractical to use to test for all chromosomal aneuploidies. However, commercially available multiple sets of probes are available that allow testing for common aneuploidies. The use of FISH with probes for chromosomes 13, 15, 16, 18, 21, 22, X and Y has detected abnormalities in 63% of miscarried specimens compared with culture and conventional karyotype that detected abnormalities in 53% of cases.[17]

Incorporating the patient's view

Pressure from patients in the UK has led to increasing the speed of diagnosis following an amniocentesis test with the widespread introduction of the use of FISH and polymerase chain reaction (PCR). The same thing has not happened for women suffering pregnancy loss. This may be because of a false impression given to women that they are suffering the loss of normal pregnancies. This then causes a desperate search for aetiology and a treatment for their miscarriages and serious emotional trauma. The full cost of failing to diagnose karotypic abnormality in repeated miscarriages is large. If women and their clinicians erroneously think that they are losing normal pregnancies when in fact they have lost trisomic pregnancies they will search for further abnormalities and treatments when in reality 'nature's quality control' is working effectively. Conversely, women who lose normal pregnancies often have to wait until they have lost three potential babies in a row before clinicians will test them for the treatable condition antiphospholipid syndrome (APS). This is in spite of a consensus statement from the International APS Society that states that one fetal loss after ten weeks of gestation and two positive tests for APS are sufficient to make the diagnosis.[18] Thus the failure to give women accurate karyotyping of their pregnancy losses has a large hidden cost. If falsely told they have lost a normal pregnancy they suffer the emotional trauma of thinking that their body has rejected a normal pregnancy instead of realising that 'nature's quality control' was working correctly. In addition, they may undergo unnecessary investigations (e.g. thrombophilia screening) and unnecessary treatments with their associated adverse effects (e.g. heparin, intravenous immunoglobulin and leucocyte transfusions). Conversely, women not investigated for APS until they have lost three normal pregnancies may suffer needless pregnancy loss because of an outdated definition. Thus analysing the miscarried products from women with repeated miscarriages using FISH is regarded as a cost-effective approach and is currently being evaluated in the Liverpool Women's Hospital. If patients were fully informed of these issues, I suggest that they would be as demanding in the processing of their samples as those receiving amniocentesis.

Structural abnormalities

Karyotyping does not detect pregnancies complicated by structural abnormalities in the presence of morphologically normal chromosomes. The newly introduced medical therapeutic abortion methodology has allowed detailed examination of undamaged first-trimester pregnancies.[19] Severe structural abnormalities likely to be incompatible with survival into the second trimester were found in 34% of specimens examined in our study.[19] Had these pregnancies continued they would have represented sporadic miscarriages. In the study[19] all women were clinically at least six weeks of gestation but 27% of intact gestation sacs had no embryo. Some had an umbilical cord but no tissue at the end of this; others had nothing. These empty sacs can also be diagnosed on high-resolution ($\pm 1\,mm$) transvaginal ultrasonography and are the worst end of the spectrum of structural abnormality as there is no embryo or fetus. As mentioned earlier, these should be called anembryonic pregnancies and any implication to the woman or her clinicians that these represent the loss of an abnormal 'pregnancy' is a fallacy.

Examination of miscarried pregnancies that have been treated medically rarely leads to useful information because of the disruption to tissues following the pregnancy loss, antiprogesterone medication, the delay in delivery, and trauma during the delivery of the tissues. To overcome these problems, an Austrian group has suggested embryoscopy using a standard hysterocope, immediately prior to evacuation of the pregnancy under general anaesthetic.[20] They found a similar pattern of disorders in first-trimester fetal deaths to those reported by Blanch and co-workers[19] from medical therapeutic abortions (Table 17.2). Importantly, Philipp and co-workers[20] found that 66% of karyotypically normal pregnancies had serious structural abnormalities. It is thus important to attempt to diagnose structural abnormality by ultrasound, embryoscopy or examination of products of conception in order to give women a reason for their pregnancy loss as well as for karyotyping the loss.

Diagnosis

It is now very important that every effort is made to inform women with miscarriages whether they have lost a normal or abnormal pregnancy. In the former case, a maternal cause should be sought. If they have lost an abnormal fetus then treating a maternal condition such as APS will make no difference because heparin does, of course, not remove extra chromosomes or put fetuses into empty anembryonic pregnancies.

Patient examination

Traditional teaching to medical students and junior doctors suggests that all women with bleeding in early pregnancy should have a vaginal examination. The aim of this should be to determine whether or not the cervical os is open or closed and to feel for adnexal masses or tenderness. However, when running the early pregnancy services at Nottingham City Hospital I found this standard advice to do physical and psychological harm. Within a period of two years the following incidents occurred:

- Junior doctors discharged three women because they found on examination that the cervical os was open, and therefore diagnosed an inevitable miscarriage. However, the women returned to a neighbouring hospital with an ectopic pregnancy.

Table 17.2. Structural abnormalities in early pregnancy reported from two different studies

	Blanch et al.[19] (n=21)	Philipp et al.[20] (n=233)	Specimens with abnormal karyotype (from Philipp et al.[20])
Reason for pregnancy loss	Medical therapeutic abortion	Fetal loss	75%
Method of examination	Binocular microscope	Embryoscopy	Culture and G banding
Normal embryos	40%	14%	48%
Anembryonic pregnancies	27%	Excluded	–
Ruptured sac	12%	Excluded	–
Growth disorganised	12%	31%	69%
Combined defects	6%	51%	86%
Isolated defects	3%	4%	60%

- On two occasions, junior doctors found masses in the adnexa on bimanual palpation, and the women then collapsed within the next 30 minutes with a ruptured ectopic pregnancy when they had been stable prior to the vaginal examination. The examination thus appeared to have precipitated rupture of the ectopic pregnancy.
- Two focus groups of ten women with spontaneous miscarriage and ten with recurrent miscarriage were held to ascertain the patients' view of our newly established nurse-led early pregnancy unit and recurrent miscarriage clinic. These were analysed by a behavioural scientist and psychologists. The patients' comments were generally positive regarding the nursing staff. However, there were frequent negative comments from the women regarding the vaginal examination. They felt that vaginal examination at the time of pregnancy loss was a physical violation and one women even said that she felt as if she had been 'raped'.

In contrast to this approach, Condous and co-workers[21] have proposed the simpler, ultrasound-based classification of bleeding in early pregnancy as 'pregnancy of known or unknown location'. With the widespread availability of high-resolution ultrasonography, it is my personal view that the potentially harmful vaginal examination of women with bleeding in early pregnancy should be abandoned except for the rare cases of maternal cervical shock thought to be caused by products of conception stuck in the cervix.

Treatment

Surgical treatment

The traditional 'gold standard' management for miscarriage was dilatation and surgical curettage of the uterus.[22] This was initiated to prevent blood loss and infection.[1] Suction curettage has replaced sharp curettage in many developed countries. Curettage was developed when ambiguity existed as to whether the pregnancy loss was spontaneous or the result of illegal abortion, a situation that still occurs in some countries today.

Advantages

Surgical management is quickly performed, has a high success rate and is relatively safe.

Disadvantages

Surgical uterine evacuation is costly[23] and it has been associated with intrauterine infection, perforation, cervical stenosis, cervical weakness,[24] bowel perforation[25] and intrauterine adhesions, and there are potential problems with general anaesthesia.

Implications for diagnosis

An increasingly important indication for surgical evacuation of the uterus is to ensure good-quality trophoblast is obtained for karyotypical diagnosis. This is particularly important if the miscarriage is the result of a treatment failure, for example in the case of a fetal loss following the administration of aspirin and heparin in a woman with

APS. If no reason is found for the treatment failure it is very difficult for the clinician to advise appropriate management for subsequent pregnancies. The current situation of the clinician's position of 'I do not know why the pregnancy failed – it could be because the fetus was abnormal but we do not know' is not acceptable for the patient.

Medical treatment

An alternative to surgical management with drugs has been developed since the early 1990s.[26] A widely used uterotonic drug is misoprostol, an inexpensive, stable analogue of prostaglandin E_1.[27] The efficacy of misoprostol alone varies from 13% to 96% depending on the type of miscarriage, the dose and the route of administration.[26,28,29] Misoprostol is most effective when given vaginally in doses of 800 μg initially.[30,31] However, in the case of ultrasound-diagnosed anembryonic, embryonic or fetal losses, priming with the antiprogesterone mifepristone has been found to produce better success rates.[32,33]

Advantages

Medical treatment may provide prompt expulsion of products, thus avoiding the costs and complications associated with surgery and the uncertainties of expectant management.[34] A higher patient satisfaction rate has been reported with medical compared with surgical treatment for miscarriage.[35]

Disadvantages

The disadvantages of medical treatment are the treatment failures that then require further doses of medication or surgical termination, the pain experienced while passing the products of conception and the adverse effects of medication. Reported adverse effects include headaches, chills, fever, nausea, vomiting, abdominal pain and heavy vaginal bleeding.[34]

Implications for diagnosis

As many women will pass an intact gestation sac in hospital with medical uterine evacuation, it is possible to examine the sac in order to ascertain any structural abnormalities.

Expectant treatment

In the developed world with widely available therapeutic abortion and rapid access to high-dose effective antibiotics and blood transfusion, the risks of serious complications arising from miscarriage are minimal. This has led to the introduction of expectant management. Women in many units can opt to miscarry their pregnancy at home, because complications can be rapidly treated in a nearby hospital if necessary.[36]

Advantages

Conservative management has been found to be a popular choice with patients.[37] In randomised controlled trials expectant management has been shown to be as effective as surgical management;[38,39] however, expectant management produced better overall patient mental health.[39]

Disadvantages

Expectant management usually results in the complete expulsion of the products of conception.[33] However, the interval between diagnosis and expulsion varies and the success rate varies depending on the type of miscarriage.[37] A success rate of 79–91% has been reported for incomplete miscarriage[38,39] but lower success rates have been seen with anembryonic pregnancy (66%)[39] and embryonic and fetal losses (25–76%).[39–41] Delay between diagnosis and expulsion of products can range from a few days to six weeks.[34] Prolonged delay of greater than two weeks is unlikely to be acceptable to all women. Other potential disadvantages of expectant management are severe pain and haemorrhage.

Implications for diagnosis

A further disadvantage of expectant management is that there is minimal chance of a karyotypical or structural abnormality being diagnosed.

Conclusions

It is clear that the current management of early pregnancy failure should involve the patient in making a fully informed choice as to the treatment option most appropriate to her situation. The lack of a diagnosis for sporadic early pregnancy loss is no longer acceptable for patients or clinicians. Obtaining an accurate aetiology should be within the capabilities of all hospital clinics and is indispensable in informing and supporting the management of miscarriage. The clinical approach needs to be consistent.

References

1. Hemminki E. Treatment of miscarriage: Current practice and rationale. *Obstet Gynecol* 1998;2:247–53.
2. Nanda K, Peloggia A, Nanda G, Grimes D. Expectant care versus surgical treatment for miscarriage (protocol for a Cochrane review). *Cochrane Database Syst Rev* 2004;(4):CD 3518.
3. Bricker L, Farquharson R. Types of loss in recurrent miscarriage: Implications for research and clinical practice. *Hum Reprod* 2002;17:1345–50.
4. Dawood F, Quenby S, Farquharson R. Recurrent Miscarriage: An overview. *Rev Gynaecol Pract* 2003;3:46–50.
5. Dawood F, Farquharson R, Quenby S. Recurrent miscarriage. *Curr Obstet Gynaecol* 2005;14:247–53.
6. McFadyen IR. Early fetal loss. In: Rodeck C, editor. *Fetal Medicine.* Oxford: Blackwell Scientific Publishers; 1989. p. 26–43.
7. Quenby S, Farquharson R, Vince G, Aplin J. Recurrent miscarriage: a defect of Nature's quality control? *Hum Reprod* 2002;17:534–8.
8. Stern JJ, Dorfmann AD, Gutierrez-Najar AJ, Cerrillo M, Coulam CB. Frequency of abnormal karyotypes among abortuses from women with and without a history of recurrent spontaneous abortion. *Fertil Steril* 1996;65:250–3.
9. Ogasawara M, Aoki K, Okada S, Suzumori K. Embryonic karyotype of abortuses in relation to the number of previous miscarriages. *Fertil Steril* 2000;73:300–4.
10. Carp H, Toder V, Aviram A, Danielle M, Mashiach S, Barkiai G. Karyotype of the abortus in recurrent miscarriage. *Fertil Steril* 2001;75:678–82.
11. Stephenson MD, Awartani KAA, Robinson WP. Cytogenetic analysis of miscarriages from couples

with recurrent miscarriage: a case–control study. *Hum Reprod* 2002;17:446–51.

12. Goddijn M, Leschot NJ. Genetic aspects of miscarriage. In: *Best Practice and Research in Obstetrics and Gynaecology*. London: Bailliere Tindall; 2000. p. 827–37.

13. Verez JR, Stern JJ, Gomez F. Frequency of abnormal karyotypes among women with a history of recurrent spontaneous abortion, assisted reproductive techniques and spontaneous pregnancy. *Fertil Steril* 1996;65:S154.

14. Daniely M, Aviram-Goldring A, Barki G, Goldman B. Detection of chromosomal aberration in fetuses arising from recurrent spontaneous abortion by comparative genomic hybridization. *Hum Reprod* 1998;13:805–9.

15. Fritz B, Hallerman C, Olert J, Fuchs B, Bruns M, Aslan M, *et al.* Cytogenetic analyses of culture failures by comparative genomic hybridisation (CGH) – Re-evaluation of chromosome aberration rates in early spontaneous abortions. *Eur J Hum Genet* 2001;9:539–47.

16. Bell KA, Van Deerlin PG, Feinberg RF, du Manoir S, Haddad BR. Diagnosis of aneuploidy in archival, paraffin-embedded pregnancy loss tissues by comparative genomic hybridization. *Fertil Steril* 2001;75:374–9.

17. Jobanputra V, Sobrino A, Kiney A, Kline J, Warburton D. Multiplex interphase FISH as a screen for common aneuploidies in spontaneous abortions. *Hum Reprod* 2002;17:1166–70.

18. Wilson WA, Gharavi AE, Koike T, Lockshin MD, Branch DW, Piette JC, *et al.* International consensus statement on preliminary classification criteria for definite antiphospholipid syndrome: report of an international workshop. *Arthritis Rheum* 1999;42:1309–11.

19. Blanch G, Quenby S, Ballantyne E, Holland K, Gosden CM, Neilson JP. Embryonic abnormalities at medical termination of pregnancy with mifepristone and misoprostol during the first trimester: observational study. *BMJ* 1998;7146:1712–14.

20. Philipp T, Philipp K, Reiner A, Beer F, Kalousek DK. Embryoscopy and cytogenetic analysis of 233 missed abortions: factors involved in the pathogenesis of developmental defects of early failed pregnancies. *Hum Reprod* 2003;18:1724–32.

21. Condous G, Okaro E, Khalid A, Timmerman D, Lu C, Zhou Y, *et al.* The use of a new logistic regression model for predicting the outcome of pregnancies of unknown location. *Hum Reprod* 2004;8:1900–10.

22. Vazquez JC, Hickey M, Neilson JP. Medical management of miscarriage (protocol for a Cochrane review). *Cochrane Database Syst Rev* 2004;(4):CD002253.

23. Hughes J, Ryan M, Hinshaw K, Henshaw R, Rispin R, Templeton A. The costs of treating miscarriage: a comparison of medical and surgical management. *BMJ* 1996;103:1217–21.

24. Hakim-Elahi E, Tovell HMM, Burnhill MS. Complications of first-trimester abortion: a report of 170,000 cases. *Obstet Gynecol* 1990;76:129–35.

25. MacKenzie J, Bibby J. Critical assessment of dilatation and curettage in 1029 women. *Lancet* 1978;ii:566–8.

26. El-Refaey H, Hinshaw K, Henshaw R, Smith N, Templeton A. Medical management of missed abortion and anembryonic pregnancy. *BMJ* 1992;305:1399–405.

27. Blandchard K, Clark S, Winikoff B, Gaines G, Ka G. Misoprostol for women's health. *Obstet Gynecol* 2002;99:316–32.

28. Crenin MD, Moyer R. Guido R. Misoprostol for medical evacuation of early pregnancy failure. *Obstet Gynecol* 1997;89:768–72.

29. De Jonge EM, Makin JD, Manefeldt E, De Wet GH, Pattinson RC. Randomised clinical trial of medical expulsion and surgical curettage for incomplete miscarriage. *BMJ* 1995;311:662–8.

30. Henshaw RC, Cooper K, el-Refaey H, Smith NC, Templeton AA. Medical management of miscarriage: non-surgical uterine evacuation of incomplete and inevitable spontaneous abortion. *BMJ* 1993;306:894–5. Erratum in: *BMJ* 1993;306:1303.

31. Chung TK, Lee DT, Cheung LP, Haines CJ, Chang AM. Spontaneous abortion: a randomized controlled trial comparing surgical evacuation with conservative management using misoprostol. *Fertil Steril* 1999;71:1054–9.

32. Wagaarachchi PT, Ashok PW, Narvekar N, Smith NC, Templeton A. Medical management of early fetal demise using a combination of mifepristone and misoprostol. *Hum Reprod* 2001;16:1845–53.

33. Neilsen S, Hahlin M, Platz-Christensen J. Randomised trial comparing expectant management with medical management for first trimester miscarriages. *Br J Obstet Gynaecol* 1999;106:804–7.

34. Gilles J, Mitchell DC, Barnhart K, Westhoff C, Fredrick MM, Zhang J. A randomised trial of saline solution-moistened misoprostol versus dry misoprostol for first-trimester pregnancy failure. *Am J Obstet Gynecol* 2004;190:389–94.

35. Demetroulis C, Saridogan E, Kunde D, Naftalin. A prospective randomized control trial comparing medical and surgical treatment for incomplete miscarriage. *Hum Reprod* 2001;16:365–9.

36. Ballagh SA, Harris HA, Demasio K. Is curettage needed for uncomplicated incomplete spontaneous abortion? *Am J Obstet Gynecol* 1998;179:1279–82.

37. Luise C, Jeremy K, May C, Costello G, Collins WP, Bourne TH. Outcome of expectant management of spontaneous first trimester miscarriage. *BMJ* 2002;324:873–5.

38. Nielsen S, Hahlin M. Expectant management of first-trimester spontaneous abortion. *Lancet* 1995;345:84–6.

39. Wieringa-De Waard M, Hartman EE, Ankum WM, Reitsma JB, Bindels PJ, Bonsel GJ. Expectant management versus surgical evacuation in first trimester miscarriage: health-related quality of life in randomized and non-randomized patients. *Hum Reprod* 2002;16:1638–42.

40. Jurkovic D, Ross JA, Nicolaides KH. Expectant management of missed miscarriage. *Br J Obstet Gynaecol* 1998;105:670–1.

41. Nagi SW, Chan YM, Tang OS, Ho PC. Vaginal misoprostol as medical treatment for first trimester spontaneous miscarriage. *Hum Reprod* 2001;7:1493–6.

Chapter 18
Recurrent miscarriage – the role of prothrombotic disorders

Arvind Vashisht and Lesley Regan

A thrombophilic defect is an abnormality in the coagulation pathways that predisposes an individual to thrombosis. Although the presence of the defect need not necessarily result in thrombosis, it may weaken the ability to deal with an additional prothrombotic insult, such as the hypercoagulable state of pregnancy. During the past few years, the antiphospholipid syndrome, an acquired thrombophilic disorder, has become established as the most important treatable cause of recurrent miscarriage. Interest has now focused on the potential role that other thrombophilic defects (both inherited and acquired) may be playing in the aetiology of recurrent early miscarriage and later pregnancy complications.

In this chapter we will develop the hypothesis that some women with a history of recurrent miscarriage (RM) are in a prothrombotic state outside of pregnancy. Further, that this state is exaggerated by the known haemostatic changes that occur during pregnancy, leading to defective placentation and pregnancy loss. The importance of reproductive haemostasis has only just started to emerge and is already proving to be an exciting new field of research and clinical investigation.

Definitions of pregnancy loss

Human reproduction is a surprisingly wasteful process. No more than 50% of all fertilised eggs result in a live birth[1] and at least 15% of clinically recognisable pregnancies end in a miscarriage.[2] Miscarriage is therefore the most common complication of pregnancy and is most frequently due to a sporadic fetal chromosomal abnormality, the risk for which rises with increasing maternal age.[3,4] In contrast to a single sporadic miscarriage, RM – defined in this chapter as the loss of three or more consecutive pregnancies – affects 1% of couples. When a definition of two or more pregnancy losses is used, the scale of the clinical problem increases to include 5% of all couples trying to achieve a successful pregnancy.[5]

There are several pieces of evidence to suggest that some cases of RM are due to an underlying systemic cause rather than repeated episodes of bad luck. A woman's risk of miscarriage is in part determined by the outcome of her previous pregnancies; the 1% observed incidence of RM is significantly higher than that expected by chance alone and furthermore women with a history of recurrent pregnancy loss have a tendency to lose chromosomally normal pregnancies.[5–7]

Aetiology of recurrent miscarriage

Historically, the causes of RM have been grouped into six main categories: genetic, anatomical, infective, endocrinological, immunological and unexplained. More recently, our understanding that thrombophilic disorders can play a part in the aetiology of recurrent pregnancy loss at various gestations has widened the scope of investigations and management options for this distressing condition.

Since miscarriage may occur at any gestational age from the time of conception until independent fetal viability, currently defined in the UK as 24 weeks, it is important to remember that there are many different causes of miscarriage and that no single investigative test or treatment can be applicable to all cases. This may seem an obvious point to the discerning reader, but it needs to be emphasised, since there has been a dramatic increase in the availability of information on reproductive issues during the last few years, both in the traditional media and via the internet. Although this can be viewed as a beneficial development in terms of disseminating valuable information to clinicians and their patients, it should be noted that much of this data has not been subjected to the rigours of peer review. Most couples who have experienced repeated pregnancy losses are desperate to improve their future chances of a successful outcome and are in an emotionally vulnerable state. All too often this may result in their being prepared or persuaded to take part in uncontrolled studies of empirical treatment.

Reproductive haemostasis

Haemostasis *in vivo* is a finely tuned balancing act between the coagulation and fibrinolytic pathways and plays a vital role in the establishment and maintenance of pregnancy. Carefully controlled fibrinolytic activity is required to facilitate ovulation and implantation of the fertilised egg into the uterine decidua. Once pregnancy has been established, maintenance of an intact placental circulation becomes the priority and during normal pregnancy the levels of many procoagulant factors increase from early in the first trimester. In addition, higher levels of systemic markers of thrombin generation such as thrombin–antithrombin (TAT) complexes and resistance to activated protein C (which inactivates factors V and VII) develop during pregnancy. However, these changes are not counteracted by increased levels of the naturally occurring anticoagulants; protein S levels are markedly reduced and fibrinolytic activity is also reduced. Levels of plasminogen activator inhibitors (PAI) 1 and 2 increase progressively during normal pregnancy, whereas the levels of the plasminogen activators remain unchanged. In addition to increased thrombin generation, an increase in platelet activation contributes to the prothrombotic state of pregnancy.[8,9] The net effect of the haemostatic changes in pregnancy is to favour coagulation. This is no accident – indeed, from an evolutionary viewpoint these changes are designed to counteract the inherent instability of haemochorial placentation and reduce blood loss from the materno–placental interface during pregnancy and at the time of delivery.

Evidence for adverse pregnancy outcome due to prothrombotic disorders

Evidence to support the hypothesis that many cases of hitherto unexplained RM are due to a disordered maternal haemostatic response in early pregnancy, resulting in thrombosis of the uteroplacental vasculature and subsequent fetal loss,[8,10] has been steadily accumulating.

Placental histology featuring the presence of microthrombi in the vasculature has been reported in many cases of RM, pre-eclampsia and intrauterine growth restriction.[11,12] Furthermore, placental infarction has been described in association with individual thrombophilic defects.[13,14]

Prospective studies have shown an increased prevalence of acquired thrombophilic disorders in women with a history of RM.[15,16] Additionally, the use of thrombo-prophylactic treatments started early in a subsequent pregnancy significantly improves pregnancy outcome for these women.[17,18] Longitudinal studies during the first trimester of pregnancy have identified haemostatic abnormalities to be present weeks before the fetal loss is declared.[19–21]

Retrospective studies have reported the risk of early and late miscarriage, stillbirth and other adverse pregnancy outcomes to be increased for women with both acquired and inherited thrombophilic defects[22–25] and even greater for women carrying multiple thrombophilic defects.[22]

However, one of the most exciting developments in this field is the growing body of evidence that some women with a history of RM are in a prothrombotic state outside of pregnancy.[21,26–28] This may result not only in an exaggerated and adverse haemostatic response during pregnancy, but also appears to increase the risk of ischaemic heart disease in later life.[29]

Lastly, the knowledge that many women with a history of RM are at greater risk of later pregnancy complications such as pre-eclampsia, fetal growth restriction and intrauterine death[30,31] suggests that these adverse pregnancy outcomes represent a spectrum of disorders which share a common origin. It would appear that the quality and depth of implantation and subsequent placental development may be adversely affected by a disordered haemostatic response in early pregnancy.

Established thrombophilic defects

The number of detectable thrombophilic defects has increased dramatically over the past few years and, as a result, we now recognise that these defects can be acquired or inherited. We shall consider both types in turn to explore the notion that there is a causal relationship between haemostatic abnormalities and adverse pregnancy outcome.

Acquired thrombophilia

Primary antiphospholipid syndrome (PAPS)

When first described, this syndrome referred to the association of antiphospholipid antibodies (aPL) with recurrent miscarriage, thrombosis or thrombocytopenia.[32] It has now become apparent that these three clinical features of PAPS are too limiting. Revised criteria for the diagnosis of PAPS recognise the importance of additional obstetric manifestations of aPL, such as a history of pre-eclampsia, intrauterine growth restriction, placental abruption and preterm labour.[33,34]

Screening for PAPS

The most clinically significant aPL are the lupus anticoagulant (LA) and the anti-cardiolipin antibodies (aCL) of the immunoglobulin G (IgG) and IgM subclasses; testing for aPL other than LA and aCL is of no proven benefit in the investigation of women with RM.[35] To diagnose PAPS, the same class of antibodies must be detected on at least two separate occasions more than six weeks apart, in order to avoid diagnostic inaccuracies resulting from temporal fluctuations and interlaboratory variation. These errors can be minimised by the use of international guidelines and by ensuring that the samples are collected in an optimal manner.[36,37] Although these aPL antibodies are also present in a proportion of women with systemic lupus erythematosus (SLE), which predisposes them to pregnancy-associated complications, women with PAPS do not have any of the clinical or serological features of SLE. A family history of thrombosis, cardiovascular disease, epilepsy or migraine may be suggestive of the presence of aPL in women presenting with RM. Those women with a personal history of thromboses are most likely to have a positive aPL status.[15]

Persistently positive aPL are present in 15% of women with RM,[15] whereas the figure is less than 2% in a normal low-risk obstetric population.[38] In women with PAPS who receive no pharmacological intervention, the miscarriage rate has been reported to be as high as 90%. In contrast, the prospective miscarriage rate in a control group of aPL-negative women with a history of RM is approximately 40%.[39] The majority of miscarriages in the aPL-positive women occurred in the first trimester after the establishment of fetal cardiac activity.

Treatment of PAPS in future pregnancies

Various treatments for PAPS have been proposed, including aspirin, heparin, steroids and immunoglobulins. The latter two have been widely disregarded, since a meta-analysis of intravenous immunoglobulin treatment reported no beneficial effect[40] and systemic steroids in pregnancy have been shown to be associated with adverse maternal and fetal morbidity, including preterm delivery and maternal diabetes.[41] Currently the gold standard for treatment of PAPS during pregnancy is a combination of low-dose aspirin and heparin from the time of the positive pregnancy test until 34 completed weeks of gestation. Reassuringly, the high live birth rate of 71% reported in the original randomised controlled trial of this drug regimen[18] has been maintained in subsequent studies by the same and other authors.[30] More recently, a meta-analysis of all available treatment studies has shown that the combined use of aspirin and heparin therapy improves the live birth rate to 54% overall.[42]

Unfractionated and low-molecular-weight heparins have been shown to be equally beneficial in the treatment of women with PAPS, the latter having the advantage of being a once-daily injection. Women may also be reassured that the modest loss in bone mineral density (BMD) observed with heparin therapy is not significantly different from the natural physiological loss in BMD seen in normal pregnancy.[43]

New insights into the pathophysiology of aPL antibodies

Although the underlying mechanism(s) accounting for the high miscarriage rate in women with aPL have traditionally centred around the development of thrombotic insults in the uteroplacental vasculature (histological evidence of infarction, perivillous fibrin deposits and chronic inflammatory lesions),[12] these placental pathologies are not universal. In addition, two important clinical observations further challenge the primacy of a thrombotic aetiology in women with RM with PAPS.

First is the later analysis of the pregnancy survival data from the randomised controlled trial by Rai *et al*.[18] in which it is evident that after 13 weeks of gestation there is no significant difference in the live birth rate among women treated with (1) combination aspirin and heparin, (2) aspirin alone, or (3) no pharmacological treatment. This suggests that the benefits of treatment are optimised when they are administered during the first trimester of pregnancy – a time at which blood flow in the intervillous circulation is minimal,[44,45] thereby precluding a conventional thrombotic aetiology. Second is the recent recognition that a small cohort of women with PAPS fail to achieve a successful outcome with aspirin and heparin, and that in subsequent pregnancies they are likely to miscarry again.[46] Collectively these data suggest that some women with PAPS are resistant to thromboprophylactic interventions and have an alternative or additional pathology underlying their repeated pregnancy losses.

Recent laboratory research supports these clinical observations. *In vitro* studies have reported that aPL also:

- exert an adverse effect on placental hormone production[47]
- impair signal transduction mechanisms controlling endometrial decidualisation[48]
- increase trophoblast apoptosis[49]
- reduce syncytiotrophoblast fusion[49,50]
- impair trophoblast invasion.[51,52]

Furthermore, all of these adverse effects have been reported to be reversed by the administration of heparin to *in vitro* culture systems.[51] Although conventionally considered as a thromboprophylactic agent, heparin and the structurally related heparan sulphate have several other properties which are important at the implantation site or materno–fetal interface. It appears that heparin is capable of binding to aPL and also of antagonising the action of the Th-1 cytokine interferon IFNγ, thereby protecting the trophoblast and maternal vascular endothelium from damage in early pregnancy. Later in pregnancy, when the intervillous circulation has been well established, the anticoagulant properties of heparin are beneficial in reducing the risk of placental fibrin deposition, thrombosis and infarction. Aspirin, by inhibiting platelet aggregation, also has a favourable thromboprophylactic effect.

Although aspirin and heparin treatment significantly reduces the severity of the defective endovascular trophoblastic invasion in women with PAPS, the underlying uteroplacental vasculopathy may still result in late pregnancy complications such as pre-eclampsia, intrauterine growth restriction, preterm birth and placental abruption in a proportion of pregnancies.[30] For example, the prevalence of placental infarction is noted to be around 8%, compared with 1% in the unselected obstetric population,[52] which emphasises the need for careful clinical surveillance of these high-risk pregnancies.

Inherited thrombophilias

Over the past decade a variety of inherited coagulation defects have been reported in the literature. Currently it is estimated that 15% of the Western population carry one or more of these thrombophilic defects, (although their risk of venous thrombo-embolism is significantly lower) and it is likely that many further defects will be identified in the future.

In addition to the knowledge that deficiencies in the endogenous anticoagulants protein C, protein S and antithrombin III have a heritable basis, three common thrombophilic gene mutations – factor V (Leiden) G1691A, factor 11 (prothrombin) G20210A and the methylene tetrahydrofolate reductase (MTHFR) thermolabile variant C677T (which leads to hyperhomocysteinaemia) – have been identified and are now firmly established causes of systemic thrombosis. However, it is only relatively recently that these defects have been implicated in the aetiology of miscarriage and later pregnancy complications.

Prevalence of inherited thrombophilic disorders in women with RM

The medical literature now contains a very large number of publications reporting the prevalence of individual coagulation defects in women with RM and later pregnancy complications. The results have been highly variable, reflecting the inherent bias introduced when studies are retrospective, include small numbers of subjects, allow selection and acquisition bias, fail to consider racial differences and employ poor matching of cases and controls in terms of previous pregnancy morbidity. Nonetheless, two meta-analyses have recently confirmed an association between the presence of factor V Leiden (FVL) and the prothrombin gene mutation with RM.[25,53]

The publications on activated protein C resistance (APCR) illustrate these shortcomings well and in the interests of brevity the following account is limited to APCR and excludes details of the other gene mutations. In 95% of cases of APCR, the coagulation disorder is due to the presence of a single point mutation in the factor V gene[54] (first discovered in a haemostasis laboratory in Leiden). This gene mutation increases the lifetime risk of systemic thrombosis among heterozygotes five-fold and in homozygotes eighty-fold. In women with RM carrying this gene mutation, histological evidence of placental infarction or thrombosis is a recognised feature[13] and is more frequently present in pregnancies in which the fetus also carries the FVL mutation.[14]

It is noteworthy, however, that the prevalence of the FVL gene mutation in the Western population is as high as 5%, and as such there are many female carriers who experience no reproductive sequelae and who proceed with an uncomplicated pregnancy. In the largest prospective cohort study available ($n = 1000$), the FVL allele frequency has been found to be similarly prevalent between women with recurrent miscarriages and parous controls. In contrast, the prevalence of acquired APCR – in which the FVL genotype is normal but the clotting cascade is disordered and may be detected by a functional coagulation-based assay – is significantly more common among both women with recurrent early miscarriage and those with late miscarriage.[16] Thus although genetic testing may reveal a definitive result for the FVL mutation, it does not provide information regarding the additional defects that contribute to phenotypic APCR, and to prothrombotic risks leading to pregnancy complications. This highlights the importance of testing for both genotypic and phenotypic causes of a hypercoagulable state.

Pregnancy outcome in women with inherited thrombophilias

In the only prospective longitudinal study of pregnancy outcome in women with a history of RM, those heterozygous for the FVL mutation had a significantly lower live birth rate than those with a normal genotype.[55] However, for some women with RM, carrying the FVL mutation was also compatible in some cases with an entirely normal pregnancy. What differentiates between these outcomes must be additional co-morbid conditions and it is becoming increasingly clear that some other factors in addition to the maternal genotype are determining the outcome of pregnancy. Currently there is no test that can discriminate between those women with RM and the FVL mutation who are destined to miscarry and those who are destined to have a successful pregnancy outcome. The varying phenotypic expression of these thrombophilias is undoubtedly due to complex interactions between acquired and inherited risk factors, and our ability to identify thrombophilic defects has outstripped our understanding of the mechanisms of fetal loss. It is well established that a combination of acquired and inherited thrombophilic factors increases the likelihood of venous thromboembolism. It may well be that a 'multi-hit' aetiology is necessary to substantially increase the likelihood of adverse pregnancy outcome in carriers of weakly prothrombotic genotypes. Indeed, one European cohort study identified a fourteen-fold increased risk of stillbirth in women with combined thrombophilic defects.[22]

Global markers of haemostatic abnormalities

Further compelling evidence of the association between haemostatic abnormalities and adverse pregnancy outcome is found in several studies demonstrating that women with RM exhibit prothrombotic tendencies outside of pregnancy. Vincent *et al*.[26] looked at levels of TAT complexes in nonpregnant women and found that these global markers of thrombin generation were significantly higher among women with a history of RM compared with age-matched fertile parous controls. This finding was independent of the gestation of previous miscarriage, and unaffected by the woman's aPL status. It may well be that in such women the hypercoagulable state of pregnancy proves to be the further 'hit' that leads to fetal loss or even a systemic thrombosis. Using alternative global markers it has also been reported that women with RM suffer from a chronic state of endothelial activation,[56] and abnormally high levels of procoagulant particles have been reported in the circulation of women with a history of hitherto unexplained early and late pregnancy miscarriage.[27,28] In addition to their direct effect on the coagulation cascade, these circulating microparticles may be exerting a proinflammatory or pro-apoptotic action resulting in a disturbance in the implantation process and subsequent damage to fetal growth.

Further evidence of the possibility of an inherent prothrombotic state outside of pregnancy in women with RM has been demonstrated using thromboelastography. The thromboelastogram (TEG) is a cheap and effective tool that assesses the kinetics, strength and stability of whole blood coagulation, and is considered a highly sensitive global test for haemostatic defects.[57] A variety of parameters scoring different stages of clot formation are registered, ranging from the initial platelet–fibrin interaction, through platelet aggregation, clot strengthening and fibrin cross-linkage to clot lysis. The great advantage of TEG testing compared with conventional coagulation assays is that it provides information about the interaction of platelets with the protein coagulation cascade. Most importantly, it is capable of identifying hypercoagulability that would only be detectable in conventional haemostasis assays when the platelet count or fibrinogen levels were markedly raised.

Among women with RM the maximal clot amplitude (MA) – a measure of the absolute strength of the fibrin clot formed and the parameter that most reliably indicates a hypercoagulable state – is significantly greater than in parous controls.[21] The prepregnancy MA has also been found to be predictive of future pregnancy outcome, being significantly higher in those women with RM whose next pregnancy ends in a further miscarriage compared with those having a live birth, further supporting the hypothesis that a subgroup of women with RM are in a prothrombotic state before pregnancy commences. Once pregnancy is declared, serial TEG testing during the first trimester is capable of identifying increases in the MA that predate the clinical evidence of impending miscarriage by several weeks.[58]

Summary

Recurrent miscarriage is a distressing condition that affects at least 1% of couples trying to achieve a successful pregnancy. The hypothesis that some cases of RM are due to a defective or exaggerated haemostatic response to pregnancy is now supported by a substantial body of robust evidence. This has led to the introduction of new treatment options that have made a significant contribution to improving pregnancy live birth rates.

For many couples presenting with RM, an underlying cause remains elusive. Undoubtedly, a proportion of these cases will be due to sporadic fetal chromosomal abnormalities, but in others there may be hitherto undiagnosed factors contributing. Although frustrating for these unfortunate couples, they should be reminded that they have a 75% chance of a successful outcome to their next pregnancy with psychological support and tender loving care alone. It is against this background that the temptation to empirically treat women, in the absence of any identifiable aetiological factor, should be resisted. These interventions may be at best unnecessary and at worst harmful. Instead, future efforts are best directed at continuing to expand and refine the ever-increasing evidence-based information available for the investigation and treatment of couples with RM.

The prevalence of thrombophilic defects among the general population is high, and the presence of a detectable defect does not necessarily preclude an uncomplicated pregnancy and term delivery. Nonetheless, recent reports have highlighted the fact that the presence of multiple prothrombotic risk factors or 'hits' are associated with poorer pregnancy outcomes. In conclusion, it appears that there is a complex interaction between the currently recognised acquired and inherited prothrombotic disorders that determine reproductive risk. The challenge for investigators in this field is the development of both global and specific measures of haemostatic abnormality that may better predict women at high risk of miscarriage and later pregnancy complications, in order that treatment can be targeted effectively.

References

1.   Kline J, Stein Z, Susser M. Conception and reproductive loss: probabilities. In: Kline J, Stein Z, Susser M, editors. *Conception to Birth: Epidemiology of Prenatal Development*. New York: Oxford University Press; 1989. p. 43–68.

2.   Regan L, Braude PR, Trembath PL. Influence of past reproductive performance on risk of

spontaneous abortion. *BMJ* 1989;299:541–5.

3. Nybo Andersen AM, Wohlfahrt J, Christens P, Olsen J, Melbye M. Maternal age and fetal loss: population based register linkage study. *BMJ* 2000;320:1708–12.

4. Hogge WA, Byrnes AL, Lanasa MC, Surti U. The clinical use of karyotyping spontaneous abortions. *Am J Obstet Gynecol* 2003;189:397–400.

5. Regan L. Sporadic and Recurrent Miscarriage. In: Grudzinskas JG, O'Brien PMS, editors. *Problems in Early Pregnancy. Advances in Diagnosis and Management*. London: RCOG Press; 1997. p. 31–52.

6. Stephenson MD, Awartani KA, Robinson WP. Cytogenetic analysis of miscarriages from couples with recurrent miscarriage: a case–control study. *Hum Reprod* 2002;17:446–51.

7. Sullivan AE, Silver RM, LaCoursiere DY, Porter TF, Branch DW. Recurrent fetal aneuploidy and recurrent miscarriage. *Obstet Gynecol* 2004;104:784–8.

8. Rai R, Regan L. Thrombophilic defects and pregnancy loss. In: Diamond MP, DeCherney AH, editors. *Infertility and Reproductive Medicine Clinics.* Volume 7. Philadelphia: WB Saunders; 1996. p. 745–58.

9. Clark P, Brennand J, Conkie JA, McCall F, Greer IA, Walker ID. Activated protein C sensitivity, protein C, protein S and coagulation in normal pregnancy. *Thromb Haemost* 1998;79:1166–70.

10. Rai R, Regan L. Thrombophilia and adverse pregnancy outcome. *Semin Reprod Med* 2000;18:369–77.

11. Rushton DI. Placental pathology in spontaneous miscarriage. In: Beard RW, Sharp F, editors. *Early Pregnancy Loss: Mechanisms and Treatment*. London: RCOG Press; 1988. p. 149–58.

12. Out HJ, Kooijman CD, Bruinse HW, Derksen RH. Histopathological findings in placentae from patients with intra-uterine fetal death and anti-phospholipid antibodies. *Eur J Obstet Gynecol Reprod Biol* 1991;41:179–86.

13. Rai RS, Regan L, Chitolie A, Donald JG, Cohen H. Placental thrombosis and second trimester miscarriage in association with activated protein C resistance. *Br J Obstet Gynaecol* 1996;103:842–4.

14. Dizon-Townson DS, Meline L, Nelson LM, Varner M, Ward K. Fetal carriers of the factor V Leiden mutation are prone to miscarriage and placental infarction. *Am J Obstet Gynecol* 1997;177:402–5.

15. Rai RS, Regan L, Clifford K, Pickering W, Dave M, Mackie I, *et al.* Antiphospholipid antibodies and beta 2-glycoprotein-I in 500 women with recurrent miscarriage: results of a comprehensive screening approach. *Hum Reprod* 1995;10:2001–5.

16. Rai R, Shlebak A, Cohen H, Backos M, Holmes Z, Marriott K, *et al.* Factor V Leiden and acquired activated protein C resistance among 1000 women with recurrent miscarriage. *Hum Reprod* 2001;16:961–5.

17. Kutteh WH. Antiphospholipid antibody-associated recurrent pregnancy loss: treatment with heparin and low-dose aspirin is superior to low-dose aspirin alone. *Am J Obstet Gynecol* 1996;174:1584–9.

18. Rai R, Cohen H, Dave M, Regan L. Randomised controlled trial of aspirin and aspirin plus heparin in pregnant women with recurrent miscarriage associated with phospholipid antibodies (or antiphospholipid antibodies). *BMJ* 1997;314:253–7.

19. Woodhams BJ, Candotti G, Shaw R, Kernoff PB. Changes in coagulation and fibrinolysis during pregnancy: evidence of activation of coagulation preceding spontaneous abortion. *Thromb Res* 1989;55:99–107.

20. Tulppala M, Viinikka L, Ylikorkala O. Thromboxane dominance and prostacyclin deficiency in habitual abortion. *Lancet* 1991;337:879–81.

21. Rai R, Tuddenham E, Backos M, Jivraj S, El'Gaddal S, Choy S, *et al.* Thromboelastography, whole-blood haemostasis and recurrent miscarriage. *Hum Reprod* 2003;18:2540–3.

22. Preston FE, Rosendaal FR, Walker ID, Briet E, Berntorp E, Conard J, *et al.* Increased fetal loss in women with heritable thrombophilia. *Lancet* 1996;348:913–16.

23. Sanson BJ, Friederich PW, Simioni P, Zanardi S, Hilsman MV, Girolami A, *et al.* The risk of abortion and stillbirth in antithrombin-, protein C-, and protein S-deficient women. *Thromb Haemost* 1996;75:387–8.

24. Kupferminc MJ, Eldor A, Steinman N, Many A, Bar-Am A, Jaffa A, *et al.* Increased frequency of genetic thrombophilia in women with complications of pregnancy. *N Engl J Med* 1999;340:9–13.

25. Rey E, Kahn SR, David M, Shrier I. Thrombophilic disorders and fetal loss: a meta-analysis. *Lancet* 2003;361:901–8.

26. Vincent T, Rai R, Regan L, Cohen H. Increased thrombin generation in women with recurrent miscarriage. *Lancet* 1998;352:116.

27. Laude I, Rongieres-Bertrand C, Boyer-Neumann C, Wolf M, Mairovitz V, Hugel B, *et al.* Circulating procoagulant microparticles in women with unexplained pregnancy loss: a new insight. *Thromb Haemost* 2001;85:18–21.

28. Carp H, Dardik R, Lubetsky A, Salomon O, Eskaraev R, Rosenthal E, *et al.* Prevalence of

circulating procoagulant microparticles in women with recurrent miscarriage: a case–controlled study. *Hum Reprod* 2004;19:191–5.

29. Smith GC, Pell JP, Walsh D. Spontaneous loss of early pregnancy and risk of ischaemic heart disease in later life: retrospective cohort study. *BMJ* 2003;326:423–4.

30. Backos M, Rai R, Baxter N, Chilcott IT, Cohen H, Regan L. Pregnancy complications in women with recurrent miscarriage associated with antiphospholipid antibodies treated with low dose aspirin and heparin. *Br J Obstet Gynaecol* 1999;106:102–7.

31. Jivraj S, Anstie B, Cheong YC, Fairlie FM, Laird SM, Li TC. Obstetric and neonatal outcome in women with a history of recurrent miscarriage: a cohort study. *Hum Reprod* 2001;16:102–6.

32. Harris EN. Syndrome of the black swan. *Br J Rheumatol* 1987;26:324–6.

33. Wilson WA, Gharavi AE, Koike T, Lockshin MD, Branch DW, Piette JC, *et al*. International consensus statement on preliminary classification criteria for definite antiphospholipid syndrome: report of an international workshop. *Arthritis Rheum* 1999;42:1309–11.

34. Backos M, Regan L. Antiphospholipid syndrome and preterm birth. In: Critchley H, Bennett P, Thornton S, editors. *Preterm Birth*. London: RCOG Press; 2004. p. 239–43.

35. Branch DW, Silver R, Pierangeli S, van Leeuwen I, Harris EN. Antiphospholipid antibodies other than lupus anticoagulant and anticardiolipin antibodies in women with recurrent pregnancy loss, fertile controls, and antiphospholipid syndrome. *Obstet Gynecol* 1997;89:549–55.

36. Guidelines on testing for the lupus anticoagulant. Lupus Anticoagulant Working Party on behalf of the BCSH Haemostasis and Thrombosis Task Force. *J Clin Pathol* 1991;44:885–9.

37. Khamashta MA, Hughes GR. ACP Broadsheet no 136: February 1993. Detection and importance of anticardiolipin antibodies. *J Clin Pathol* 1993;46:104–7.

38. Lockwood CJ, Romero R, Feinberg RF, Clyne LP, Coster B, Hobbins JC. The prevalence and biologic significance of lupus anticoagulant and anticardiolipin antibodies in a general obstetric population. *Am J Obstet Gynecol* 1989;161:369–73.

39. Rai RS, Clifford K, Cohen H, Regan L. High prospective fetal loss rate in untreated pregnancies of women with recurrent miscarriage and antiphospholipid antibodies. *Hum Reprod* 1995;10:3301–4.

40. Daya S, Gunby J, Porter F, Scott J, Clark DA. Critical analysis of intravenous immunoglobulin therapy for recurrent miscarriage. *Hum Reprod Update* 1999;5:475–82.

41. Laskin CA, Bombardier C, Hannah ME, Mandel FP, Ritchie JW, Farewell V, *et al*. Prednisone and aspirin in women with autoantibodies and unexplained recurrent fetal loss. *N Engl J Med* 1997;337:148–53.

42. Empson M, Lassere M, Craig JC, Scott JR. Recurrent pregnancy loss with antiphospholipid antibody: a systematic review of therapeutic trials. *Obstet Gynecol* 2002;99:135–44.

43. Backos M, Rai R, Thomas M, Murphy M, Dore C, Regan L. Bone density changes in pregnant women treated with heparin: a prospective, longitudinal study. *Hum Reprod* 1999;14:2876–80.

44. Jurkovic D, Jauniaux E, Kurjak A, Hustin J, Campbell S, Nicolaides KH. Transvaginal color Doppler assessment of the uteroplacental circulation in early pregnancy. *Obstet Gynecol* 1991;77:365–9.

45. Burton GJ, Jauniaux E, Watson AL. Maternal arterial connections to the placental intervillous space during the first trimester of human pregnancy: the Boyd collection revisited. *Am J Obstet Gynecol* 1999;181:718–24.

46. Regan L, Rai R. Unpublished data.

47. Di Simone N, De Carolis S, Lanzone A, Ronsisvalle E, Giannice R, Caruso A. *In vitro* effect of antiphospholipid antibody-containing sera on basal and gonadotrophin releasing hormone-dependent human chorionic gonadotrophin release by cultured trophoblast cells. *Placenta* 1995;16:75–83.

48. Mak IY, Brosens JJ, Christian M, Hills FA, Chamley L, Regan L, *et al*. Regulated expression of signal transducer and activator of transcription, Stat5, and its enhancement of PRL expression in human endometrial stromal cells *in vitro*. *J Clin Endocrinol Metab* 2002;87:2581–8.

49. Bose P, Black S, Kadyrov M, Weissenborn U, Neulen J, Regan L, *et al*. Heparin and aspirin attenuate placental apoptosis *in vitro*: implications for early pregnancy failure. *Am J Obstet Gynecol* 2005;192:23–30.

50. Lyden TW, Vogt E, Ng AK, Johnson PM, Rote NS. Monoclonal antiphospholipid antibody reactivity against human placental trophoblast. *J Reprod Immunol* 1992;22:1–14.

51. Bose P, Black S, Kadyrov M, Bartz C, Shlebak A, Regan L, *et al*. Adverse effects of lupus anticoagulant positive blood sera on placental viability can be prevented by heparin *in vitro*. *Am J Obstet Gynecol* 2004;191:2125–31.

52. Sebire NJ, Backos M, El Gaddal S, Goldin RD, Regan L. Placental pathology, antiphospholipid antibodies, and pregnancy outcome in recurrent miscarriage patients. *Obstet Gynecol* 2003;101:258–63.

53. Kovalevsky G, Gracia CR, Berlin JA, Sammel MD, Barnhart KT. Evaluation of the association between hereditary thrombophilias and recurrent pregnancy loss: a meta-analysis. *Arch Intern Med* 2004;164:558–63.

54. Bertina RM, Koeleman BP, Koster T, Rosendaal FR, Dirven RJ, de Ronde H, *et al.* Mutation in blood coagulation factor V associated with resistance to activated protein C. *Nature* 1994;369:64–7.

55. Rai R, Backos M, Elgaddal S, Shlebak A, Regan L. Factor V Leiden and recurrent miscarriage–prospective outcome of untreated pregnancies. *Hum Reprod* 2002;17:442–5.

56. Gris JC, Ripart-Neveu S, Maugard C, Tailland ML, Brun S, Courtieu C, *et al.* Respective evaluation of the prevalence of haemostasis abnormalities in unexplained primary early recurrent miscarriages. The Nimes Obstetricians and Haematologists (NOHA.) Study. *Thromb Haemost* 1997;77:1096–103.

57. Mallett SV, Cox DJ. Thrombelastography. *Br J Anaesth* 1992;69:307–13.

58. Rai R, Tuddenham E, Backos M, Regan L. Pre-pregnancy thrombophilic abnormalities are associated with subsequent spontaneous abortion. *Hum Reprod* 2000;15:168(A).

Chapter 19
Reproductive disorders and pregnancy outcome

Jan J Brosens, Luca Fusi, Robert Pijnenborg and
Ivo A Brosens

Summary

The formation of a functional placenta is dependent upon highly coordinated interactions between the invading trophoblast and differentiating uterine tissues. In most species, the remodelling of the maternal tissues required for placenta formation, a process termed decidualisation, is triggered by the implanting blastocyst. However, in a handful of species, including humans, this decidual process occurs independently of pregnancy and is initiated in the secretory phase of each menstrual cycle. This raises the possibility that reproductive disorders that affect the preconceptual endometrial milieu predispose for impaired trophoblast invasion in pregnancy. Defective deep placentation, characterised predominantly by inadequate physiological transformation of the spiral arteries, is associated with a spectrum of feto-maternal complications, including miscarriage, pre-eclampsia, fetal growth restriction and preterm labour. In recent years, several large studies have shown that subfertile women are at increased risk of poor pregnancy outcome, thereby providing epidemiological evidence for a pathological link between reproductive disorders and pregnancy complications. However, the molecular defects in differentiating endometrium that predispose for poor trophoblast invasion are largely undefined. Furthermore, well-conducted, prospective, randomised trials are urgently needed to evaluate the efficacy of periconceptual medical intervention in the prevention of early and late pregnancy complications.

Introduction

The increased incidence of feto-maternal complications in infertile women is usually attributed to certain patient characteristics, such as older age or primiparity, or to the higher incidence of multiple pregnancy after fertility treatment. While this may be so, recent studies support the view that subfecundity, or delayed time to conception, is an independent risk factor for poor feto-maternal outcome. This would suggest that certain pathological processes involved in subfecundity also predispose for a spectrum of pregnancy complications such as spontaneous miscarriage, preterm delivery, pre-eclampsia and fetal growth restriction. This chapter reviews the evidence in support of such a pathological link and discusses the implications for clinical management.

Subfecundity and adverse feto-maternal outcome

Several studies have reported that infertile couples are at increased risk of poor obstetric outcome when compared with fertile couples.[1–6] In a large population-based case–control study, Draper and co-workers[7] found that women with a history of infertility, whether treated or not, were at increased risk of perinatal death. This association could not be explained by confounding factors such as multiple pregnancies. Similarly, an earlier study by Venn and Lumley[8] also reported increased perinatal mortality in women with a history of infertility, irrespective of maternal age or parity, when compared with the general population. A large cohort study published in 2003 found that singleton pregnancies in subfertile women are also at increased risk of preterm delivery, fetal growth restriction and caesarean section, even if the women conceived without treatment.[9] The association between infertility and preterm delivery reported in this study was not a consequence of increased incidence of pre-eclampsia. It is important to note that several population studies have indicated that infertility treatment *per se* is unlikely to be a major factor in adverse obstetric outcome.

Taking 'time to pregnancy' (TTP) as a criterion, several studies have shown that a long inter-pregnancy interval is associated with an increased risk of pre-eclampsia.[10–12] A large study based on the Danish National Birth Cohort confirmed that the risk of pre-eclampsia increases with conception delay.[13] It has been estimated that in the first pregnancy the risk of pre-eclampsia increases by 50% if the TTP exceeds six months whereas for multiparous women the risk increases if TTP is 12 months or longer. Several studies have shown that a pregnancy, even if it ends in a miscarriage, decreases the subsequent risk of pre-eclampsia.[14–16] However, Skjaerven *et al.*[12] reported that this protective effect is transient and calculated that after a ten-year inter-pregnancy interval the risk of pre-eclampsia is comparable to that of a nulliparous woman. Furthermore, the authors found that, after adjustment for the interval between births, a change of partner is not associated with an increased risk of pre-eclampsia. Subfertility has also been associated with an increased risk of miscarriage although the available data are not very strong.[17] After adjustment for other variables, Joffe and Li[4] found that pregnancies that ended in miscarriage tended to take 23% longer to conceive. However, a large population-based study reported in 2004 that a history of recurrent miscarriage, defined in this study as two or more first-trimester spontaneous losses, is associated with cervical weakness, preterm premature rupture of membranes (PPROM) and preterm labour, independently from the effects of other risk factors.[18] These epidemiological studies provide support for the notion that a common aetiology underpins subfertility, early pregnancy failure and late obstetric complications.

In vitro fertilisation and pregnancy outcome

Several epidemiological studies have investigated pregnancy outcome in singleton pregnancy after *in vitro* fertilisation/intracytoplasmic sperm injection (IVF/ICSI). In a systematic review of a series of controlled studies, Helmerhorst *et al.*[19] concluded that singleton pregnancies from assisted reproduction have a significantly worse perinatal outcome than spontaneously conceived singleton pregnancies. The perinatal risks included preterm delivery, small for gestational age, caesarean section and perinatal mortality. Surprisingly, in twin pregnancies, the perinatal mortality was found to be approximately 40% lower after assisted conception when compared with natural conception.[19] A large nationwide US study found that singleton pregnancies conceived after IVF/ICSI have a higher incidence of small-for-gestation-age and very-small-for-gestation-age infants.[20] For term babies conceived after IVF/ICSI, the risk was increased by 2.5 times (OR 2.5; 95% CI 2.4–2.6).[20]

The lack of appropriate matched control groups in these studies makes it difficult to determine unequivocally whether the adverse pregnancy outcome associated with assisted reproduction technologies is the result of the treatment or is the consequence of the underlying condition in infertile women.[21] It is, however, interesting to note that gestational carriers or women who conceived after ICSI for strict male infertility were not found to be at increased risk of fetal growth restriction.[20]

Reproductive disorders and adverse pregnancy outcome

The lack of consensus diagnostic criteria and the heterogeneous nature of contemporary infertility investigations make it difficult to define the risk of adverse pregnancy outcome in relation to specific reproductive disorders, such as endometriosis or polycystic ovary syndrome (PCOS). At least a quarter of all infertile couples in the UK have unexplained infertility.[22] Pandian *et al.*[23] analysed the obstetric history and perinatal outcome of 498 couples with unexplained infertility, defined as having normal semen parameters, ovulatory cycles and bilateral tubal patency. After adjusting for age, parity and multiple pregnancies, the authors found a significantly higher incidence of pre-eclampsia, placental abruption and preterm labour in women with unexplained infertility compared with the general obstetric population.

It is likely that, when laparoscopy is not part of the fertility exploration, a substantial proportion of women with unexplained infertility have minimal or mild endometriosis. Indeed, Akande *et al.*[24] reported in 2004 that the time to natural conception in women with unexplained infertility is significantly prolonged when minor endometriosis is found but not treated at the time of diagnostic laparoscopy. However, a Finnish matched case–control study[25] reported no apparent negative effect of endometriosis on subsequent obstetric outcome, although it is unclear from this report to what extent the endometriosis had been treated surgically or medically prior to conception. It is important to note that endometriosis, like other reproductive disorders, comprises a spectrum of lesions, from active and haemorrhagic lesions to 'burnt-out' disease, characterised by fibrosis and adhesions. Hence, a straightforward relationship between specific reproductive disorders and pregnancy outcome is unlikely to exist. The risk of pregnancy complication is more likely determined by the effect of the disease on biological systems critical for pregnancy, such as the immune, haemostatic and endocrine systems.

Defective deep placentation and adverse pregnancy outcome

In humans, the formation of a functional placenta requires invasion of fetal trophoblast not only into the maternal decidua and inner myometrium (interstitial invasion) but also into the maternal spiral arteries (endovascular invasion).[26] In early pregnancy, the invading endovascular trophoblast effectively blocks perfusion to the developing fetus.[27,28] This 'plugging' of the spiral arteries by trophoblast is thought to be critical to protect the early conceptus from exposure to excessive amount of reactive oxygen species.[27,28] Later in pregnancy, the invading endovascular trophoblast replaces the endothelial lining and most of the musculo–elastic wall of the spiral arteries, thereby creating a high-flow, low-resistance circulation devoid of maternal vasomotor control. The process of 'disappearance of the normal muscular and elastic structures of the arteries and their replacement by fibrinoid material in which trophoblast cells are embedded' was first described in 1967 and termed 'physiological transformation' of the spiral arteries.[26] There is general agreement that spiral artery remodelling reduces maternal blood flow resistance and increases uteroplacental perfusion to meet the requirements of the developing fetus.[29]

Defective deep placentation, characterised by the absence of physiological transformation of the myometrial spiral arteries in the placental bed, was first described in pre-eclampsia.[30] The abnormality is manifested by the absence of large 'sinusoidal' vessels and the persistence of spiral arteries with a musculo–elastic wall in the inner third of the myometrium. Examination of hysterectomy specimens with the placenta *in situ* obtained from patients with pre-eclampsia and associated fetal growth restriction demonstrated that physiological transformation of the spiral arteries was limited to just a few vessels in the centre of the placental bed. Furthermore, hypertensive vascular lesions, such as thrombosis, acute atherosis and arteriosclerosis, were apparent in endometrial spiral and basal arterioles in and outside the placental bed. Variable degrees of defective physiological transformation of the spiral arteries have now been found in placental bed biopsy specimens from women with pre-eclampsia without fetal growth restriction, nonproteinuric pregnancy-induced hypertension, chronic hypertension without superimposed pre-eclampsia, fetal growth restriction without associated pre-eclampsia, placental abruption, and preterm labour with and without intact membranes.[31–37]

Failure of physiological transformation is thought to increase the vascular resistance in the placental bed and to reduce the blood flow to the intervillous space. It is intriguing that there are pre-eclamptic pregnancies without fetal growth restriction infants and yet the uteroplacental remodelling in these pregnancies is as defective as observed in pregnancies complicated by intrauterine growth restriction (Table 19.1). A note of caution is that these studies have been largely based on biopsy material obtained blindly from the uterine wall after removal of the placenta. As the depth of arterial remodelling decreases towards the periphery of the placenta, a random biopsy from the placental bed may not be entirely representative. Furthermore, defective physiological changes do not necessarily hamper uteroplacental blood flow sufficiently to cause clinical symptoms. It appears increasingly likely that additional factors such as genetic predisposition (e.g. genetic thrombophilias), environmental factors (e.g. hormone disruptors) and pre-existing vascular pathology modify the threshold for the clinical manifestations of defective deep placentation. Although pregnancy-induced hypertension and pre-eclampsia are likely to be multifactorial disorders, there is strong clinical evidence to suggest that the degree of vascular resistance in the placental bed determines the feto-maternal outcome in these women.[38]

Defective physiological changes of the terminal spiral arteries in the decidua have been associated with recurrent miscarriage of fetuses with normal chromosomes in the presence or absence of circulating antiphospholipid antibodies.[37,39] Analysis of a large series of archived miscarriage specimens by Hustin *et al.*[40] suggested that haemorrhage at the feto-maternal interface could be the consequence of failure of endovascular trophoblast to invade and plug the endometrial arterioles. The authors postulated that premature onset of the maternal intervillous blood circulation could

Table 19.1. Physiological changes of the myometrial segment of placental bed spiral arteries; based on combined data from Brosens *et al.*[30] and Dommisse and Tiltman[33]

Clinical presentation	*n*	Physiological changes
NT AGA	28	93%
NT SGA	42	43%
PE AGA	19	0%
PE SGA	47	2%

NT = normotensive; AGA = adequate-for-gestational-age newborns; PE = pre-eclampsia; SGA = small-for-gestational-age newborns

be noxious for the fetus. Hempstock *et al.*[28] recently found morphological and immunohistochemical evidence of cellular stress, damage and apoptosis in tissues obtained from delayed miscarriages. A variety of markers, including enhanced expression of heat shock protein 70, formation of nitrotyrosine residues and lipid peroxidation, indicated that the tissues had been exposed to oxidative stress that was far greater than the antioxidant defence systems could handle. The authors concluded that, although spontaneous fetal loss may have multiple causes, placental oxidative stress with resultant damage to the syncytiotrophoblast, secondary to premature onset of the maternal circulation, could be a final common mechanism.[28]

Defective trophoblast invasion or defective decidualisation?

Defective deep placentation is frequently attributed to impaired trophoblast invasiveness. Intuitively, this seems a logical explanation that appears to be supported by experiments in mice demonstrating that ablation of a variety of genes results in impaired trophoblast differentiation along the various cell lineages (for a review see Red-Horse *et al.*[41]). However, there is little or no evidence in humans to suggest that primary defects in trophoblast cells are a common cause of defective deep placentation. It has been reported that the invading trophoblast in pre-eclamptic pregnancies has a different phenotype, characterised by aberrant expression of integrins and cell adhesion molecules, but this was not confirmed by subsequent studies.[7,42-44] Arguably, a primary trophoblast defect should impair not only endovascular but also interstitial trophoblast invasion in pre-eclamptic pregnancies, but this is not the case.[45]

An alternative explanation is that a hostile endometrial milieu results in patho-logical decidual–trophoblast interactions. The term 'decidua' is often used synonymously for a differentiated endometrial stromal compartment. However, the decidualisation process extends to all cellular compartments and includes altered local immune cell populations, characterised predominantly by influx of uterine natural killer (uNK) cells, and remodelling of the spiral arteries independently of invading trophoblast. In humans, decidualisation is first apparent approximately ten days after the luteinising hormone (LH) surge in stromal cells around the spiral arterioles and capillaries of the superficial layer.[46] The differentiating stromal cells become rounded, acquire myofibroblast characteristics, and secrete a variety of phenotypic antigens, including prolactin, tissue factor and insulin-like growth factor binding protein-1.[45-48]

In vitro studies have revealed that decidual transformation of endometrial stromal cells involves extensive reprogramming of many cell functions, including altered steroid hormone receptor expression and steroid metabolism, remodelling of the extracellular matrix and cytoskeleton, altered expression of intracellular enzymes, growth factors and cytokines and their receptors, and induction of apoptosis modulators and decidua-specific transcription factors.[49,50]

Ramsey *et al.*[51] pointed out in 1976 that in primate species the depth of trophoblast invasion in the placental bed is apparently related to the degree of decidualisation, suggesting a critical role for this process in limiting trophoblast invasion. However, emerging evidence suggests that this extensive cellular differentiation process is also critical for tissue haemostasis prior to and during pregnancy and that it confers cellular resistance to oxidative stress and inflammatory cytokines.[52–55] Furthermore, the decidualisation process plays an integral role in ensuring immunotolerance towards the semi-allogeneic feto-placental unit while simultaneously protecting mother and fetus against pathogens. For instance, the post-ovulatory rise in progesterone levels induces expression of macrophage inflammatory protein 1β and interleukin 15 by differentiating endometrial stromal cells, which in turn provide the chemotactic and proliferative signals for the recruitment of CD56+, CD16− uNK cells.[56–58] Recent gene expression studies of human uNK cells reported high expression of immuno-modulatory molecules such as galectin-1 and glycodelin A.[59] Galectin-1 is known to inhibit T cell proliferation and survival and attenuates expression of proinflammatory cytokines by activated T cells. Similarly, glycodelin A (also termed placental protein 14) potently inhibits T cell activation through its ability to interact with the tyrosine phosphatase receptor CD45 on the T cell surface.[60–62] The decidua, like syncytio-trophoblast, also expresses the tryptophan-catabolising enzyme indoleamine 2,3-dioxygenase (IDO).[63,64] Tryptophan is a rare but essential amino acid required for cell proliferation. Studies in mice revealed an essential role for IDO in pregnancy. Treatment of mothers with an IDO inhibitor, 1-methyl-tryptophan, induces extensive inflammation, massive complement deposition, and haemorrhagic necrosis at the feto-maternal interface, resulting in the resorption of semi-allogeneic fetuses. However, no inflammatory reaction is observed when syngeneic mothers are given the IDO inhibitor and the pregnancy is not lost.[65–68] These data strongly suggest that IDO activity protects the fetus by suppressing T cell-dependent inflammatory responses to fetal alloantigens.

Reproductive disorders and adverse uterine milieu

The post-ovulatory rise in progesterone is the master signal for endometrial remodelling. However, the cellular responses to progesterone are complex and regulated at many levels. Uterine target cells express various complements of membrane and nuclear progesterone receptors, each capable of differentially responding to hormonal activation. Furthermore, progesterone signalling in the reproductive tract is invariably intertwined with other hormones, cytokine or growth factor signalling.[69] For instance, there is compelling evidence to suggest that decidual transformation in the secretory phase of the cycle coincides with the expression of a variety of factors, such activin A, relaxin, prostaglandin E_2 and corticotrophin-releasing hormone, capable of elevating cytoplasmic cyclic adenosine monophosphate (cAMP) levels in stromal cells. As a consequence of elevated cAMP levels, a repertoire of specific transcription factors, such as FOXO1A, C/EBP beta, HOXA10, and STAT5, are either induced or activated in endometrial stromal cells.[70–73] Emerging evidence suggests that many of these 'subsidiary' transcription factors physically interact with the progesterone receptor, thereby modifying the genomic response to progesterone. A major advantage of this system is that a single hormonal signal (progesterone) can elicit a highly coordinated cascade of cellular responses. A major disadvantage, however, is that a variety of aberrant signals can potentially disrupt the formation of these specific progesterone-dependent transcriptional complexes necessary for normal endometrial differentiation.[46]

Among couples with subfecundity, the uterine microenvironment has been most extensively investigated in woman with endometriosis. There is now abundant evidence indicating that endometriosis is associated with impaired tissue responses to progesterone.[74,75] This is characterised by attenuated expression of progesterone-dependent genes during the secretory phase of the cycle as well as impaired repression of other gene sets, such as metalloproteinases. The concept of relative progesterone insensitivity of the eutopic endometrium in women with endometriosis is further supported by the observation that progesterone treatment of mice inoculated with human eutopic endometrium inhibits development of endometriotic lesions when derived from disease-free women but not from affected patients.[76] The underlying mechanism of relative progesterone insensitivity in endometriosis is not well understood although there are strong experimental data to suggest that inflammation and activation of proinflammatory transcription factors, such as nuclear factor kappa B (NFκB) and STAT1, interfere with progesterone receptor-dependent gene expression.[55,73,77] Similarly, elevated androgens and antiphospholipid antibodies have been shown to impair decidual transformation of the endometrial cells, thereby providing a potential explanation for the increased incidence of reproductive failure associated with PCOS and primary antiphospholipid syndrome (APS), respectively.[70,78,79]

Certain pathological processes underpin both reproductive disorders and pregnancy complications. For instance, oxidative stress is a component of any inflammatory reaction, including endometriosis and pre-eclampsia.[80,81] This is manifested in the endometrium by the altered expression of enzymes such as manganese superoxide dismutase and glutathion peroxidase that are involved in the defence against oxidative stress. Murphy *et al.*[82,83] highlighted the analogies between endometriosis and arteriosclerosis. Both diseases are characterised by oxidative stress, the presence of tissue macrophages that express scavenger receptors, increased levels of oxidised lipoproteins, and the presence of inflammatory cytokines and growth factors. Many *et al.*[80] showed an association between impaired trophoblast invasion and oxidative stress in pre-eclamptic women, as indicated by altered xanthine oxidase and superoxide dismutase expression as well as tissue accumulation of nitrotyrosine residues. Macrophages are involved in both oxidative stress and inhibition of trophoblast invasion.[84] Furthermore, the characteristic foam cells in atherotic spiral and basal arterioles in pre-eclampsia are macrophage-derived.[31] Finally, antioxidant treatment in a group of women with increased risk of pre-eclampsia showed a potential benefit in the prevention of pre-eclampsia, possibly by antagonising the negative effects of a poorly adapted uterine microenvironment.[85,86]

Periconceptual manipulation of the uterine milieu

There is evidence to suggest that manipulation of the uterine microenvironment can improve pregnancy rates and outcome. In rodents, the decidual process can be triggered by local application of oil drops or tissue injury in the presence of elevated progesterone levels.[87] In humans, there is evidence indicating that an inflammatory endometrial response may be beneficial for subsequent pregnancy and that this effect persists in subsequent cycles. For instance, randomised studies have shown an increased pregnancy rate in subfertile women following hysterosalpingography with oil-soluble contrast medium.[88] Similarly, Barash and co-workers[89] reported that an endometrial biopsy prior to IVF treatment doubles the chance of a take-home baby. Conversely, suppression of inflammatory processes by gonadotrophin-releasing hormone (GnRH) agonist therapy for three months has also been reported to improve IVF pregnancy in certain women.[90] Ishihara et al.[91] have recently demonstrated that prolonged treatment with GnRH agonists inhibits endometrial aromatase P450 expression in women with fibroids and endometriosis, emphasising that the type of downregulation and stimulation protocols used in IVF should be tailored to specific patient groups.[91]

Certain treatment modalities, including prednisolone, paternal leucocyte immunisation and intravenous immunoglobulin (IVIG), have been shown to be ineffective or even dangerous in randomised controlled studies and should no longer be offered to women at risk of early pregnancy failure or late obstetric complications.[92–95] Other pharmacological interventions during the periconception period, including progesterone, heparin, metformin and antioxidant therapy with vitamins C and E, warrant further evaluation in well-controlled clinical trials.

A major challenge in clinical practice is to refine our diagnostic tests so that medical intervention is not random but targets the underlying pathology. A case in point is the periconceptual use of progesterone for the prevention of early pregnancy failure. Besides its direct effect on decidual transformation, progesterone has important local and systemic immunomodulatory properties (reviewed in Dosiou and Guidice[96]). Furthermore, emerging evidence suggests that immune-mediated pregnancy failure not only involves the local induction of inflammatory processes at the feto-maternal interface but also the inhibition of ovarian steroidogenesis.[97] Despite these lines of evidence, the pharmacological use of progesterone during the luteal phase and in early pregnancy has fallen into disrepute, largely because it has been shown to be ineffective in the prevention of threatened sporadic miscarriage.[98] However, in women with three or more consecutive miscarriages, in whom an underlying immunological cause is much more likely, progesterone treatment has been shown to decrease the miscarriage rate significantly compared with placebo or no treatment (OR 0.39; 95% CI 0.17–0.91).[99] Similarly, progesterone support improves pregnancy outcome after IVF treatment and two recent randomised trials have reported that progesterone also markedly reduces the incidence of preterm labour in at-risk women.[100–102] Interestingly, heparin, which is widely used for the prevention of recurrent miscarriage associated with antiphospholipid antibodies, has also been shown to suppress NK cell cytotoxicity, to antagonise interferon γ signalling and to inhibit complement activation, in addition to its anticoagulant effects.[103–105]

Conclusions

It has taken many years to realise that successful treatment of subfertility is not pregnancy but the birth of a single, healthy, term baby. The epidemiological evidence for a pathological link between subfertility and poor feto-maternal outcome raises a number of important challenges and opportunities in clinical practice. First, the data emphasise the importance of periconceptual care for the prevention of not only early pregnancy loss but also late obstetric complications such as pre-eclampsia and preterm labour. Remodelling of uterine tissues prior to and during early pregnancy is critical for successful deep haemochorial placentation. The corollary of this observation is that medical intervention aimed at preventing late obstetric complications is likely to be effective only if initiated during the periconceptual period. Second, treatment should be targeted and much more effort should be placed on defining the biochemical perturbations in the endometrial milieu prior to pregnancy. Microarray and proteomic technologies raise the possibility that diagnostic 'fingerprints' will be discovered in endometrial or blood samples of women at risk of pregnancy complications. Finally, there is an urgent need for a national or international framework that coordinates large, well-conducted, prospective, randomised trials assessing the safety and effectiveness of periconceptual medical treatments.

Acknowledgement

This work was supported by a St Mary's Hospital Special Trustees research grant.

References

1. Ghazi HA, Spielberger C, Kallen B. Delivery outcome after infertility – a registry study. *Fertil Steril* 1991;55:726–32.
2. Li TC, MacLeod I, Singhal V, Duncan SL. The obstetric and neonatal outcome of pregnancy in women with a previous history of infertility: a prospective study. *Br J Obstet Gynaecol* 1991;98:1087–92.
3. Olivennes F, Rufat P, Andre B, Pourade A, Quiros MC, Frydman R. The increased risk of complication observed in singleton pregnancies resulting from in-vitro fertilization (IVF) does not seem to be related to the IVF method itself. *Hum Reprod* 1993;8:1297–300.
4. Joffe M, Li Z. Association of time to pregnancy and the outcome of pregnancy. *Fertil Steril* 1994;62:71–5.
5. Sundstrom I, Ildgruben A, Hogberg U. Treatment-related and treatment-independent deliveries among infertile couples, a long-term follow-up. *Acta Obstet Gynecol Scand* 1997;76:238–43.
6. Henriksen TB, Baird DD, Olsen J, Hedegaard M, Secher NJ, Wilcox AJ. Time to pregnancy and preterm delivery. *Obstet Gynecol* 1997;89:594–9.
7. Draper ES, Kurinczuk JJ, Abrams KR, Clarke M. Assessment of separate contributions to perinatal mortality of infertility history and treatment: a case–control analysis. *Lancet* 1999;353:1746–9.
8. Venn A, Lumley J. Births after a period of infertility in Victorian women 1982–1990. *Aust N Z J Obstet Gynaecol* 1993;33:379–84.
9. Basso O, Baird DD. Infertility and preterm delivery, birthweight, and caesarean section: a study within the Danish National Birth Cohort. *Hum Reprod* 2003;18:2478–84.
10. Lie RT, Rasmussen S, Brunborg H, Gjessing HK, Lie-Nielsen E, Irgens LM. Fetal and maternal contributions to risk of pre-eclampsia: population based study. *BMJ* 1998;316:1343–7.
11. Conde-Agudelo A, Belizan JM. Maternal morbidity and mortality associated with interpregnancy interval: cross sectional study. *BMJ* 2000;321:1255–9.
12. Skjaerven R, Wilcox AJ, Lie RT. The interval between pregnancies and the risk of preeclampsia. *N Engl J Med* 2002;346:33–8.
13. Basso O, Weinberg CR, Baird DD, Wilcox AJ, Olsen J. Subfecundity as a correlate of preeclampsia: a study within the Danish National Birth Cohort. *Am J Epidemiol* 2003;157:195–202.
14. Eskenazi B, Fenster L, Sidney S. A multivariate analysis of risk factors for preeclampsia. *JAMA* 1991;266:237–41.
15. Eras JL, Saftlas AF, Triche E, Hsu CD, Risch HA, Bracken MB. Abortion and its effect on risk of preeclampsia and transient hypertension. *Epidemiology* 2000;11:36–43.
16. Sibai BM, Ewell M, Levine RJ, Klebanoff MA, Esterlitz J, Catalano PM, et al. Risk factors associated with preeclampsia in healthy nulliparous women. The Calcium for Preeclampsia Prevention (CPEP) Study Group. *Am J Obstet Gynecol* 1997;177:1003–10.
17. Gray RH, Wu LY. Subfertility and risk of spontaneous abortion. *Am J Public Health* 2000;90:1452–4.
18. Hammoud A, Bujold E, Krapp M, Diamond M, Baumann P. Recurrent miscarriages and risks of preterm birth. *Fertil Steril* 2004;82(Suppl 2):S18.
19. Helmerhorst FM, Perquin DA, Donker D, Keirse MJ. Perinatal outcome of singletons and twins after assisted conception: a systematic review of controlled studies. *BMJ* 2004;328:261.

20. Schieve LA, Meikle SF, Ferre C, Peterson HB, Jeng G, Wilcox LS. Low and very low birth weight in infants conceived with use of assisted reproductive technology. *N Engl J Med* 2002;346:731–7.
21. Kovalevsky G, Rinaudo P, Coutifaris C. Do assisted reproductive technologies cause adverse fetal outcomes? *Fertil Steril* 2003;79:1270–2.
22. Templeton AA, Penney GC. The incidence, characteristics, and prognosis of patients whose infertility is unexplained. *Fertil Steril* 1982;37:175–82.
23. Pandian Z, Bhattacharya S, Templeton A. Review of unexplained infertility and obstetric outcome: a 10 year review. *Hum Reprod* 2001;16:2593–7.
24. Akande VA, Hunt LP, Cahill DJ, Jenkins JM. Differences in time to natural conception between women with unexplained infertility and infertile women with minor endometriosis. *Hum Reprod* 2004;19:96–103.
25. Kortelahti M, Anttila MA, Hippelainen MI, Heinonen ST. Obstetric outcome in women with endometriosis – a matched case–control study. *Gynecol Obstet Invest* 2003;56:207–12.
26. Brosens I, Robertson WB, Dixon HG. The physiological response of the vessels of the placental bed to normal pregnancy. *J Pathol Bacteriol* 1967;93:569–79.
27. Jauniaux E, Watson AL, Hempstock J, Bao YP, Skepper JN, Burton GJ. Onset of maternal arterial blood flow and placental oxidative stress. A possible factor in human early pregnancy failure. *Am J Pathol* 2000;157:2111–22.
28. Hempstock J, Jauniaux E, Greenwold N, Burton GJ. The contribution of placental oxidative stress to early pregnancy failure. *Hum Pathol* 2003;34:1265–75.
29. Kaufmann P, Black S, Huppertz B. Endovascular trophoblast invasion: implications for the pathogenesis of intrauterine growth retardation and preeclampsia. *Biol Reprod* 2003;69:1–7.
30. Brosens IA, Robertson WB, Dixon HG. The role of the spiral arteries in the pathogenesis of preeclampsia. *Obstet Gynecol Annu* 1972;1:177–91.
31. Hanssens M, Pijnenborg R, Keirse MJ, Vercruysse L, Verbist L, Van Assche FA. Renin-like immunoreactivity in uterus and placenta from normotensive and hypertensive pregnancies. *Eur J Obstet Gynecol Reprod Biol* 1998;81:177–84.
32. Pijnenborg R, Anthony J, Davey DA, Rees A, Tiltman A, Vercruysse L, *et al.* Placental bed spiral arteries in the hypertensive disorders of pregnancy. *Br J Obstet Gynaecol* 1991;98:648–55.
33. Dommisse J, Tiltman AJ. Placental bed biopsies in placental abruption. *Br J Obstet Gynaecol* 1992;99:651–4.
34. Khong TY, De Wolf F, Robertson WB, Brosens I. Inadequate maternal vascular response to placentation in pregnancies complicated by pre-eclampsia and by small-for-gestational age infants. *Br J Obstet Gynaecol* 1986;93:1049–59.
35. Kim YM, Chaiworapongsa T, Gomez R, Bujold E, Yoon BH, Rotmensch S, *et al.* Failure of physiologic transformation of the spiral arteries in the placental bed in preterm premature rupture of membranes. *Am J Obstet Gynecol* 2002;187:1137–42.
36. Kim YM, Bujold E, Chaiworapongsa T, Gomez R, Yoon BH, Thaler HT, *et al.* Failure of physiologic transformation of the spiral arteries in patients with preterm labor and intact membranes. *Am J Obstet Gynecol* 2003;189:1063–9.
37. Khong TY, Liddell HS, Robertson WB. Defective haemochorial placentation as a cause of miscarriage: a preliminary study. *Br J Obstet Gynaecol* 1987;94:649–55.
38. Aardema MW, Saro MC, Lander M, De Wolf BT, Oosterhof H, Aarnoudse JG. Second trimester Doppler ultrasound screening of the uterine arteries differentiates between subsequent normal and poor outcomes of hypertensive pregnancy: two different pathophysiological entities? *Clin Sci (Lond)* 2004;106:377–82.
39. Sebire NJ, Fox H, Backos M, Rai R, Paterson C, Regan L. Defective endovascular trophoblast invasion in primary antiphospholipid antibody syndrome-associated early pregnancy failure. *Hum Reprod* 2002;17:1067–71.
40. Hustin J, Jauniaux E, Schaaps JP. Histological study of the materno–embryonic interface in spontaneous abortion. *Placenta* 1990;11:477–86.
41. Red-Horse K, Zhou Y, Genbacev O, Prakobphol A, Foulk R, McMaster M, *et al.* Trophoblast differentiation during embryo implantation and formation of the maternal–fetal interface. *J Clin Invest* 2004;114:744–54.
42. Zhou Y, Damsky CH, Chiu K, Roberts JM, Fisher SJ. Preeclampsia is associated with abnormal expression of adhesion molecules by invasive cytotrophoblasts. *J Clin Invest* 1993;91:950–60.
43. Zhou Y, Damsky CH, Fisher SJ. Preeclampsia is associated with failure of human cytotrophoblasts to mimic a vascular adhesion phenotype. One cause of defective endovascular invasion in this syndrome? *J Clin Invest* 1997;99:2152–64.
44. Lyall F, Bulmer JN, Duffie E, Cousins F, Theriault A, Robson SC. Human trophoblast invasion and spiral artery transformation: the role of PECAM-1 in normal pregnancy, preeclampsia, and fetal growth restriction. *Am J Pathol* 2001;158:1713–21.
45. Brosens JJ, Pijnenborg R, Brosens IA. The myometrial junctional zone spiral arteries in normal and abnormal pregnancies: a review of the literature. *Am J Obstet Gynecol* 2002;187:1416–23.
46. Gellersen B, Brosens J. Cyclic AMP and progesterone receptor cross-talk in human endometrium: a decidualizing affair. *J Endocrinol* 2003;178:357–72.
47. Brosens JJ, Takeda S, Acevedo CH, Lewis MP, Kirby PL, Symes EK, *et al.* Human endometrial fibroblasts immortalized by simian virus 40 large T antigen differentiate in response to a

decidualization stimulus. *Endocrinology* 1996;137:2225–31.

48. Brosens JJ, Hayashi N, White JO. Progesterone receptor regulates decidual prolactin expression in differentiating human endometrial stromal cells. *Endocrinology* 1999;140:4809–20.

49. Brar AK, Kessler CA, Handwerger S. An Ets motif in the proximal decidual prolactin promoter is essential for basal gene expression. *J Mol Endocrinol* 2002;29:99–112.

50. Popovici RM, Kao LC, Giudice LC. Discovery of new inducible genes in *in vitro* decidualized human endometrial stromal cells using microarray technology. *Endocrinology* 2000;141:3510–13.

51. Ramsey EM, Houston ML, Harris JW. Interactions of the trophoblast and maternal tissues in three closely related primate species. *Am J Obstet Gynecol* 1976;124:647–52.

52. Schatz F, Krikun G, Caze R, Rahman M, Lockwood CJ. Progestin-regulated expression of tissue factor in decidual cells: implications in endometrial hemostasis, menstruation and angiogenesis. *Steroids* 2003;68:849–60.

53. Lockwood CJ, Krikun G, Hausknecht V, Wang EY, Schatz F. Decidual cell regulation of hemostasis during implantation and menstruation. *Ann N Y Acad Sci* 1997;828:188–93.

54. Schatz F, Krikun G, Hausknecht V, Ziegler D, Caze R, Lockwood CL. Physiological and clinical implications of decidualization-associated protease activity. *Ann N Y Acad Sci* 1997;828:175–9.

55. Zoumpoulidou G, Jones MC, de Mattos SF, Francis JM, Fusi L, Lee YS, *et al.* Convergence of interferon-gamma and progesterone signaling pathways in human endometrium: role of PIASy (protein inhibitor of activated signal transducer and activator of transcription-y). *Mol Endocrinol* 2004;18:1988–99.

56. Okada H, Nakajima T, Sanezumi M, Ikuta A, Yasuda K, Kanzaki H. Progesterone enhances interleukin-15 production in human endometrial stromal cells *in vitro*. *J Clin Endocrinol Metab* 2000;85:4765–70.

57. Kitaya K, Nakayama T, Okubo T, Kuroboshi H, Fushiki S, Honjo H. Expression of macrophage inflammatory protein-1beta in human endometrium: its role in endometrial recruitment of natural killer cells. *J Clin Endocrinol Metab* 2003;88:1809–14.

58. Croy BA, He H, Esadeg S, Wei Q, McCartney D, Zhang J, *et al.* Uterine natural killer cells: insights into their cellular and molecular biology from mouse modelling. *Reproduction* 2003;126:149–60.

59. Koopman LA, Kopcow HD, Rybalov B, Boyson JE, Orange JS, Schatz F, *et al.* Human decidual natural killer cells are a unique NK cell subset with immunomodulatory potential. *J Exp Med* 2003;198:1201–12.

60. Logdberg L, Wester L. Immunocalins: a lipocalin subfamily that modulates immune and inflammatory responses. *Biochim Biophys Acta* 2000;1482:284–97.

61. Rabinovich GA, Baum LG, Tinari N, Paganelli R, Natoli C, Liu FT, *et al.* Galectins and their ligands: amplifiers, silencers or tuners of the inflammatory response? *Trends Immunol* 2002;23:313–20.

62. Rachmilewitz J, Borovsky Z, Riely GJ, Miller R, Tykocinski ML. Negative regulation of T cell activation by placental protein 14 is mediated by the tyrosine phosphatase receptor CD45. *J Biol Chem* 2003;278:14059–65.

63. Kudo Y, Hara T, Katsuki T, Toyofuku A, Katsura Y, Takikawa O, *et al.* Mechanisms regulating the expression of indoleamine 2,3-dioxygenase during decidualization of human endometrium. *Hum Reprod* 2004;19:1222–30.

64. Kudo Y, Boyd CA, Spyropoulou I, Redman CW, Takikawa O, Katsuki T, *et al.* Indoleamine 2,3-dioxygenase: distribution and function in the developing human placenta. *J Reprod Immunol* 2004;61:87–98.

65. Mellor AL, Munn DH. Immunology at the maternal–fetal interface: lessons for T cell tolerance and suppression. *Annu Rev Immunol* 2000;18:367–91.

66. Mellor AL, Chandler P, Lee GK, Johnson T, Keskin DB, Lee J, *et al.* Indoleamine 2,3-dioxygenase, immunosuppression and pregnancy. *J Reprod Immunol* 2002;57:143–50.

67. Munn DH, Zhou M, Attwood JT, Bondarev I, Conway SJ, Marshall B, *et al.* Prevention of allogeneic fetal rejection by tryptophan catabolism. *Science* 1998;281:1191–3.

68. Munn DH, Shafizadeh E, Attwood JT, Bondarev I, Pashine A, Mellor AL. Inhibition of T cell proliferation by macrophage tryptophan catabolism. *J Exp Med* 1999;189:1363–72.

69. Brosens JJ, Tullet J, Varshochi R, Lam EW. Steroid receptor action. *Best Pract Res Clin Obstet Gynaecol* 2004;18:265–83.

70. Mak IY, Brosens JJ, Christian M, Hills FA, Chamley L, Regan L, *et al.* Regulated expression of signal transducer and activator of transcription, Stat5, and its enhancement of PRL expression in human endometrial stromal cells *in vitro*. *J Clin Endocrinol Metab* 2002;87:2581–8.

71. Christian M, Zhang X, Schneider-Merck T, Unterman TG, Gellersen B, White JO, *et al.* Cyclic AMP-induced forkhead transcription factor, FKHR, cooperates with CCAAT/enhancer-binding protein beta in differentiating human endometrial stromal cells. *J Biol Chem* 2002;277:20825–32.

72. Christian M, Pohnke Y, Kempf R, Gellersen B, Brosens JJ. Functional association of PR and CCAAT/enhancer-binding protein beta isoforms: promoter-dependent cooperation between PR-B and liver-enriched inhibitory protein, or liver-enriched activatory protein and PR-A in human endometrial stromal cells. *Mol Endocrinol* 2002;16:141–54.

73. Christian M, Marangos P, Mak I, McVey J, Barker F, White J, *et al.* Interferon-gamma modulates prolactin and tissue factor expression in differentiating human endometrial stromal cells. *Endocrinology* 2001;142:3142–51.

74. Kao LC, Tulac S, Lobo S, Imani B, Yang JP, Germeyer A, et al. Global gene profiling in human endometrium during the window of implantation. *Endocrinology* 2002;143:2119–38.
75. Kao LC, Germeyer A, Tulac S, Lobo S, Yang JP, Taylor RN, et al. Expression profiling of endometrium from women with endometriosis reveals candidate genes for disease-based implantation failure and infertility. *Endocrinology* 2003;144:2870–81.
76. Bruner-Tran KL, Eisenberg E, Yeaman GR, Anderson TA, McBean J, Osteen KG. Steroid and cytokine regulation of matrix metalloproteinase expression in endometriosis and the establishment of experimental endometriosis in nude mice. *J Clin Endocrinol Metab* 2002;87:4782–91.
77. Kalkhoven E, Wissink S, van der Saag PT, van der Burg B. Negative interaction between the RelA(p65) subunit of NF-kappaB and the progesterone receptor. *J Biol Chem* 1996;271:6217–24.
78. Jakubowicz DJ, Essah PA, Seppala M, Jakubowicz S, Baillargeon JP, Koistinen R, et al. Reduced serum glycodelin and insulin-like growth factor-binding protein-1 in women with polycystic ovary syndrome during first trimester of pregnancy. *J Clin Endocrinol Metab* 2004;89:833–9.
79. Cermik D, Selam B, Taylor HS. Regulation of HOXA-10 expression by testosterone *in vitro* and in the endometrium of patients with polycystic ovary syndrome. *J Clin Endocrinol Metab* 2003;88:238–43.
80. Many A, Hubel CA, Fisher SJ, Roberts JM, Zhou Y. Invasive cytotrophoblasts manifest evidence of oxidative stress in preeclampsia. *Am J Pathol* 2000;156:321–31.
81. Van Langendonckt A, Casanas-Roux F, Donnez J. Oxidative stress and peritoneal endometriosis. *Fertil Steril* 2002;77:861–70.
82. Murphy AA, Palinski W, Rankin S, Morales AJ, Parthasarathy S. Macrophage scavenger receptor(s) and oxidatively modified proteins in endometriosis. *Fertil Steril* 1998;69:1085–91.
83. Murphy AA, Palinski W, Rankin S, Morales AJ, Parthasarathy S. Evidence for oxidatively modified lipid-protein complexes in endometrium and endometriosis. *Fertil Steril* 1998;69:1092–4.
84. Reister F, Frank HG, Kingdom JC, Heyl W, Kaufmann P, Rath W, et al. Macrophage-induced apoptosis limits endovascular trophoblast invasion in the uterine wall of preeclamptic women. *Lab Invest* 2001;81:1143–52.
85. Chappell LC, Seed PT, Briley AL, Kelly FJ, Lee R, Hunt BJ, et al. Effect of antioxidants on the occurrence of pre-eclampsia in women at increased risk: a randomised trial. *Lancet* 1999;354:810–6.
86. Chappell LC, Seed PT, Kelly FJ, Briley A, Hunt BJ, Charnock-Jones DS, et al. Vitamin C and E supplementation in women at risk of preeclampsia is associated with changes in indices of oxidative stress and placental function. *Am J Obstet Gynecol* 2002;187:777–84.
87. Finn CA, Martin L. Endocrine control of the timing of endometrial sensitivity to a decidual stimulus. *Biol Reprod* 1972;7:82–6.
88. Mackey RA, Glass RH, Olson LE, Vaidya R. Pregnancy following hysterosalpingography with oil and water soluble dye. *Fertil Steril* 1971;22:504–7.
89. Barash A, Dekel N, Fieldust S, Segal I, Schechtman E, Granot I. Local injury to the endometrium doubles the incidence of successful pregnancies in patients undergoing *in vitro* fertilization. *Fertil Steril* 2003;79:1317–22.
90. Surrey ES, Silverberg KM, Surrey MW, Schoolcraft WB. Effect of prolonged gonadotropin-releasing hormone agonist therapy on the outcome of *in vitro* fertilization-embryo transfer in patients with endometriosis. *Fertil Steril* 2002;78:699–704.
91. Ishihara H, Kitawaki J, Kado N, Koshiba H, Fushiki S, Honjo H. Gonadotropin-releasing hormone agonist and danazol normalize aromatase cytochrome P450 expression in eutopic endometrium from women with endometriosis, adenomyosis, or leiomyomas. *Fertil Steril* 2003;79 Suppl 1:735–42.
92. Laskin CA, Bombardier C, Hannah ME, Mandel FP, Ritchie JW, Farewell V, et al. Prednisone and aspirin in women with autoantibodies and unexplained recurrent fetal loss. *N Engl J Med* 1997;337:148–53.
93. Jeng GT, Scott JR, Burmeister LF. A comparison of meta-analytic results using literature vs individual patient data. Paternal cell immunization for recurrent miscarriage. *JAMA* 1995;274:830–6.
94. Daya S, Gunby J, Porter F, Scott J, Clark DA. Critical analysis of intravenous immunoglobulin therapy for recurrent miscarriage. *Hum Reprod Update* 1999;5:475–82.
95. Christiansen OB, Pedersen B, Rosgaard A, Husth M. A randomized, double-blind, placebo-controlled trial of intravenous immunoglobulin in the prevention of recurrent miscarriage: evidence for a therapeutic effect in women with secondary recurrent miscarriage. *Hum Reprod* 2002;17:809–16.
96. Dosiou C, Giudice LC. Natural killer cells in pregnancy and recurrent pregnancy loss: endocrine and immunologic perspectives. *Endocr Rev* 2005;26:44–62.
97. Erlebacher A, Zhang D, Parlow AF, Glimcher LH. Ovarian insufficiency and early pregnancy loss induced by activation of the innate immune system. *J Clin Invest* 2004;114:39–48.
98. Sotiriadis A, Papatheodorou S, Makrydimas G. Threatened miscarriage: evaluation and management. *BMJ* 2004;329:152–5.
99. Oates-Whitehead RM, Haas DM, Carrier JA. Progestogen for preventing miscarriage. *Cochrane Database Syst Rev* 2003;(4):CD003511.
100. Daya S, Gunby J. Luteal phase support in assisted reproduction cycles. *Cochrane Database Syst Rev* 2004;(3):CD004830.

101. da Fonseca EB, Bittar RE, Carvalho MH, Zugaib M. Prophylactic administration of progesterone by vaginal suppository to reduce the incidence of spontaneous preterm birth in women at increased risk: a randomized placebo-controlled double-blind study. *Am J Obstet Gynecol* 2003;188:419–24.
102. Meis PJ, Klebanoff M, Thom E, Dombrowski MP, Sibai B, Moawad AH, *et al.* Prevention of recurrent preterm delivery by 17 alpha-hydroxyprogesterone caproate. *N Engl J Med* 2003;348:2379–85.
103. Yamamoto H, Fuyama S, Arai S, Sendo F. Inhibition of mouse natural killer cytotoxicity by heparin. *Cell Immunol* 1985;96:409–17.
104. Johann S, Zoller C, Haas S, Blumel G, Lipp M, Forster R. Sulfated polysaccharide anticoagulants suppress natural killer cell activity *in vitro. Thromb Haemost* 1995;74:998–1002.
105. Fritchley SJ, Kirby JA, Ali S. The antagonism of interferon-gamma (IFN-gamma) by heparin: examination of the blockade of class II MHC antigen and heat shock protein-70 expression. *Clin Exp Immunol* 2000;120:247–52.

Chapter 20
Risk factors for first-trimester miscarriage: summary of results from the National Women's Health Study

Noreen Maconochie and Pat Doyle

Background

Miscarriage is a common event but is remarkably difficult to study epidemiologically. Most investigations report that around one in five clinical pregnancies will end in miscarriage (fetal death before 24 weeks),[1,2] while prospective studies of conception and early pregnancy have reported fetal loss rates approaching one-third.[3-5] Well-established risk factors for miscarriage include increased maternal age,[6] previous history of miscarriage, and infertility,[7,8] but the interaction between age, parity, infertility and previous pregnancy loss is complex and not entirely understood. Furthermore, several behavioural and social risk factors have been reported as increasing the risk of miscarriage but most remain controversial or unconfirmed.

Methods

The National Women's Health Study was a population-based, two-stage, postal survey of reproductive histories of adult women living in the UK in 2001, sampled from the electronic electoral roll.[9] In Stage 1 a short 'screening' questionnaire was sent to over 60 000 randomly selected women in order to identify those aged below 56 years who had ever been pregnant or ever attempted to achieve a pregnancy. A brief reproductive history was requested and the data on stillbirth, multiple birth and maternal age were compared with national data in order to assess response bias.

Stage 2 involved a more lengthy questionnaire requesting detailed information on every pregnancy (and fertility problems), and including questions relating to sociodemographic, behavioural and other factors for the most recent pregnancy in order to examine risk factors for miscarriage. Cases in this analysis consisted of all women whose most recent pregnancy had resulted in a first-trimester miscarriage (< 13 completed weeks), or, if the most recent pregnancy had not resulted in miscarriage, who had had a miscarriage since 1995. Controls comprised all women whose most recent pregnancy (including pregnancies current at the time of survey) continued beyond 13 or more weeks of gestation. The association between miscarriage and each risk factor was explored using logistic regression analysis, calculating odds ratios and 95% confidence intervals for each factor.

Results

A total of 26 050 questionnaires were returned in Stage 1, a response rate of 49%. Comparison of key reproductive indicators (stillbirth and multiple birth rates and maternal age at first birth) with national statistics showed that the data look remarkably similar to the general population. Among all women who had ever been pregnant, 21% reported ever having had a miscarriage. Most women had only had one miscarriage in their reproductive lifetime: lifetime risk for women aged 35 years and over at survey was 16% for one miscarriage, 4% for two, and just 1.4% for three or more. The majority (77%) of those reporting one or more miscarriage had subsequently had at least one live birth.

The response rate was 73% for the more targeted Stage 2 questionnaire. Six hundred and three cases and 6116 controls were included in the case–control analysis of risk factors for first-trimester miscarriage. After adjusting for year of conception, maternal age, previous miscarriage and previous livebirth, we found the results listed below.

Factors associated with an increased risk of first-trimester miscarriage:

- maternal age over 35 years
- previous miscarriage
- previous termination of pregnancy for non-medical reasons
- time to conception
- infertility problems
- assisted conception
- not living with the father of the baby
- being underweight
- being stressed or anxious
- experiencing one or more stressful/traumatic events
- changing partners
- paternal age over 45 years.

Factors associated with a decreased risk of first-trimester miscarriage:

- previous live birth
- nausea
- taking vitamins (in particular folic acid, iron or pregnancy preparations)
- eating fresh fruit and vegetables daily
- feeling happy and relaxed.

Factors with no effect on the risk of first-trimester miscarriage:

- social class
- caffeine consumption (after accounting for nausea)
- smoking
- moderate alcohol consumption (after accounting for nausea)
- strenuous exercise
- full-time work
- pregnancy order, irrespective of previous pregnancy outcome.

Conclusions

This study has enabled the assembly of a very large data set of women's reproductive histories that appears to be unbiased compared with the general UK population. It is unique in being truly population-based, allowing investigation of adverse outcomes, such as early miscarriage and infertility, that are often not routinely captured via medical records. We were also able to obtain information on each woman's lifetime experience of reproductive events and outcomes.

The results of this case–control study have confirmed some well-established risk factors, including increased maternal age and previous history of miscarriage and infertility, as well as the protective effect of nausea. We found that the relationship with pregnancy order is complex, and that having a live birth is more predictive of 'success' in a future pregnancy than pregnancy order itself. We are currently investigating the interaction between age, pregnancy order and pregnancy outcome in more detail. This study found no evidence for the commonly held beliefs that risk of early miscarriage varies by social class, employment status during pregnancy or strenuous exercise.

The reduced risks associated with taking vitamins, consumption of fresh fruit and vegetables and feeling happy and relaxed during pregnancy are perhaps not surprising, but further work is needed to establish causal pathways and whether these results can be explained by selection or reporting biases.

Our findings of increased risk associated with previous termination, stress and traumatic events in pregnancy, change of partner, increased father's age and low prepregnancy weight are novel. We suggest that further work be initiated to confirm these findings in other study populations.

References

1. Garcia-Enguidanos A, Calle ME, Valero J, Luna S, Dominguez-Rojas V. Risk factors in miscarriage: a review. *Eur J Obstet Gynecol Reprod Biol* 2002;102:111–19.
2. Savitz DA, Hertz-Picciotto I, Poole C, Olshan AF. Epidemiologic measures of the course and outcome of pregnancy. *Epidemiol Rev* 2002;24:91–101.
3. Zinaman MJ, Clegg ED, Brown CC, O'Connor J, Selevan SG. Estimates of human fertility and pregnancy loss. *Fertil Steril* 1996;65:503–9.
4. Ellish NJ, Saboda K, O'Connor J, Nasca PC, Stanek EJ, Boyle C. A prospective study of early pregnancy loss. *Hum Reprod* 1996;11:406–12.
5. Wilcox AJ, Weinberg CR, O'Connor JF, Baird DD, Schlatterer JP, Canfield RE, et al. Incidence of early loss of pregnancy. *N Engl J Med* 1988;319:189–94.
6. Nybo Andersen AM, Wohlfahrt J, Christens P, Olsen J, Melbye M. Maternal age and fetal loss: population based register linkage study. *BMJ* 2000;320:1708–12.
7. Hakim RB, Gray RH, Zacur H. Infertility and early pregnancy loss. *Am J Obstet Gynecol* 1995;172:1510–17.
8. Roman E, Doyle P, Beral V, Alberman E, Pharoah P. Fetal loss, gravidity, and pregnancy order. *Early Hum Dev* 1978;2:131–8.
9. Maconochie N, Doyle P, Prior S. The National Women's Health Study: assembly and description of a population-based reproductive cohort. *BMC Public Health* 2004;4:35.

Chapter 21
Single-embryo transfer

Siladitya Bhattacharya and Zabeena Pandian

Introduction

In vitro fertilisation (IVF) is the treatment of choice in couples with persistent infertility. In the UK, over 25 000 IVF cycles were performed in a 12-month period between 2000 and 2001.[1] In recent years, advances in clinical and laboratory skills have led to increased pregnancy rates of 30–40% per cycle of treatment.[2] At the same time, routine transfer of multiple embryos has amplified the risk of multiple pregnancy. Over half of all infants born as a result of IVF are twins, triplets or higher order multiples. In the USA, where three embryos are still commonly transferred, the multiple pregnancy rate is 39%.[3] In Europe, wider acceptance of a two embryo transfer policy has resulted in fewer triplets but the current twin pregnancy rate of 25% remains unacceptably high when compared with a population-based incidence of 1.25%.[4,5]

Consequences of twin pregnancy

Twin pregnancies are associated with higher maternal and perinatal morbidity and mortality.[6] In comparison with singletons, twins face a six-fold increased risk of mortality[7] and permanent handicap[8] owing to cerebral palsy, chronic lung dysfunction, blindness, learning difficulties and behavioural disorders. Maternal complications such as miscarriage, pregnancy-induced hypertension, gestational diabetes, premature labour and abnormal delivery are also more common.[9] Stress associated with rearing twins[10] and increased costs of prenatal and neonatal intensive care are also significant health service issues.[11,12] Daily hospital charges have been shown to increase from $591 for a singleton delivery to $996 for each twin.[11] In 1995 the cost of hospital services in the UK for IVF-related multiple births was estimated at £4.3 million.[13] In view of these potential complications, iatrogenic multiple pregnancy has been identified as the biggest single threat to the future safety and success of IVF.[5] Elective transfer of two embryos has substantially reduced triplet and higher order multiple births, but has had no impact on the incidence of twin pregnancies. This has underlined the need to develop a practical effective strategy to minimise twin pregnancies resulting from IVF.

Strategies for prevention of twins

Suggested options for the elimination of multiple pregnancies include selective fetal reduction, single blastocyst transfer and elective single-embryo transfer (eSET).

Selective fetal reduction

Selective fetal reduction carries a risk of miscarriage and poses serious ethical and legal questions.[14] It is thus difficult to justify its routine use as a method of preventing twin births.

Single blastocyst transfer

Routine embryo transfer is usually undertaken on day 2 or day 3 post-insemination. Blastocyst transfer, on the other hand, involves transferring fewer, but higher quality embryos that have survived in culture up to the blastocyst stage (day 5). This technique requires special expertise and cannot be routinely offered by all laboratories. Failure to grow to blastocyst stage can limit the number of embryos available for fresh and frozen transfers. This, in turn, can compromise the live birth rate per cycle started. In addition, universally agreed criteria for the selection of blastocysts for transfer are yet to be clarified.[15] Most importantly, a Cochrane review[16] failed to show any advantage of blastocyst transfer over conventional (day 2–3) transfer, in terms of pregnancy rate per woman. The combined odds ratio (OR) in favour of day 2–3 transfer was 0.80 (95% CI 0.57–1.29).

Elective single-embryo transfer

Primary prevention of twin pregnancies by limiting the number of embryos transferred would appear to be a simple and potentially effective strategy. The clear benefits of such an approach have to be weighed up against the possible risk of lowering success rates. An obvious solution is to consider an individualised embryo transfer policy based on factors associated with a higher embryo implantation rate. It has been shown that where more than four embryos are available for transfer, transferring two rather than three reduces the risk of multiple gestation without affecting the live birth rate.[17] This policy does take into account the effect of varying embryo quality on the chances of live birth.[18] A retrospective analysis of 35 554 IVF procedures suggested that embryo quality was a key prognostic factor for live birth, but not for multiple pregnancy rates.[19] On the other hand, a second study, based on a series of 1736 IVF cycles, indicated that the risk of multiple pregnancy was related not just to the number of transferred embryos but also to their quality.[20] Studying the effect of embryo quality on treatment outcome is further complicated by the imprecise nature of embryo assessment. Although morphological criteria are used to predict the likelihood of successful implantation,[21,22] many embryos that appear 'normal' may have chromosomal anomalies.[23] Nevertheless, the ability to select suitable embryos remains an important factor influencing the outcome of IVF.[17,24,25] Thus a practical way to eliminate iatrogenic twin pregnancies without undermining pregnancy rates would appear to lie with elective transfer of carefully selected embryos in women at significant risk of multiple gestation.[5,26–28]

Evidence in favour of single-embryo transfer

Observational studies

The reluctance of many clinicians to perform SET for fear of compromising pregnancy rates is based on published results of non-elective SET where only one embryo was available. In the absence of choice, the implantation potential of the only available embryo is usually poor, yielding clinical pregnancy rates of around 10%.[29–34] It is worth noting that pregnancy rates are poor, even for multiple embryo transfers, if the transferred embryos are the only ones available.[35]

An early observational study[36] from Finland reported a pregnancy rate of 20.2% in 94 women where only one embryo was available for transfer, compared with a pregnancy rate of 29.7% following eSET. The cumulative pregnancy rate after frozen/thawed embryo transfers in the second group was 47.3% per oocyte retrieval. In comparison, the pregnancy rate for double embryo transfer (DET) was 29.4%, and 23.9% of these were twin pregnancies.[36]

Data on eSET from initial studies suggest that, by using strict embryo selection criteria in specific groups of women, a pregnancy rate of 30–40% per fresh treatment cycle can be achieved and twin pregnancies virtually eliminated. The outcome is enhanced by a policy of repeated transfer of thawed cryopreserved spare embryos leading to a cumulative pregnancy rate comparable with that associated with DET (47–53%).[37]

Randomised trials

A systematic review of randomised trials comparing the effectiveness of eSET with DET has recently been undertaken by our group.[38] MEDLINE and EMBASE databases were searched from 1970 to 2003 and 1985 to 2003, respectively. The following medical subject headings (MeSH terms) and all combinations of these words were used: embryo transfer, multiple pregnancy, IVF, in vitro fertil$, ICSI, intra-cytoplasmic sperm injection, infertility, subfertility, single/one embryo, two/double embryo, three/four/multiple embryos, effectiveness, ART, assisted reprod$ techn$, randomised controlled trial, clinical trial. All women undergoing IVF and intracytoplasmic sperm injection (ICSI) were included. Studies on embryo transfer at the blastocyst stage were excluded.

In addition, a hand search was performed through appropriate conference proceedings and bibliographies from the identified studies. Where necessary, additional data were sought by contacting authors. The review used the search strategy developed for the Cochrane Menstrual Disorders and Subfertility Group. Relevant trials were identified from the group's specialised register of controlled trials (searched 25 June 2003) and the Cochrane Central Register of Controlled Trials (Cochrane Library Issue 4, 2003).

Three trials comparing eSET with elective DET were identified.[2,25,39] All involved women who had undergone embryo transfer in a fresh IVF/ICSI cycle. One study also presented data from subsequent frozen replacement cycles.[2] The study population in the three trials displayed some clinical differences. The upper age limit varied from 34 years[25] to 35 years.[39] In the only multicentre trial to be included in this review, variable upper age limits were used by different participating clinics.[2] There were also minor variations in laboratory and clinical protocols among the trials. While elective transfer of 'good quality' embryos was performed in all, precise morphological characteristics used to define such embryos were unclear in one of the reported trials.[39] The use of standard embryo culture media and catheters for embryo transfer was enforced in two of the trials.[2,25] Frozen embryo transfers were carried out in both natural and artificially stimulated cycles.[2] One of the trials (only reported in abstract form) failed to include any details about methods used for ovarian stimulation, oocyte recovery, embryo transfer or luteal phase support.[39] The timing of embryo transfer varied from 46–50 hours[2] to 64–67 hours[25,39] after insemination.

In the absence of demonstrable statistical heterogeneity, aggregated data were used to study clinical pregnancy rate, live birth rate and multiple pregnancy rate per fresh cycle of IVF treatment (per woman). The clinical pregnancy rate following DET was significantly higher in comparison with eSET (OR 2.08; 95% CI 1.24–3.50; test for overall effect $P = 0.006$) (Figure 21.1), as was the live birth rate per woman (OR 1.90; 95% CI 1.12–3.22; test for overall effect $P = 0.02$) (Figure 21.2). The risk of multiple pregnancy (twins) was nearly ten times higher in women who had undergone DET (OR 9.97; 95% CI 2.61–38.19; $P = 0.0008$) (Figure 21.3). Data from a single study[2] failed to reveal a difference in miscarriage rates between eSET and DET (OR 3.27; 95% CI 0.33–32.17; $P = 0.3$) (Figure 21.4). These results suggest that while eSET reduces the risk of twins substantially, it also halves the live birth rate per fresh IVF treatment cycle.

These results are based on relatively few trials, with small sample sizes. Three trials contributed a total of 122 women in the SET group and 126 in the DET group. It is thus possible that clinically significant differences in treatment effects could have remained undetected. The methodological quality of the studies was poor. Only one trial[2] used a computer-generated random number table balanced in sets of ten. Two of the studies[25,39] did not describe the method of randomisation. Measures used for concealment of allocation were described explicitly in a single trial.[25] None of the trials included a formal power calculation, analysis by intention to treat or a clear description of the number of withdrawals (including cancellations and dropouts).

In terms of limiting multiple pregnancy rates, the effect is strikingly in favour of SET. Given that nearly all the multiples were twins, the potential benefits of eliminating this risk may not be apparent to all.[12] The definite reduction in success rates per fresh IVF treatment may seem to be a major disadvantage of eSET. These results do not reflect the outcome per woman following first fresh and subsequently frozen transfers using embryos generated from a single oocyte retrieval. None of the trials reported cumulative live birth rates per woman (i.e. data from fresh and subsequent frozen embryo transfers). One of the trials[2] presented data relating to outcome after transfer of frozen embryos in a subgroup which suggest comparable cumulative outcomes for eSET and DET. Unfortunately, there was no enforcement of the randomisation schedule for frozen transfers, making it difficult to interpret the final results.

Pregnancy and live birth rates per woman/fresh treatment cycle are important outcomes to be measured; however future trials should also estimate cumulative live birth rates (fresh eSET as well as subsequent frozen SET). This outcome is perhaps more meaningful, as the principal benefit of single-embryo transfer is its ability to offer comparable cumulative live birth rates while eliminating twins. In this context, Cox proportional hazard regression analysis (a form of survival analysis) can be used to evaluate cumulative live birth rates following multiple treatments.[40] It is important to include all cycles in the denominator as excluding those with poor outcomes can exaggerate the effectiveness of the intervention.

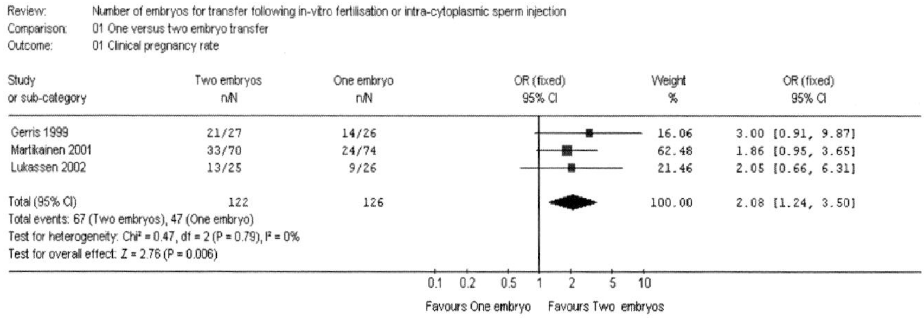

Review: Number of embryos for transfer following in-vitro fertilisation or intra-cytoplasmic sperm injection
Comparison: 01 One versus two embryo transfer
Outcome: 01 Clinical pregnancy rate

Study or sub-category	Two embryos n/N	One embryo n/N	OR (fixed) 95% CI	Weight %	OR (fixed) 95% CI
Gerris 1999	21/27	14/26		16.06	3.00 [0.91, 9.87]
Martikainen 2001	33/70	24/74		62.48	1.86 [0.95, 3.65]
Lukassen 2002	13/25	9/26		21.46	2.05 [0.66, 6.31]
Total (95% CI)	122	126		100.00	2.08 [1.24, 3.50]

Total events: 67 (Two embryos), 47 (One embryo)
Test for heterogeneity: Chi² = 0.47, df = 2 (P = 0.79), I² = 0%
Test for overall effect: Z = 2.76 (P = 0.006)

0.1   0.2   0.5   1   2   5   10
Favours One embryo   Favours Two embryos

Figure 21.1. Clinical pregnancy rate: one versus two embryo transfer; reproduced with permission from Pandian *et al.*[38] (*The Cochrane Database of Systematic Reviews*, © 2004 Cochrane Library)

Review: Number of embryos for transfer following in-vitro fertilisation or intra-cytoplasmic sperm injection
Comparison: 01 One versus two embryo transfer
Outcome: 02 Livebirth rate

Study or sub-category	Two embryos n/N	One embryo n/N	OR (fixed) 95% CI	Weight %	OR (fixed) 95% CI
Gerris 1999	20/27	10/26		13.11	4.57 [1.42, 14.71]
Martikainen 2001	28/70	22/74		63.72	1.58 [0.79, 3.14]
Lukassen 2002	8/25	7/26		23.17	1.28 [0.38, 4.27]
Total (95% CI)	122	126		100.00	1.90 [1.12, 3.22]

Total events: 56 (Two embryos), 39 (One embryo)
Test for heterogeneity: Chi² = 2.87, df = 2 (P = 0.24), I² = 30.2%
Test for overall effect: Z = 2.39 (P = 0.02)

0.1   0.2   0.5   1   2   5   10
Favours one embryo   Favours Two embryos

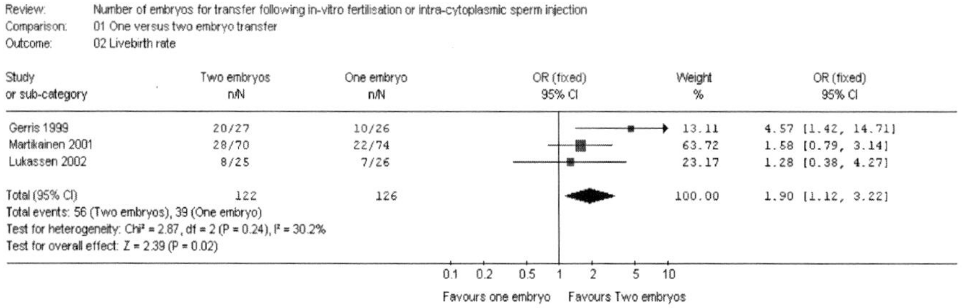

Figure 21.2. Live birth rate: one versus two embryo transfer; reproduced with permission from Pandian *et al.*[38] (*The Cochrane Database of Systematic Reviews*, © 2004 Cochrane Library)

Subsequent to the completion of this review, the initial results of a large multicentre randomised controlled trial of eSET versus DET[41] have become available in abstract form. In this trial, involving three Scandinavian countries, 661 women were recruited from a total of 11 clinics. All were younger than 36 years, were in their first or second cycle of IVF, and possessed two or more good quality embryos for transfer. The women were randomised to receive either:

1. a fresh eSET, followed by a single frozen SET in the absence of a live birth
2. a single fresh DET.

Three hundred and thirty women were randomised to the eSET group and 331 women to the DET group. The mean age of the women at fresh transfer was 30.9 and 30.8 years, respectively, in the two groups. The cumulative continuing live birth rate was 131/330 (40%) in the eSET group and 144/331 (44%) in the DET group. The rate of continuing multiple pregnancies was 52/144 (36%) in the DET group. In

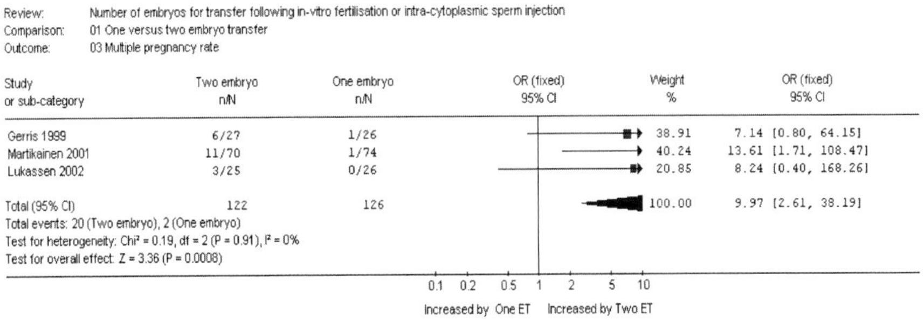

Review: Number of embryos for transfer following in-vitro fertilisation or intra-cytoplasmic sperm injection
Comparison: 01 One versus two embryo transfer
Outcome: 03 Multiple pregnancy rate

Study or sub-category	Two embryo n/N	One embryo n/N	OR (fixed) 95% CI	Weight %	OR (fixed) 95% CI
Gerris 1999	6/27	1/26		38.91	7.14 [0.80, 64.15]
Martikainen 2001	11/70	1/74		40.24	13.61 [1.71, 108.47]
Lukassen 2002	3/25	0/26		20.85	8.24 [0.40, 168.26]
Total (95% CI)	122	126		100.00	9.97 [2.61, 38.19]

Total events: 20 (Two embryo), 2 (One embryo)
Test for heterogeneity: Chi² = 0.19, df = 2 (P = 0.91), I² = 0%
Test for overall effect: Z = 3.36 (P = 0.0008)

0.1 0.2 0.5 1 2 5 10
Increased by One ET   Increased by Two ET

Figure 21.3. Multiple pregnancy rate: one versus two embryo transfer; reproduced with permission from Pandian *et al.*[38] (*The Cochrane Database of Systematic Reviews*, © 2004 Cochrane Library)

Review: Number of embryos for transfer following in-vitro fertilisation or intra-cytoplasmic sperm injection
Comparison: 01 One versus two embryo transfer
Outcome: 04 Miscarriage rate

Study or sub-category	Two embryos n/N	One embryo n/N	OR (fixed) 95% CI	Weight %	OR (fixed) 95% CI
Martikainen 2001	3/70	1/74		100.00	3.27 [0.33, 32.19]
Total (95% CI)	70	74		100.00	3.27 [0.33, 32.19]

Total events: 3 (Two embryos), 1 (One embryo)
Test for heterogeneity: not applicable
Test for overall effect: Z = 1.01 (P = 0.31)

0.1 0.2 0.5 1 2 5 10
Increased by one ET   Increased by Two ET

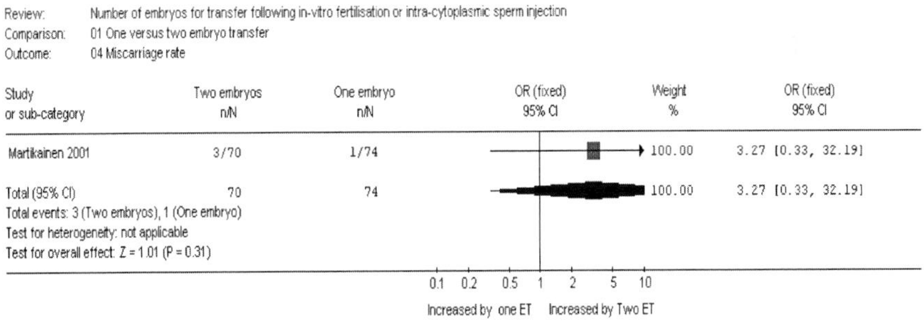

Figure 21.4. Miscarriage rate: one versus two embryo transfer; reproduced with permission from Pandian *et al.*[38] (*The Cochrane Database of Systematic Reviews*, © 2004 Cochrane Library)

the eSET group there was a single twin pregnancy. This trial showed clearly that a policy of elective fresh and frozen SET produced live birth rates comparable with those after DET but with a very low risk of multiples. As the results of this trial have yet to be published as a full paper, it is difficult to comment on the quality of the trial. In the absence of separate outcomes for fresh and frozen cycles, it was not possible to incorporate these data within the Cochrane review at this stage. The strength of this trial lies in its numbers, which exceed the combined sample size on which the Cochrane meta-analysis is based. It therefore provides the strongest evidence so far in favour of eSET in a selected population of young women with a good prognosis.

Implementation

It is clear that in a selected population the cumulative outcome of eSET is comparable with that of DET while virtually eliminating multiple pregnancies. However, wider implementation of this strategy is likely to be challenged by a number of barriers.

Lack of convincing proof of effectiveness and acceptability

The evidence presented so far supports the hypothesis that replacing embryos singly, in a combination of fresh and frozen cycles, will virtually eliminate twins and yet offer live birth rates comparable with a single fresh DET. Although prevention of twin pregnancies is a certainty, we do not have sufficient trial data on cumulative live birth rates per woman following either eSET or DET. We also have little data from prospective trials on the cumulative cost per live birth, including costs of cryopreservation and patient costs. Most importantly, we do not have any data on couples' views on the acceptability of the alternative strategies or whether eSET offers 'value for money'. This is crucial as, globally, the majority of IVF treatments are funded by couples themselves.

The need for improvements in the laboratory

Embryo selection

As a process, IVF is relatively inefficient. A large number of oocytes is required in order to provide a chance of producing a few good quality embryos. Expressed as birth per oocyte collected, the success rate of IVF is ten times lower than that seen in nature.[42] The ratio of retrieved oocytes to live birth is 1/40. Only 24% of transferred embryos develop into pregnancies[43] and half of all embryos cultured *in vitro* show arrested pre-implantation development.[15] Morphological assessment of embryo quality is far from ideal and our inability to select embryos with good implantation potential is one of the reasons behind the tradition of multiple embryo transfer. While there have been marked improvements in the laboratory over the years, more needs to be done in terms of refining techniques of embryo culture and noninvasive tests of embryo viability in order to create a climate where transfer of a single well-selected embryo will have a high chance of a pregnancy and transfer of two such embryos will inevitably lead to twins. A constant source of frustration is failure of implantation despite the replacement of 'good quality' embryos. Suggested methods of improving the quality of transferred embryos include culturing embryos to the blastocyst stage[44] and pre-implantation genetic screening.[45,46] There is currently little convincing evidence from randomised trials to support routine use of either technique.

Cryopreservation

The outcome of an eSET policy can be substantially enhanced in conjunction with an efficient and reliable embryo cryopreservation programme.[37,47] However, while human IVF embryos can be frozen successfully, the rates of survival after thawing vary substantially from clinic to clinic and live birth rates are reduced in frozen cycles. Methods used to freeze human embryos are based on empirically developed protocols for the cryopreservation of rabbit, mouse and cattle embryos. There are no controlled data to show that the protocol favoured by most clinics is optimal. It is therefore important to investigate modification of the commonly used freezing protocols in order to increase the proportion of embryos that survive cryopreservation and to enhance the viability of the survivors. Most clinics freeze pronucleate and early cleavage stage embryos and report that 30–80% survive thawing. Such damage is not inconsistent with development to term but intact embryos have a greater potential for implantation and development.[48] There is a need to develop alternative cryopreservation protocols that will lead to improved outcome in frozen cycles.

Selectivity of an SET policy

A major drawback of eSET is our inability to implement it as a universal policy in all women undergoing IVF. Available data indicate that SET should be reserved only for women who are at significant risk of multiple gestation.[41] This includes those who are relatively young, are in their first or second IVF cycle, and possess a number of good quality embryos.[28] The precise definition of this subgroup of 'twin-prone' couples has varied from centre to centre. This issue will need greater clarification if SET is to become part of routine IVF, instead of being the preserve of a few.

In addition, there are uncertainties about the optimum laboratory protocol with regard to embryo transfer. Many workers will ensure that only the 'top' embryo, i.e. one with potentially the best chance of implantation, is transferred, in order to optimise the chance of pregnancy in a fresh treatment cycle. Observing embryos in culture in order to select the best for transfer[49] can potentially limit the number of embryos available for cryopreservation. Such a policy may not be compatible with plans to achieve high cumulative pregnancy rates by maximising multiple single-embryo transfers after an initial oocyte retrieval.[37,41] In fact, two clear eSET strategies are evident. The first involves multiple fresh cycles with repeated transfer of top quality (single) embryos; the other is based on the availability of multiple embryos for cryopreservation and an efficient freezing programme.

Defining success in IVF

The decision to opt for SET is influenced by the perception of success associated with treatment. It is the definition of 'success' in this context that has generated a degree of controversy. Outcomes in IVF are conventionally expressed in terms of a live birth per fresh cycle. Outcomes of subsequent frozen cycles are reported separately. It comes as no surprise that expressing outcomes per fresh cycle underestimates the success of SET by half. This is a serious deterrent to couples and clinics considering eSET. It has been suggested that expressing outcomes as live birth per woman makes better practical and statistical sense.[50] In contrast to other types of fertility treatment, such as ovulation induction, the two outcomes are often similar in IVF, as most trials report on a single fresh IVF cycle in a woman. Proponents of SET have argued that the best outcome should be either singleton live birth or term singleton live birth.[51] While both underline the importance of a healthy singleton birth as the desired outcome of fertility treatment, they still focus on the cycle (treatment) rather than the woman as the denominator.

Expressing the outcome of treatment in terms of live birth per oocyte retrieval may be more logical. This would include results after fresh and frozen embryo transfer of all embryos created as a result of a single fresh treatment cycle.[47,52] Although logical, this is not without some potential problems. Expressing the outcome as live birth per couple/oocyte recovery will mean a prolonged period of follow-up, as not all couples will use their spare embryos within a constant and predictable period of time. It will also introduce further complexities if women have multiple pregnancies from the same set of embryos created from a single oocyte retrieval process.

Perception of risk and consumer choice

Clinicians may feel that a high twin rate in IVF is unacceptable[53] but couples may have different views.[12] Some women, especially mothers of IVF twins, may actually see twins as a desirable outcome.[54,55] Others who are paying for their own treatment may feel that having twins represents a cost-effective way of completing their family. Many are willing to take risks in order to achieve this goal. This may be due, in part, to insufficient information about the risks of a twin pregnancy. Yet improved methods of communicating risks to couples does not always change couples' opinions.[56] Fewer than a third of UK women in their early 30s embarking on their first IVF cycle felt that a hypothetical policy of eSET was acceptable if it meant slightly reduced pregnancy rates.[56] Just over half would consider eSET, provided they were not charged for cryopreservation and subsequent replacement of spare embryos.

Financial arrangements

Couples who are charged either for multiple fresh IVF cycles (resulting in a transfer of the single best embryo) or for freezing and thawing embryos are understandably reluctant to consider eSET. Elective SET has worked well in European settings where IVF is subsidised. In the case of Belgium, prior to 2002, 75% of the costs of IVF were reimbursed. In 2002, infertility officially gained recognition as a medical condition and the Belgian Society for Reproductive Medicine (BSRM) proposed a move to abolish triplets and reduce twins by 50%. Under these new proposals, women under 42 years would be eligible for six fully funded cycles of IVF with a policy of SET in place for the first and second cycles for women under 35 years. Assuming 1750 pregnancies from 7000 cycles in Belgium, the additional costs of treatment would be €8.4 million. These costs would be offset completely by €9.1 million saved by eliminating triplets and minimising twins.[57] The existing system in the UK, where many couples pay for IVF treatment while neonatal care is free, is apt to discourage couples from SET.

Regulation

It is clear from the European experience that legislation is a potent factor in changing practice in IVF. This is backed up by the results of a qualitative study[59] which suggest that while many couples undergoing IVF are unsure about opting for eSET they would have little difficulty with complying with any legal requirements enforcing it. However, if legislation is considered as the final step in implementing SET, this will need to be backed up with adequate funding for multiple treatments.[55]

Conclusion

Twin pregnancies resulting from IVF treatment are associated with higher maternal and perinatal morbidity. There is now some evidence to suggest that eSET, in a selected population of women, can eliminate twins without jeopardising cumulative live birth rates. This is ideally combined with effective methods of embryo selection and cryopreservation. Currently, eSET is mainly confined to settings where there is financial support or strict legislation in place to support such a policy. More data from pragmatic trials are needed to demonstrate whether a policy of eSET is effective, acceptable and financially viable in other clinical settings.

References

1. Human Fertilisation and Embryology Authority. *Patients' Guides: National Data Statistics (2000–2001)*. London: HFEA; 2002 [http://www.hfea.gov.uk/HFEAPublications/PatientsGuides].

2. Martikainen H, Tiitinen A, Candido T, Tapamainen J, Orava M, Tuomivaara L, *et al*. One versus two embryo transfer after IVF and ICSI: a randomised study. *Hum Reprod* 2001;16:1900–3.

3. Society for Assisted Reproductive Technology (SART) and American Society for Reproductive Medicine (ASRM). Assisted reproductive technology in the United States: 1997 results generated from the ASRM/SART registry. *Fertil Steril* 2000;74:4–11.

4. Bhattacharya S, Templeton A. In treating infertility, are multiple pregnancies unavoidable? *N Engl J Med* 2000;343:58–9.

5. ESHRE Campus Report. Prevention of twin pregnancies after IVF/ICSI by single embryo transfer. *Hum Reprod* 2001;16:790–800.

6. Bergh T, Ericson A, Hillensjo T, Nygren KG, Wennerholm UB. Deliveries and children born after in-vitro fertilisation in Sweden 1982–95: a retrospective cohort study. *Lancet* 1999;354:1579–85.

7. Luke B, Keith LG. The contribution of singletons, twins and triplets to low birth weight, infant mortality and handicap in the United States. *J Reprod Med* 1992;37:661–6.

8. Yokoyama Y, Shimizu T, Hayakawa K. Incidence of handicaps in multiple births and associated factors. *Acta Genet Med Gemellol (Roma)* 1995;44:81–91.

9. Seoud MA, Toner JP, Kruithoff C, Muasher SJ. Outcome of twin, triplet and quadruplet in-vitro fertilisation pregnancies: the Norfolk experience. *Fertil Steril* 1992;57:825–34.

10. Garel M, Blondel B. Assessment at one year of the psychological consequences of having triplets. *Hum Reprod* 1992;7:729–32.

11. Callahan TL, Hall JE, Ettner SL, Christiansen CL, Greene MF, Crowley WF Jr. The economic impact of multiple gestation pregnancies and the contribution of assisted reproduction techniques to their incidence. *N Engl J Med* 1994;331:244–9.

12. Goldfarb J, Kinzer DJ, Boyle M, Kurit D. Attitudes of *in vitro* fertilisation and intrauterine insemination couples towards multiple gestation pregnancy and multifetal pregnancy reduction. *Fertil Steril* 1996;65:815–20.

13. Mugford M, Henderson J. Resource implications of multiple births. In: Ward HR, Whittle M, editors. *Multiple Births*. London: RCOG; 1995. p. 334–45.

14. Berkowitz RL, Lynch L, Stone J, Alvarez M. The current status of multifetal pregnancy reduction. *Am J Obstet Gynecol* 1996;174:1265–72.

15. Bavister BD, Boatman DE. The neglected human blastocyst revisited. *Hum Reprod* 1997;12:1606–18.

16. Blake D, Proctor M, Johnson N, Olive D. Cleavage stage versus blastocyst stage embryo transfer in assisted conception. *Cochrane Database Syst Rev* 2002;(2):CD002118.

17. Templeton A, Morris JK. Reducing the risk of multiple births by transfer of two embryos after *in vitro* fertilization. *N Engl J Med* 1998;339:573–7.

18. Abdalla HI, Gearon C, Wren M. Swedish in-vitro fertilisation study. *Lancet* 2000;355:844–5.

19. Schieve LA, Peterson HB, Meikle SF, Jeng G, Danel I, Burnett NM, *et al*. Live-birth rates and multiple-birth risk using *in vitro* fertilization. *JAMA* 1999;282:1832–8.

20. Bassil S, Wyns C, Toussaint-Demylle D, Abdelnour W, Donnez J. Predictive factors for multiple pregnancy in *in vitro* fertilization. *J Reprod Med* 1997;42:761–6.

21. Steer CV, Mills CL, Tan SL, Campbell S, Edwards RG. The cumulative embryo score: a predictive embryo scoring technique to select the optimal number of embryos to transfer in an *in vitro* fertilization and embryo transfer programme. *Hum Reprod* 1992;7:117–19.

22. Shulman A, Ben-Nun I, Ghetler Y, Kaneti H, Shilon M, Beyth Y. Relationship between embryo morphology and implantation rate after *in vitro* fertilization treatment in conception cycles. *Fertil Steril* 1993;60:123–6.

23. Munné S, Alikani M, Tomkin G, Grifo J, Cohen J. Embryo morphology, developmental rates and maternal age are correlated with chromosome abnormalities. *Fertil Steril* 1995;64:382–91.

24. Staessen C, Camus M, Bollen N, Devroey P, Van Steirteghem AC. The relationship between embryo quality and the occurrence of multiple pregnancies. *Fertil Steril* 1992;57:626–30.

25. Gerris J, De Neubourg D, Mangelschots K, Van Royen E, Van de Meerssche M, Valkenburg M. Prevention of twin pregnancy after in-vitro fertilisation or intracytoplasmic sperm injection based on strict embryo criteria: a prospective randomized clinical trial. *Hum Reprod* 1999;14:2581–7.

26. Coetsier T, Dhont M. Avoiding multiple pregnancies in in-vitro fertilization: Who's afraid of single embryo transfer? *Hum Reprod* 1998;13:2663–4.

27. Templeton A. Avoiding multiple pregnancies in ART. Replace as many embryos as you like – one at a time. *Hum Reprod* 2000;15:1662–5.

28. Hunault CC, Eijkemans MJC, Pieters MHEC, te Velde ER, Habbema JDF, Fauser BCJM, *et al.* A prediction model for selecting patients undergoing *in vitro* fertilisation for elective single embryo transfer. *Fertil Steril* 2002;77:725–32.

29. FIVNAT (French In Vitro National). Pregnancies and births resulting from in vitro fertilization: French national registry, analysis of data 1986 to 1990. *Fertil Steril* 1995;64:746–56.

30. Giorgetti C, Terriou P, Auquier P, Hans E, Spach JL, Salzmann J, *et al.* Embryo score to predict implantation after in-vitro fertilization: based on 957 single embryo transfers. *Hum Reprod* 1995;10:2427–31.

31. Preutthipan S, Amso N, Curtis P, Shaw RW. The influence of number of embryos transferred on pregnancy outcome in women undergoing *in vitro* fertilization and embryo transfer (IVF-ET). *J Med Assoc Thai* 1996;79:613–17.

32. Lieberman, B. An embryo too many? *Hum Reprod* 1998;13:2664–6.

33. Yaron Y, Amit A, Kogosowski A, Peyser MR, David MP, Lessing JB. The optimal number of embryos to be transferred in shared oocyte donation: walking the thin line between low pregnancy rates and multiple pregnancies. *Hum Reprod* 1997;12:699–702.

34. Westergaard HB, Johansen AM, Erb K, Andersen AN. Danish National IVF Registry 1994 and 1995. Treatment, pregnancy outcome and complications during pregnancy. *Acta Obstet Gynecol Scand* 2000;79:384–9.

35. Ludwig M, Schopper B, Katalinic A, Sturm R, Al-Hasani S, Diedrich K. Experience with the elective transfer of two embryos under the conditions of the German embryo protection law: results of a retrospective data analysis of 2573 transfer cycles. *Hum Reprod* 2000;15:319–24.

36. Vilska S, Tiitinen A, Hyden-Granskog C, Hovatta O. Elective transfer of one embryo results in an acceptable pregnancy rate and eliminates the risk of multiple birth. *Hum Reprod* 1999;14:2392–5.

37. Tiitinen A, Halttunen M, Harkki P. Elective single embryo transfer: the value of cryopreservation. *Hum Reprod* 2001;16:1140–4.

38. Pandian Z, Bhattacharya S, Ozturk O, Serour G, Templeton A. Number of embryos for transfer following in-vitro fertilisation or intra-cytoplasmic sperm injection. *Cochrane Database Syst Rev* 2004;(4):CD003416.

39. Lukassen HGM, Braat DDM, Zeilhuis, Adang EM, Kremer JAM. 2X1 versus 1X2, a randomized study. *Hum Reprod* 2002;(17) Abstract Book 1:1.

40. Cohlen BJ, Hughes E, te Velde ER. Intrauterine insemination for unexplained subfertility. *Cochrane Database Syst Rev* 1999;(4):CD001838.

41. Thurin A, Hausken J, Hillensjo T, Jablonowska B, Pinborg A, Strandell A, *et al.* Elective single embryo transfer in IVF, a randomized study. 20th Annual Meeting of the ESHRE, 27–30 June 2004, Berlin, Germany. Abstract O-170:i60.

42. Dhont M. Single-embryo transfer. *Semin Reprod Med* 2001;19:251–8.

43. Hardy K. Development of human blastocysts *in vitro*. In: Bavister B, editor. *Preimplantation Embryo Development*. New York: Springer-Verlag; 1993. p. 184–99.

44. Gardner MK, Lane M. Culture and selection of viable human blastocysts: a feasible proposition for human IVF? *Hum Reprod Update* 1997;3:367–82.

45. Gianaroli L, Magli MC, Munné S, Fiorentino A, Montanaro N, Ferraretti AP. Will pre-implantation genetic diagnosis assist patients with a poor prognosis to achieve pregnancy? *Hum Reprod* 1997;12:1762–7.

46. Gianaroli L, Magli MC, Ferraretti AP, Munné S. Pre-implantation diagnosis for aneuploidies in patients undergoing *in vitro* fertilisation with a poor prognosis: identification of the categories for which it should be proposed. *Fertil Steril* 1999;72;837–44.

47. Tiitinen A, Hyden-Granskog C, Gissler M. What is the most relevant standard of success in assisted reproduction?: The value of cryopreservation on cumulative pregnancy rates per single oocyte retrieval should not be forgotten. *Hum Reprod* 2004;19:2439–41.

48. Van den Abeel E, Camus M, Van Wasesberghe L, Devrey P, Van Steirtenghem AC. Viability of partially damaged human embryos after cryopreservation. *Hum Reprod* 1997;12:2006–10.

49. Van Royen E, Mangelschots K, De Neubourg D, Valkenburg M, Van de Meerssche M, Ryckaert G, *et al.* Characterization of a top quality embryo, a step towards single-embryo transfer. *Hum Reprod* 1999;14:2345–9.

50. Vail A, Gardener E. Common statistical errors in the design and analysis of subfertility trials. *Hum Reprod* 2003;18:1000–4.

51. Min JK, Breheny SA, MacLachlan V, Healy DL. What is the most relevant standard of success in assisted reproduction? The singleton, term gestation, live birth rate per cycle initiated: the BESST endpoint for assisted reproduction. *Hum Reprod* 2003;19:3–7.

52. Ozturk O, Bhattacharya S, Templeton A. Avoiding multiple pregnancies in ART: evaluation and implementation of new strategies. *Hum Reprod* 2001;16:1319–21.

53. Hazekamp J, Bergh C, Wennerholm UB, Hovatta O, Karlstrom PO, Selbing A. Avoiding multiple pregnancies in ART, Consideration of new strategies. *Hum Reprod* 2000;15:1217–19.
54. Gleicher N, Campbell DP, Chan CL, Karande V, Rae R, Balin M, *et al.* The desire for multiple births in couples with infertility problems contradicts present practice patterns. *Hum Reprod* 1995;10:1079–84.
55. Pinborg A, Loft A, Schmidt L, Andersen AN. Attitudes of IVF/ICSI-twin mothers towards twins and single embryo transfer. *Hum Reprod* 2003;18:621–7.
56. Murray S, Shetty A, Rattray A, Taylor V, Bhattacharya S. A randomized comparison of alternative methods of information provision on the acceptability of elective single embryo transfer. *Hum Reprod* 2004;19:911–16.
57. Bhattacharya S, Templeton A. What is the most relevant standard of success in assisted reproduction? Redefining success in the context of elective single embryo transfer: evidence, intuition and financial reality. *Hum Reprod* 2004;19:1939–42.
58. Olofsson JI, Borg K, Hardarson T, Hillensjo T, Reismer U, Selleskog U, *et al.* (2004). Effects of novel legislation on embryo transfer policy, results and pregnancy outcome in a Swedish IVF unit. 20th Annual Meeting of the ESHRE, 27–30 June 2004, Berlin, Germany. Abstract O-169:i59.
59. Porter MA, Bhattacharya S. Qualitative investigation of staff and patients' opinions of a proposed trial of elective single embryo transfer. British Fertility Society Annual Meeting, 2004, Cheltenham. Abstract 018:34.

Chapter 22
Paediatric outcome after assisted reproductive technology

Alastair G Sutcliffe

It's hardly a Darwinian way of reproducing.

DAVE, NOTTINGHAM TAXI DRIVER

Before overviewing the literature concerning paediatric follow-up of children conceived by assisted reproductive technology (ART), it is worth considering the difficulties facing researchers in this area. When trying to establish an international study of pre-implantation genetic diagnosis (PGD) outcome the author travelled around PGD centres to try to get the study under way. The vast majority of ill effects arise from the birth of children from twin, triplet, quadruplet or higher multiple pregnancies. Fifty per cent of twins are born at less than 38 weeks of gestation and at less than 2500 g. The birth rate of twins has doubled in most western countries over the past 25 years (and this is approximately 90% due to ART.)

An anecdote from one clinic visited in the USA, concerning multiple births and the relationship between a fertility team and a neonatal team, comes to mind. The head of neonates invited the fertility clinicians to visit the unit to see some of the premature babies born of higher order birth after fertility treatments. When no one visited he raised the stakes by offering to nail a silver dollar to the door frame outside the main entrance to the neonatal unit (in the style of Moby Dick.) Still no one visited. This may not represent every view but certainly represents denial. The birth of children from higher order births after ART is still its *prima facie* risk to the expectant parents. Fortunately, at the time of writing, there is generally positive legislation being developed in many countries to stop the replacement of more than one embryo, thus substantially improving the potential short- and long-term morbidity after ART.

Difficulties with outcome studies looking at quality of life in children after ART conception

Treatment effects and impairments from a history of infertility confound the evaluation of the safety of ART. While reports are continually emerging that question the safety of ART (on the basis of often retrospective child outcome studies), the ideal study has yet to be performed because of methodological difficulties.

What are the limitations on an ideal study being conducted?

The main limitations are:

- prospective study design, in which the unit of analysis, such as per cycle, or per couple, is defined
- appropriate use of statistical techniques with due correlates to treatment exposure
- data collected at appropriate times, such as before treatment, at treatment and post-treatment.

Longitudinal studies established in this manner will potentially overcome the lingering doubts concerning the safety, or not, of ART, for the child outcome.

However, in practice there could still be difficulties and these are best exemplified by the experience of the long-term follow-up for children treated with leukaemia in the UK. One would expect that families whose children had been cured from leukaemia would be grateful to the medical profession and allied professions for that cure. Yet despite very thorough, attentive follow-up of these children, it is the experience of one of the leaders in the field of child cancer follow-up, Dr Mike Hawkins, in Birmingham, that these children are still not always brought to five-year, ten-year and fifteen-year follow-up appointments. Thus, it is the nature of longitudinal studies, where the data has to be collected directly from the family, that some children can 'disappear' from the cohort over time. However, these studies are necessary and there seems to be a culture of change, in which a lot of countries, as well as international organisations, are trying to encourage robust and appropriate outcome studies, especially where there are clinical trials, involving the introduction of novel forms of fertility treatments.

When considering prospective study design further, the correct unit of analysis and also the timescale need to be carefully established in advance. A good example where things may become confused is intracytoplasmic sperm injection (ICSI), which was initially used for male factor subfertility. It is now used, in some countries, such as Belgium, for most treatment cycles.

Finally, in the context of child studies the following endpoints are important:

- plurality at birth
- birth size
- birth defects
- developmental difficulties
- cancer
- future sexual maturation
- future fertility.

All these endpoints need to be addressed by prospective studies.

Brief overview of concepts

Plurality at birth

This issue is of prime importance and is the single most significant determinant of paediatric outcome after ART. The types of treatment used, such as *in vitro* fertilisation (IVF), ICSI, blastocyst transfer and others, become mere subtleties when faced with the birth of triplets. The Western Australian triplet study[1] showed an up to 30 times increased risk of cerebral palsy and this is only one of the severest forms of morbidity these children can potentially suffer – there are many others. On the subject of triplets, it is worth recollecting a Parisian triplet study in which couples with ART-conceived triplets were interviewed.[2] They were asked if they were counselled as to the risk of triplets when being offered or suggesting replacement of more than two embryos. One parent said that she was warned about the risk but at the time (she had waited more than ten years for a pregnancy) she did not believe the counsellor. A calculation has been done to estimate how many hours per week it takes to provide routine care for triplets. This number worked out at the figure of 186 hours – obviously there is an incompatibility here! Parents are thus faced with the difficulty of feeling guilty that they are not providing adequate care for their much-wanted babies.

Birth size

The balance of known literature considering ART outcome shows that singleton ART-conceived children from any type of ART are consistently, even at term, a little lighter for dates than their naturally conceived (NC) peers.[3] Why this is so is unclear (possibly related to the history of infertility) and probably of little significance for individual children.

Birth defects

There is probably a continuum of risk between standard IVF (a well-established and long-standing form of ART) and the more recent ICSI, with even more invasive forms of ART such as ICSI with testicular sperm aspiration (TESA) being of higher risk for the birth of children with birth defects. However, again this has to be put in context. The risk of birth defects after IVF is in the region of 1.2–1.5 times that of the background population and for ICSI this figure rises to up to twice that of the background population.[3]

Developmental difficulties

There is no convincing evidence that ART *per se* is associated with neurodevelopmental difficulties when high-risk groups such as preterm babies are excluded. In the latter group, however, like in any preterm babies, that risk is magnified for every day born less mature. In terms of other areas of psychosocial development, the definitive European study published this year has some clear messages.[4] Firstly, ART families find parenting more rewarding and work less rewarding than a comparable matched group of naturally conceiving parent. Secondly, there appear to be no distorting factors (as a result of the stress of going through the ART process) in the relationship between the couple (the dyadic relationship) or between parent and child. However, it is important not to misinterpret these findings. In this study all families had normal values and it was only the comparison which showed a difference. This does not mean that ART parents make better parents.

Childhood cancer

There is only one report,[5] from the Netherlands, suggesting an association between ART and childhood cancer. This suggested an increased risk of retinoblastoma.

However, the data have not been confirmed. Other studies have looked at children born to mothers after ovulation induction, and cancer rates in children after IVF conception, with no other reports suggesting negative outcomes. The perfect study has not been done. Attempts to conduct a linkage study looking at this have failed largely because of the restrictions on usage of the Human Fertilisation and Embryology Authority (HFEA) database.

Future sexual maturation and fertility

This will prove to be one of the most sensitive areas to investigate. There is not yet any literature on this topic because of the relative youth of the population involved.

Special subgroups

Embryo cryopreservation

There are a limited number of studies on the specific outcome of pregnancies after embryo cryopreservation. These conclude that there is nothing specific about these children as distinguished from the population of children born after ART.

PGD

Very little is known here and the outcome data available is uncontrolled and from modest numbers of births.

Twins

Separate reports concerning the health of ART-conceived twins are slowly emerging. When compared with non-ART twins, they have the same risks as twin births *per se,* plus slightly increased risk of neonatal death, ventilation and time on neonatal units than their NC control twins.

Literature review

Developmental outcome studies of ART-conceived children

An overview of developmental outcome studies for conventional IVF is provided in Table 22.1 and for ICSI in Table 22.2.

ICSI-CFO was an international collaborative study of ICSI child and family outcomes and was by far the largest (and most recent) study on IVF/ICSI children. It was performed in five European countries and comprised approximately 500 singleton ICSI, 500 IVF and 500 NC children aged 5 years in groups each assessed with observer blinding to conception status. Confounders were avoided by ensuring that all children were > 32 weeks of gestation, singleton, matched for sex and social class, and Caucasian. These children were assessed in detailed protocol by experienced paediatricians and psychologists, the latter of whom were blinded to conception status. This study showed no effect whatsoever of conception status on neurodevelopment.[1,3,6] There was, however, greater use of health service resources by ICSI and IVF children in comparison with NC children (more use of therapy, more surgery especially genitourinary surgery and more use of medication.) However,

Table 22.1. Developmental outcome studies for conventional IVF children; modified from an unpublished thesis of C Peters with kind permission

Authors	Study group	Study type	Outcome	Key results	Comments
D'Souza et al. (1997)[41]	278 IVF and 278 naturally conceived UK children. IVF singletons mean 25.5 months (SD 7.9). IVF multiple births mean 24.8 months (SD 5.1)	Prospective case–control study, matched for sex and social class	Results of Griffiths scales of development	Mean developmental quotient (DQ); IVF singletons 116.9 (SD 12.6) IVF multiple births 106.9 (SD 10.9) Not stated for controls Developmental delay (DQ < 70) noted in 2 multiple birth IVF children only	46% IVF children from multiple births; al controls were singleton; no matching for prematurity, birthweight or gestation
Cederblad et al. (1996)[42]	99 Swedish IVF children (age 33–85 months)	Single cohort compared with Swedish and American norms	Results of Griffiths scales of development	DQ above Swedish norm	No matched control group; high numbers of multiple births and prematurity
Brandes et al. (1992)[43]	116 Israeli (Hebrew speaking) IVF children and 116 matched non-IVF children (age 12–45 months)	Case–control study, matched for birthweight, gestational age, birth order, order in multiple births, mode of delivery, sex, age, maternal age and education	Bayley scales for infants up to 30 months Stanford–Binet scales for children >30 months Scales mean 100 ± 16	MDI Bayley scores: IVF 106 ± 19.6 non-IVF 110.6 ± 19.3 Composite Index for Stanford–Binet: IVF 106.2 ± 8 non-IVF 104.4 ± 10.2	No correction for prematurity because children all > 12 months
Morin et al. (1989)[44]	83 IVF children from Norfolk, USA and 93 matched non-IVF children (age 12–30 months)	Case–control study, matched for age, sex, race, multiple births and maternal age	Results of Bayley scales: MDI and PDI mean score 100	MDI scores: non-IVF 111 ± 13 PDI scores: IVF 114 ± 14 non-IVF 108 ± 15	Study had power of 99% to detect difference; strongly suggests no difference; however, scores corrected for prematurity
Mushin et al. (1985)[7]	33 Australian children (age 12–37 months)	Single cohort from first 52 infants conceived at Monash IVF centre, no matched controls	Results of Bayley scales One child (37 months) assessed using McCarthy scales	Overall MDI of 111 (SD 15) and PDI of 105 (SD 23) Four children with physical and developmental problems had lower scores	High numbers of multiple births and prematurity; of 4 children with poor scores, 2 were VLBW and 1 had severe CHD
Yovich et al. (1986)[45]	20 Australian children (age 12–13 months)	Single cohort of first 20 infants conceived after IVF in Western Australia	Results of Griffiths scales of development	General developmental quotient (GQ) was greater than mean of 100 in 19/20 children after correction for gestational age	No matched control group; increased rate of multiple births, IUGR, prematurity and caesarean section

MDI = mean developmental index; PDI = physical developmental index; VLBW = very low birthweight; CHD = congenital heart disease; IUGR = intrauterine growth restriction

Table 22.2. Developmental outcome studies for ICSI children; modified from an unpublished thesis of C Peters with kind permission

Authors	Study group	Study type	Outcome	Key results	Comments
Bonduelle, et al. (2005)[3]	1515 children: 538 natural (NC), 437 IVF, 540 ICSI; aged 5 years	Population control study, singleton, >32 weeks, Cauacasian	Results of WPPSI, McCarthy motor scales, laterality, full physical check, growth, audiometry, ophthalmic checks	Normal IQ, normal laterality, normal motor skills, taller than NC peers, higher anomalies	The most important study in the medical literature. Ability at 5 is predictive of ability at adult life.
Sutcliffe et al. (2001)[17]	208 UK children conceived after ICSI compared with 221 NC controls. Age 12–24 months	Case–control study, matched for social class, maternal educational level, region, sex and race	Results of Griffiths scales of infant development	Griffiths quotients: ICSI 98.08 (SD10.93) controls 98.69 (SD 9.99)	No correction for gestational age in Griffiths scales Single observer 90% follow-up
Bowen et al. (1998)[8] 89	Australian ICSI children compared with 84 conventional IVF children and 80 NC. Assessed at birth and at corrected age of 12 months	Prospective case–control study, matched for parental age, parity and multiplicity of the pregnancy Conventional and IVF children were recruited through separate study	Results of Bayley scales of infant development	98% follow-up at 1 year MDI Bayley scores: ICSI 95.9 (SD 10.7) IVF 101.8 (SD 8.5) non-IVF 102.5 (SD 7.6)	Included frozen embryos (39% ICSI, 31% IVF) Lack of blinding and differences in sociodemographic factors, particularly between the parents of the ICSI group and other groups
Bonduelle et al. (1998)[12]	201 Belgian (Dutch speaking) ICSI children compared with 131 conventional IVF children. Assessment age 22–26 months	Blinded prospective case–control trial	Results of Bayley scales. Test results scored by subtracting chronological age from test age. Test age calculated from subset of 1283 Dutch children aged 2–30 months	Scored mean age differences: ICSI singleton +2.11 (SD 3.12) IVF singleton +2.30 (SD 2.63) ICSI twin +1.67 (SD 3.06) IVF twin +0.31 (SD 3.75) Lower scores for triplets, with males scoring lower than females	No correction for gestational age Higher scores for singletons Matching not discussed in this letter Single observer 60% follow-up

WPPSI = Wechsler preschool and primary scale of intelligence when examined in a comprehensive manner 'top to toe', these children were not found to be physically different from NC children, with the exception of congenital anomalies where they had double the rates of the NC group. We specifically excluded children who had had circumcision and found that there were children who were more likely to have an ectopic kidney, duplex systems or vesico-ureteric reflux in this group.

Developmental differences in an ICSI-conceived group of children when compared with conventional IVF and NC controls were reported in 1998.[7,8] This Sydney group found an increase in mild developmental delay using the Bayley scales of infant development[9] to derive a mental development index. However, the study used comparison groups of IVF and NC children that were already enrolled in a separate study and had differing demographics to the ICSI group. There was also no blinding of the assessors and the number of participants in the study was small with 89 ICSI-conceived children.

Bonduelle et al.[10–15] have published several papers investigating congenital malformation rates and physical development of ICSI children. Several of these papers allude to the fact that developmental milestones were assessed, but formal assessments of these children, undertaken in the period 1995–98, were published in a research letter to *The Lancet* in 1998.[12] This article reported 201 ICSI children and 131 IVF children who were assessed using the Bayley scales and the results were compared with a subset of children representing the Dutch population. The age of the children was not corrected for gestational age, but the ICSI and IVF children were found to have similar scores to the general population. The twins scored slightly lower than the singletons.

Sutcliffe et al.[16,17] studied 208 singleton ICSI-conceived children at around 18 months and compared them with a matched NC control group. The children were assessed by a single observer using the Griffiths scales of mental development.[18] No differences in developmental outcome were found between the two groups.

Embryo cryopreservation

The limited literature here shows that these children are not any different in any areas from ART-conceived children as a whole.[17,19,20] They will not be discussed separately any further in this brief overview.

Physical assessments other than for congenital anomalies

Use of medical services

IVF children are more likely to need neonatal care, primarily because of the prematurity related to multiple pregnancies.

Initial reports suggested that IVF children did not require extra medical attention after the neonatal period.[21,22] Leslie studied 95 IVF children and compared them with 79 NC children matched for maternal age and parity. IVF children were also less likely to be breastfed by the time of discharge. However ICSI-CFO has disagreed with these findings and has clearly shown higher use of medical resources among IVF/ICSI children, including surgery.[3]

The point to emphasise here is that the ICSI-CFO study was performed with older children and was 10 times as large as any of these early studies and thus far more likely to detect a difference.

Growth

Saunders *et al.*[22] published a case-matched control study of children conceived after ART and found that the physical outcomes of weight, head circumference and malformation rates were no different between groups. The IVF group had a greater mean length centile and the twins in each group had poorer physical outcomes with an increase in prematurity and lower birthweights, and reduced height and weight at age two when compared with singletons in each group. This finding needs verification but is somewhat alarming as so far no one has accurately charted growth of ART children and so far larger children have been 'buried' in the effects of prematurity and higher order births. Studies are currently in progress to investigate whether there has been a change in the Ponderal index of ART children between birth and later years.

Retinopathy of prematurity

The increase in multiple births and premature births related to assisted conception has led to an increase in conditions such as retinopathy that are directly related to early births and low birthweights.[23,24]

Anteby *et al.*[25] reported the ocular manifestations in children born after IVF and referred for ophthalmological assessment. Major ocular malformations were found in 12 (26%) of the small cohort of 47 children studied. Seven major malformations were listed, including congenital cataract, optic atrophy and retinoblastoma. The study was limited in power owing to the small numbers of children involved and, because the study was conducted in a tertiary hospital, it is possible that the numbers were skewed as a result of the type of patients referred.

Childhood cancer

There have been case reports[26,27] of children conceived after assisted conception developing neuroectodermal tumours but no large study has confirmed this finding. Bruinsma *et al.*[28] used a record-linkage cohort design to link ART births to a population-based cancer registry in Australia. This study included 5249 births and found no increase in the incidence of cancers in the assisted reproduction groups. However, these groups were relatively small and underpowered for the outcomes measured. The mean length of follow-up was only 3 years 9 months, although neuroblastomas do tend to occur within the first year of life. These findings were supported by a smaller, similar Israeli study.[29]

More recently, Klip *et al.*[30] examined a large population-based historical cohort, established to investigate gynaecological disorders in women undergoing IVF. This cohort included 9484 children whose mothers had been given IVF or related fertility treatments and 7532 children whose mothers were subfertile but had conceived naturally. The mothers were mailed questionnaires enquiring about cancer in their children. There was a 67% response rate and no difference between the groups was noted, implying that IVF and related treatments do not increase the cancer risk to the child.

The cancer incidence in IVF children studied for the UK Medical Research Council (MRC) working party[31] and a Swedish national cohort study of IVF children[32] also found no increase in cancer rates, but the power of these studies was limited by too small a number of children studied. Doyle *et al.*[31] estimated that 20 000 children would be required to observe a doubling or halving of the risk of childhood cancer in children conceived after ART compared with the general population. This would provide 95% significance and 90% power if children were followed up for 5 years.

Neurological outcomes

There has been some suggestion from a Swedish study[33] that children born after IVF have an increased risk of developing neurological problems, particularly cerebral palsy. They found a four-fold increase in risk of cerebral palsy in children born after IVF compared with matched controls (OR 3.7; 95% CI 2.0–6.6). The risk in singletons was nearly three times (OR 2.8; 95% CI 1.3–5.8). After adjusting for birthweight and a gestation of > 37 weeks, the risk remained with an odds ratio of 2.5 (95% CI 1.1–5.2). The authors admitted that the frequency of cerebral palsy in controls was lower than the Swedish norm. Calculations using their data indicate a prevalence of cerebral palsy in the control group as 1.5/1000 compared with an accepted prevalence rate of 2.0–2.5/1000.[34] The increased risk was shown to be mainly with multiple births and was associated with low birthweight and low gestational age. Leviton and colleagues[35] noted that there was some over-aggregation of the data, with children less than 30 weeks of gestation grouped together. This does not allow for the effect of decreasing risk of cerebral palsy with increasing gestation, particularly in those infants born after 30 weeks.[35] Also, in a commentary by Sutcliffe,[16] it was noted that the study used proxy measures for disability and that it was unexplained why the rate of problems seemed higher in the singleton group than the IVF group, in contradiction to the entire twin literature.

Genomic imprinting

Genomic imprinting is the mechanism that determines the expression or repression of genes from maternal or paternal chromosomes. This modification of genetic material is epigenetic, i.e. reversible between generations and is not a mutation. Maternal and paternal germlines confer an imprint or sex-specific mark on certain chromosome regions. Therefore, although the sequence of the genes on these chromosomes could be identical, they are not functionally equivalent.

Over 40 imprinted genes have now been characterised. They have been shown to influence embryonic growth and development and are implicated in the inactivation of tumour suppressor genes resulting in some childhood cancers, e.g. Wilms tumour, embryonal rhabdomyosarcoma, osteosarcoma and bilateral retinoblastoma. These are thought to occur by the 'two-hit' hypothesis of cancer. The first inactivation of a tumour suppressor allele would occur by imprinting rather than mutation. Wilms tumour appears to have two different tumour precursor lesions. One type is thought to be due to an imprinting defect of the gene for insulin-like growth factor 2 (IGF2). The second subtype occurs after a mutation of the *WT1* gene.[36]

There is evidence that several syndromes are also caused by imprinting disorders, such as Prader–Willi, Angelman, Russell–Silver, Beckwith–Wiedemann and McCune–Albright syndromes, and transient neonatal diabetes and pseudohypoparathyroidism.

Two recent studies have suggested that there may an increased incidence of Beckwith–Wiedemann syndrome after assisted conception.[37,38] Although small, these studies support previous findings. Olivennes *et al.*[39] reported a boy with Beckwith–Wiedemann syndrome in a cohort of 73 children conceived after IVF. An earlier study by Sutcliffe *et al.*[19] in 1995 also reported a child with Beckwith–Wiedemann syndrome in a cohort of 91 children born after replacement of frozen embryos.

Angelman syndrome is caused by a loss of the maternal allele function secondary to uniparental disomy of the paternal allele, a mutation of the maternal allele, or a sporadic genetic imprinting error causing a paternal imprint on a maternal chromosome.[40] A report of two children with Angelman syndrome, conceived after ICSI, suggested that an inherited defect was unlikely in these cases and therefore the defect was possibly caused at a post-zygotic stage.

Conclusion

Generally, ART-conceived children who are born singleton and at term are similar in most longer term outcomes to naturally conceived children (with the exception of congenital anomalies.) They do, however, appear to use more health service resources. There are some questions that are unresolved concerning their progress into adult life:

- Are there longer term risks of imprintable disorders and cancer?
- Will these children be fertile when they are sexually mature?

ART-conceived children will be a significant client group as they grow up (at least 1% of the population in rich countries.) If their ART conception has exposed them to undue risk because these factors were not studied, when the techniques were introduced, they may well take a very different view of the justifications for ART than the readers of this chapter. Further studies need to be performed – the ideal one has yet to be conducted.

Further reading

Sutcliffe AG. *IVF Children: The First Generation*. 1st ed. London: Parthenon; 2002.

References

1. Petterson B, Nelson KB, Watson L, Stanley F. Twins, triplets, and cerebral palsy in births in Western Australia in the 1980s. *BMJ* 1993;307:1239–43.
2. Australian Multiple Births Association. *Proposal Submitted to the Federal Government Concerning 'Act of Grace' Payments for Triplet and Quadruplet Families*. Coogee: AMBA; 1984.
3. Bonduelle M, Wennerholm UB, Loft A, Tarlatzis BC, Peters C, Henriet S, *et al*. A multi-centre cohort study of the physical health of 5-year-old children conceived after intracytoplasmic sperm injection, *in vitro* fertilization and natural conception. *Hum Reprod* 2005;20:413–9.
4. Barnes J, Sutcliffe AG, Kristoffersen I, Loft A, Wennerholm U, Tarlatzis BC, *et al.*; European Study. The influence of assisted reproduction on family functioning and children's socio-emotional development: results from a European study. *Hum Reprod* 2004;19:1480–7.
5. Moll AC, Imhof SM, Cruysberg JR, Schouten-van Meeteren AY, Boers M, van Leeuwen FE. Incidence of retinoblastoma in children born after in-vitro fertilisation. *Lancet* 2003;361:309–10.
6. Ponjaert-Kristoffersen I, Bonduelle M, Barnes J, Nekkebroeck J, Loft A, Wennerholm UB, *et al*. International collaborative study of intracytoplasmic sperm injection-conceived, *in vitro* fertilization-conceived, and naturally conceived 5-year-old child outcomes: cognitive and motor assessments. *Pediatrics* 2005;115:e283–9.
7. Mushin D, Spensley J, Barreda-Hanson M. Children of IVF. *Clin Obstet Gynaecol* 1985;12:865–76.

8. Bowen JR, Gibson FL, Leslie GI, Saunders DM. Medical and developmental outcome at 1 year for children conceived by intracytoplasmic sperm injection. *Lancet* 1998;351:1529–34.

9. Bayley N. *Bayley Scales of Infant Development*. 2nd ed. San Antonio, TX: The Psychological Corporation; 1993.

10. Bonduelle M, Legein J, Buysse A, Van Assche E, Wisanto A, Devroey P, *et al.* Prospective follow-up study of 423 children born after intracytoplasmic sperm injection. *Hum Reprod* 1996;11:1558–64.

11. Bonduelle M, Wilikens A, Buysse A, Van Assche E, Wisanto A, Devroey P, *et al.* Prospective follow-up study of 877 children born after intracytoplasmic sperm injection (ICSI), with ejaculated epididymal and testicular spermatozoa and after replacement of cryopreserved embryos obtained after ICSI. *Hum Reprod* 1996;11 Suppl 4:131–55; discussion 156–9.

12. Bonduelle M, Joris H, Hofmans K, Liebaers I, Van Steirteghem A. Mental development of 201 ICSI children at 2 years of age. *Lancet* 1998;351:1553.

13. Bonduelle M, Camus M, De Vos A, Staessen C, Tournaye H, Van Assche E, *et al.* Seven years of intracytoplasmic sperm injection and follow-up of 1987 subsequent children. *Hum Reprod* 1999;14 Suppl 1:243–64.

14. Bonduelle M, Liebaers I, Deketelaere V, Derde MP, Camus M, Devroey P, *et al.* Neonatal data on a cohort of 2889 infants born after ICSI (1991–1999) and of 2995 infants born after IVF (1983–1999). *Hum Reprod* 2002;17:671–94.

15. Bonduelle M, Aytoz A, Wilikens A, Buysse A, Van Assche E, Devroey P, *et al.* Prospective follow-up study of 1,987 children born after intracytoplasmic sperm injection (ICSI). In: Silicori M, Flamigni C, editors. *Treatment of Infertility: The New Frontiers*. Princeton: Communication Media for Education; 1998. p. 445–61.

16. Sutcliffe AG, Taylor B, Li J, Thornton S, Grudzinskas JG, Lieberman BA. Children born after intracytoplasmic sperm injection: population control study. *BMJ* 1999;318:704–5.

17. Sutcliffe AG, Taylor B, Saunders K, Thornton S, Lieberman BA, Grudzinskas JG. Outcome in the second year of life after in-vitro fertilisation by intracytoplasmic sperm injection: a UK case–control study. *Lancet* 2001;357:2080–4.

18. Griffiths R. *The Griffiths Mental Development Scales 1996 Revision*, revised by Huntley M. Henley: Association for Research in Infant and Child Development, Test Agency; 1996.

19. Sutcliffe AG, D'Souza SW, Cadman J, Richards B, McKinlay IA, Lieberman B. Outcome in children from cryopreserved embryos. *Arch Dis Child* 1995;72:290–3.

20. Wennerholm UB, Albertsson-Wikland K, Bergh C, Hamberger L, Niklasson A, Nilsson L, *et al.* Postnatal growth and health in children born after cryopreservation as embryos. *Lancet* 1998;351:1085–90.

21. Leslie GI, Gibson FL, McMahon C, Tennant C, Saunders DM. Infants conceived using in-vitro fertilization do not over-utilize health care resources after the neonatal period. *Hum Reprod* 1998;13:2055–9.

22. Saunders K, Spensley J, Munro J, Halasz G. Growth and physical outcome of children conceived by *in vitro* fertilization. *Pediatrics* 1996;97:688–92.

23. McKibbin M, Dabbs TR. Assisted conception and retinopathy of prematurity. *Eye* 1996;10:476–8.

24. Watts P, Adams GG. *In vitro* fertilisation and stage 3 retinopathy of prematurity. *Eye* 2000;14:330–3.

25. Anteby I, Cohen E, Anteby E, BenEzra D. Ocular manifestations in children born after *in vitro* fertilization. *Arch Ophthalmol* 2001;119:1525–9.

26. White L, Giri N, Vowels MR, Lancaster PA. Neuroectodermal tumours in children born after assisted conception. *Lancet* 1990;336:1577.

27. Kobayashi N, Matsui I, Tanimura M, Nagahara N, Akatsuka J, Hirayama T, *et al.* Childhood neuroectodermal tumours and malignant lymphoma after maternal ovulation induction. *Lancet* 1991;338:955.

28. Bruinsma F, Venn A, Lancaster P, Speirs A, Healy D. Incidence of cancer in children born after in-vitro fertilization. *Hum Reprod* 2000;15:604–7.

29. Lerner-Geva L, Toren A, Chetrit A, Modan B, Mandel M, Rechavi G, *et al.* The risk for cancer among children of women who underwent *in vitro* fertilization. *Cancer* 2000;88:2845–7.

30. Klip H, Burger CW, de Kraker J, van Leeuwen FE; OMEGA-project group. Risk of cancer in the offspring of women who underwent ovarian stimulation for IVF. *Hum Reprod* 2001;16:2451–8.

31. Doyle P, Bunch KJ, Beral V, Draper GJ. Cancer incidence in children conceived with assisted reproduction technology. *Lancet* 1998;352:452–3.

32. Bergh T, Ericson A, Hillensjo T, Nygren KG, Wennerholm UB. Deliveries and children born after in-vitro fertilisation in Sweden 1982–95: a retrospective cohort study. *Lancet* 1999;354:1579–85.

33. Stromberg B, Dahlquist G, Ericson A, Finnstrom O, Koster M, Stjernqvist K. Neurological sequelae in children born after in-vitro fertilisation: a population-based study. *Lancet* 2002;359:461–5.

34. Healy DL, Saunders K. Follow-up of children born after in-vitro fertilisation. *Lancet* 2002;359:459–60.
35. Leviton A, Stewart JE, Allred EN, Dammann O, Kuban K. Neurological sequelae in in-vitro fertilisation babies. *Lancet* 2002;360:718.
36. Reeve AE, Becroft DM, Morison IM, Fukuzawa R. Insulin-like growth factor-II imprinting in cancer. *Lancet* 2002;359:2050–1.
37. DeBaun MR, Niemitz EL, Feinberg AP. Association of *in vitro* fertilization with Beckwith–Wiedemann syndrome and epigenetic alterations of LIT1 and H19. *Am J Hum Genet* 2003;72:156–60.
38. Maher ER, Afnan M, Barratt CL. Epigenetic risks related to assisted reproductive technologies: epigenetics, imprinting, ART and icebergs? *Hum Reprod* 2003;18:2508–11.
39. Olivennes F, Mannaerts B, Struijs M, Bonduelle M, Devroey P. Perinatal outcome of pregnancy after GnRH antagonist (ganirelix) treatment during ovarian stimulation for conventional IVF or ICSI: a preliminary report. *Hum Reprod* 2001;16:1588–91.
40. Cox GF, Burger J, Lip V, Mau UA, Sperling K, Wu BL, *et al.* Intracytoplasmic sperm injection may increase the risk of imprinting defects. *Am J Hum Genet* 2002;71:162–4..
41. D'Souza SW, Rivlin E, Cadman J, Richards B, Buck P, Lieberman BA. Children conceived by *in vitro* fertilisation after fresh embryo transfer. *Arch Dis Child Fetal Neonatal Ed* 1997;76:F70–4.
42. Cederblad M, Friberg B, Ploman F, Sjoberg NO, Stjernqvist K, Zackrisson E. Intelligence and behaviour in children born after in-vitro fertilization treatment. *Hum Reprod* 1996;11:2052–7.
43. Brandes JM, Scher A, Itzkovits J, Thaler I, Sarid M, Gershoni-Baruch R. Growth and development of children conceived by *in vitro* fertilization. *Pediatrics* 1992;90:424–9.
44. Morin NC, Wirth FH, Johnson DH, Frank LM, Presburg HJ, Van de Water VL, *et al.* Congenital malformations and psychosocial development in children conceived by *in vitro* fertilization. *J Pediatr* 1989;115:222–7.
45. Yovich JL, Parry TS, French NP, Grauaug AA. Developmental assessment of twenty *in vitro* fertilization (IVF) infants at their first birthday. *J In Vitro Fert Embryo Transf* 1986;3:253–7.

SECTION 5
CONSENSUS VIEWS

Chapter 23
Consensus views arising from the 48th Study Group: Implantation and Early Development

Future research

Endometrial receptivity

1. The process of embryonic implantation is still something of a black box. A molecular definition of endometrial receptivity is needed. This would not only allow researchers to focus on a well-defined process but might also lead to the development of new therapeutic targets and diagnostic tools, and to the use of a multidisciplinary systems biology approach (involving clinicians, scientists and other stakeholders) to achieve a better understanding of implantation, placentation and early development. Understanding of this process should improve the treatment of disorders such as pre-eclampsia, miscarriage and infertility.
2. Given the constraints on investigating early human pregnancy, there is a need to continue to take an enlightened approach to embryo research and the use of animal models for functional studies (within an appropriate ethical and legal framework and whilst pursuing a policy of reduction, refinement and replacement).
3. Further basic studies should address the complexity of the endometrial vasculature, including the key 'what, where and when' questions relating to factors that affect endothelial cells (including assessment of regional differences in vascular function within the uterus, and extension of the observations into early pregnancy using appropriate models).

Embryo–endometrial interaction

4. The multidisciplinary systems biology approach that is needed to assess endometrial receptivity should also be used to understand the reciprocal dialogue between the embryo and the decidualised endometrium. This will include a continued focus on human embryo research and the development of appropriate functional models of implantation that will allow the investigation of molecules mediating blastocyst–endometrial/decidual interaction. Ultimately, this should lead to novel targeted therapies to treat implantation defects.

5. Extrauterine (ectopic) pregnancy is a life-threatening event and is not uncommon in humans. The precise reason why implantation occurs in a site distant to the uterus is still unknown. Ectopic pregnancy could be considered as a model to study the failure or the absence of mechanisms that limit implantation. A molecular understanding of the aetiology of ectopic pregnancy could advance our knowledge of how implantation is regulated in normal pregnancy.

Gamete and embryo biology

6. Further work is required to determine the link between oocyte quality and embryo development. Pivotal to this will be an understanding of the role of epigenetic modification during the later phases of oocyte maturation. Experience with cell nuclear replacement has identified the key role of cytoplasmic and nuclear factors for normal embryonic development. A cautious approach should be adopted in relation to the clinical application of oocyte *in vitro* maturation (IVM) until the mechanisms governing epigenetic modification have been more clearly determined.
7. More sophisticated tests are required to assess the contribution of the male gamete to fertility and embryo development. The conventional measurements of sperm concentration, motility and morphology only act as surrogate markers of fertility. These surrogate markers should be assessed in relation to more definitive outcomes, including population live birth data.
8. The role of epigenetic modification in early embryo development needs to be more clearly defined, again by the application of a multidisciplinary systems biology approach. We still need to understand what makes an 'implantation-competent blastocyst' that will give rise to a normal baby. Furthermore, large-scale follow-up studies will be required to determine the impact of such epigenetic modification on long-term health and disease.

Early pregnancy failure

9. There is a need for a national framework responsible for coordinating clinical trials assessing the efficacy of pharmacological interventions in patients with recurrent pregnancy failure.
10. Women miscarrying one normal pregnancy should ideally be investigated for maternal causes for their loss. However, there is a need for a comprehensive economic and cost evaluation assessment to see whether such an approach would be feasible in practice.
11. Further research is needed to establish the contribution that inherited thrombotic disorders make to reproductive failure.
12. The number and activity of natural killer (NK) cells in peripheral blood show no correlation with reproductive success. There are no controlled data to support the current use of these tests in clinical practice.
13. There is no scientific rationale for offering women with infertility or recurrent pregnancy loss treatment with steroids, white cell infusions or intravenous immunoglobulin. The use of these interventions cannot be recommended in normal healthy women because of the incidence of well-recognised and potentially severe adverse effects.

Translation into clinical practice

14. More data from randomised trials are needed to demonstrate whether a single-embryo transfer policy would be effective, acceptable and financially viable in the UK.
15. Parents of children born following embryo biopsy should be encouraged to take part in follow-up studies of the health and development of their children (including into adult life).
16. Further work is needed to identify appropriate criteria for recommending pre-implantation genetic screening (PGS) and, through appropriately structured research, an assessment should be made of its efficacy per treatment cycle.

Clinical practice

1. New treatments should not be introduced into clinical practice until they have undergone rigorous evaluation and have been shown to be effective by adequately designed clinical trials.

Management of early pregnancy loss

2. Antiphospholipid syndrome is an established cause of fetal loss. Treatment with aspirin and heparin during pregnancy significantly improves the live birth rate.
3. There is no evidence to support the notion that couples should wait three months before trying to conceive again following early pregnancy loss.

Pre-implantation testing

4. Pre-implantation genetic diagnosis (PGD) should be carried out by specialist centres that have a multidisciplinary genetic support infrastructure including genetic counselling, and CPA (Clinical Pathology Accreditation) qualified cyto-genetics and molecular genetics laboratories.

Assisted reproduction

5. Elective single-embryo transfer substantially reduces the risk of twins following *in vitro* fertilisation.
6. There are no data to support the practice of endometrial biopsy as part of the pretreatment assessment for assisted conception.

Health policy/education

1. One to two per cent of children born in developed societies are now the result of assisted conception-related technologies. There is an urgent need to coordinate large-scale (national) follow-up studies of mothers and their children to audit the safety and long-term outcomes of these treatments.
2. As outlined in the clinical practice section above, new treatments should only be introduced when they have undergone rigorous evaluation and have been shown to be effective by adequately designed clinical trials. For example, the possible risks of oocyte *in vitro* maturation (IVM) need to be further evaluated.

Similarly, studies are required to assess the potential teratogenic effects of the high concentrations of cytotoxic chemicals employed during the process of vitrification.

3. Funding of PGD should be considered outside the remit of normal infertility purchasing as the procedure is not aimed specifically at alleviating infertility but at preventing genetic disease. On the other hand (if appropriate), PGS might be considered as part of infertility service provision.

4. Despite certain methodological limitations, epidemiological studies are useful for determining both genetic and environmental risk factors for reproductive health. There is a strong public heath argument for being able to link national databases (such as those held by the National Cancer Registry and the Human Fertilisation and Embryology Authority).

5. Children born after assisted reproduction are usually healthy. However, multiple pregnancy is the single biggest cause of perinatal morbidity and mortality in pregnancies conceived following assisted conception treatments.

6. Our understanding of developmental biology continues to proceed at a rapid rate. Regulators and policy-makers should therefore scan the horizon to be aware of possible future developments in assisted conception (such as *in vitro* maturation of gametes, germinal vesicle transfer or the creation of artificial gametes).

Index

acetylation, histone H4 143–4, 147
actin
    early embryo cells 133–4
    invading trophoblast 95, 96
activated protein C resistance (APCR)
    230, 234
activator protein 1 (AP1) 72–3, 74
activins 110
acyl-coenzyme A:acyltransferase
    (ACAT) 86
ADAM17/TACE 51
adhesion molecules
    in embryonic compaction 130
    in implantation 9, 49–60, 92
        candidates 51–3
        clinical implications 55
        endometrial transcriptome and
            54–5
        mouse genetic models 53–4
    in infertile women 55
Affymetrix arrays 204
age, maternal
    ART outcome and 156–7
    pre-implantation genetic screening
        and 177
allele drop-out (ADO) 174, 175
Alox15 207–9
androgen receptors (AR) 4, 5, 109
androgens

action within ovary 108, 109–10
    endometrial regulation 5
anembryonic pregnancy 220, 222
aneuploidy screening, pre-
    implantation see pre-implantation
    genetic screening
Angelman syndrome (AS) 156, 162,
    277
angiogenesis
    endometrial receptivity and 63–4
    key factors regulating 64–6
    in luteal growth 61
    regulation by COX/prostanoids
        9–10
    sprouting 63–4
angiopoietin 1 (ANG1) 65
angiopoietin 2 (ANG2) 24, 65
angiopoietins 63, 65–6
animal–vegetal (AV) egg polarity 137
anticardiolipin antibodies (aCL) 232
antigen-presenting cells (APCs)
    16–18, 22
antiphospholipid antibodies (aPL)
    231, 232–3
antiphospholipid syndrome (APS),
    primary (PAPS) 229, 231–3
    adverse uterine milieu 246
    management 232, 285
    pathophysiology 232–3

screening 222, 232
apolipoprotein D 86
apolipoprotein E 92
apoptosis, in implantation 11
arachidonic acid (AA) 6, 7
Arg-Gly-Asp (RGD) adhesion
    sequence 123
ASIP/PAR3 133
aspirin, in antiphospholipid syndrome
    232, 233
assisted reproductive technology
    (ART)
    consensus views 285, 286
    epigenetics and genomic
        imprinting 161–3
    oocyte quality and 103
    paediatric outcome 268–79
    pregnancy outcomes 156, 241–2
    pre-implantation genetic testing
        169, 172
    risk factors for adverse outcomes
        156–61
    risks 113, 155–68, 286
    sperm functional demands 119,
        120
    see also intracytoplasmic sperm
        injection; in vitro fertilisation
autocrine regulation, implantation
    process 3, 6–11
autoimmune diseases 22
5-aza-2'-deoxycytidine 148

basigin (EMMPRIN; CD147) 6, 52,
    54
Beckwith–Wiedemann syndrome
    (BWS) 113, 155, 156, 162–3,
    276–7
BERKO (ERβ knockout) mice 109
birth defects
    after embryo biopsy 176
    after in vitro culture 155, 160
    ART-conceived babies 270, 274
birth size, ART-conceived babies 270
blastocoel formation 129, 133, 134
blastocyst(s) 129

adhesion/attachment 9, 51, 92
    adhesion molecules 52, 53–4
    solid-phase assays 93, 94
axis determination 137
biopsy, for genetic testing 169–70
cell lineages see cell lineages, early
    embryo
chemokine receptors 80, 81
endometrial cell co-cultures 94–7
ICM immunosurgery 134–6
invasiveness 71
leptin secretion 83–4
three-dimensional co-cultures 97,
    98
transfer, single 257
see also embryo
blastomeres
    asymmetric divisions 130–3
    cell contacts 134–6
    cell polarisation 130
    intercellular adhesion 130
    lineage diversification see cell
        lineages, early embryo
bleeding in early pregnancy, patient
    examination 223–4
blighted ovum 219
blood vessels, endometrial see
    vasculature, endometrial
B lymphocytes 16
    uterine mucosal 21
bone morphogenetic protein 2
    (BMP2) 195
bone morphogenetic protein 4
    (BMP4) 195
bone morphogenetic protein 15
    (BMP15) 107, 110
bone morphogenetic proteins (BMPs)
    110

cadherins 52
calcitonin 4, 50, 207
calcium (Ca²⁺), intracellular 50, 130,
    134
cancer, ART-conceived children
    270–1, 275–6

capillaries, endometrial 62
catecholoestrogen 50
β-catenin 130
CCR2B 80, 81
CCR5 80, 81
CD3⁺ T cells 22
CD44 52, 53
CD56⁺ cells, uterine 24
  see also natural killer (NK) cells,
    uterine
CD94/NKG2A 24, 25, 26, 27
CD147 *see* basigin
cDNA microarrays 204–5
  see also DNA microarrays
Cdx2 137
cell differentiation
  plasticity 148–50
  potential of somatic cells 148
cell hybridisation studies 149
cell lineages, early embryo 129–40
  cell contacts and dynamic
    regulation 134–6
  egg polarity, cell polarity and cell
    interactions 137
  epigenetic regulation 143, 144
  origin of fetal and extra-
    embryonic 130–3
  transcriptional factors and
    diversification 136–7
  trophectoderm differentiation
    133–4
cell polarity, blastomeres 130
cerebral palsy 276
chemokine receptors 79–81
  blastocyst 80, 81
  endometrial 80, 81
chemokines 79–80, 211
child outcome *see* paediatric outcome
chromatin 141–2
  condensation, in cloned embryos
    146
  modifications, in cloned embryos
    146–8
  priming, before nuclear transfer
    147–8

chromosomal abnormalities
  ICSI-related 159–60
  maternal age-related 156–7
  miscarriage and 221, 222
  pre-implantation diagnosis 173,
    174
  pre-implantation screening 177
cingulin 136
claudins 86, 134
clinical practice, consensus views 285
clomiphene citrate 157
cloning, animal
  nuclear reprogramming after
    144–8
  by nuclear transfer 142
clot, maximal amplitude (MA) 236
collagenases 40, 71
collagens 52, 54
compaction, embryonic 130, 132, 133
comparative genomic hybridisation
  (CGH) 179, 221
congenital defects *see* birth defects
connexins 50
consensus views 283–6
  clinical practice 285
  future research 283–5
  health policy/education 285–6
corpus luteum, growth 61
costs
  pre-implantation genetic diagnosis
    171
  single-embryo transfer 262, 264
  twin pregnancy 256
cryopreservation
  embryo *see* embryo
cryopreservation
  pregnancy outcomes 160–1
CXCR1 80, 81
CXCR4 80, 81
cyclic adenosine 3',5'-monophosphate
  (cAMP) 4, 44, 109, 245–6
cyclooxygenase 1 (COX1) 6, 7–8
cyclooxygenase 2 (COX2) 6
  LIF-mediated regulation 189,
    195, 196

regulation of implantation 6–11
cyclooxygenase (COX)/prostaglandin
biosynthetic pathway 6–11
  in blastocyst adhesion and invasion
    9
  paracrine signalling in
    implantation 8–9
  programmed cell death and 11
  regulation of angiogenesis 10–11
  role in implantation 7–8, 50
cytokeratin filaments 95, 96
cytokines, regulation of trophoblast
  invasion 72, 74
cytoplasmic extracts, nuclear
  reprogramming of somatic cells
  149–50
cytoplasmic transfer, pregnancy
  outcomes after 158–9
cytoskeleton, early embryo cells 133–4
cytotrophoblast 19
cytotrophoblastic (CTB) cells 71
  MMP9 gene regulation 72–5, 76
  MMP and TIMP secretion 71–2

danger model, Matzinger's 17, 18
DAP12 25
decidualisation 21, 62–3, 70, 185
  defective 244–5
  endocrine regulation 4
  haemostasis and vascular stability
    and 32–48
  role of LIF 188–9, 195
  therapeutic manipulation 246–7
decorin 54
de-differentiation, somatic cells 149
dendritic cells 21, 22
desmin 195
desmosomes 192
development
  epigenetics in 141–54
  role of LIF in peri-implantation
    195–7
developmental difficulties, ART-
  conceived children 270, 271–4
Dickkopf 86

diethylstilboestrol 189–91
differentially methylated region
  (DMR) 161–2
differentiation, cell *see* cell
  differentiation
DNA
  methylation 142–3, 147, 161–2
  mitochondrial (mtDNA) 158–9
  quality, sperm 125–6
  structure 141–2
DNA microarrays 6, 92, 203–15
  clinical implications 213–14
  endometrial receptivity 54–5,
    85–7, 92, 205–12
  endometriosis 212–13
  limitations 213
  pre-implantation genetic diagnosis
    179–80
  techniques 204–5
double-embryo transfer (DET) 256,
  258–61
DP receptors 6

early pregnancy loss 55–6
  cloned embryos 144
  management 285
  preventive therapy 247, 284
  research needs 284
  sporadic 219–28
  terminology 219–21, 229
  timing of implantation and 49
  see also miscarriage
E-cadherin 9, 130
ectopic pregnancy 223, 224, 284
eggs
  animal–vegetal (AV) polarity 137
  cytoplasmic extracts for nuclear
    reprogramming 150
  see also oocytes
embryo
  attachment *see* blastocyst(s),
    adhesion/attachment
  biology, research needs 284
  cell lineages *see* cell lineages, early
    embryo

cloned, nuclear reprogramming
144–8
compaction 130, 132, 133
DNA methylation 143
hatching 50
histone H4 acetylation 143–4
in vitro culture *see in vitro* culture
research, consensus view 283
sex determination 170, 172–3
sex selection *see* sex selection
see also blastocyst(s)
embryo biopsy
pregnancy outcomes 176
pre-implantation genetic screening
177
research needs 285
techniques 169–70
embryo cryopreservation 161
paediatric outcome 271, 274
single-embryo transfer and 262
embryo–endometrial
dialogue/interface 49–50, 79–89
adhesion molecules 51–5
chemokine receptors 79–81
in vitro models 90–9
leptin and leptin receptors 82–4
relaxin and relaxin receptor LGR7
84–5
research needs 283–4
tissue remodelling 70–8
embryonic loss 219–20
embryonic period 219
embryonic stem (ES) cells 129
somatic cell de-differentiation into
149
transcription factors regulating
136–7
embryo quality 55, 56
in vitro assessment 95–7
IVF outcome and 257
single-embryo transfer and 262
embryoscopy, in miscarriage 223
embryo transfer
double (DET) 256, 258–61
multiple 256

single *see* single-embryo transfer
to surrogates 157
EMMPRIN *see* basigin
endocrine regulation, endometrium
3–5
endometrial biopsy 247, 285
endometrial cell–blastocyst co-
cultures 94–7
endometrial cell–blastocyst three-
dimensional co-cultures 97, 98
endometrial endothelial cells *see*
endothelial cells, endometrial
endometrial epithelial cells (EEC)
chemokine receptors 81
leptin and leptin receptors 83
endometrial epithelium
barrier function 50–1, 71
blastocyst adhesion *see*
blastocyst(s), adhesion/attachment
endometrial luminal epithelium (LE)
185
LIF-induced molecular changes
192–4
LIF-induced ultrastructural
changes 192, 193
LIF targets 188–9
endometrial receptivity 3, 49, 71,
185, 205–6
adhesion molecules and 51–5
clinical and therapeutic aspects
55, 56
endocrine and paracrine
regulation 3–12
in fertile and infertile women 55
LIF and 186, 192
microarray studies 85–7, 92,
205–12
adhesion molecules 54–5
difficulties in comparing
studies 211
mifepristone in women
211–12
progesterone-regulated genes
in mice 207–9
in women 209–11

research needs 283
vascular growth and modelling
and 61–2, 63–4
endometrial stromal cells
decidualisation 62–3
defective decidualisation 244–5
human *see* human endometrial
stromal cells
IL1β-stimulated, microarray study
204, 206
LIF actions 192, 195
endometriosis
adverse uterine milieu 246
microarray studies 212–13
pregnancy outcome 242
endometrium
chemokine receptors 80, 81
DNA microarrays *see* DNA
microarrays
embryo interactions *see*
embryo–endometrial
dialogue/interface
endocrine and paracrine signalling
3–15
haemostasis and vascular stability
32–48
leptin and leptin receptors (OB-
R) 83
LIF expression 186–8
relaxin receptor LGR7 85
vasculature *see* vasculature,
endometrial
endosalpinx, sperm contact 121, 122,
123–4
endothelial cells, endometrial 61–2
COX2/prostaglandin-mediated
regulation 10–11
endocrine regulation 5
key factors regulating 64–6
proliferation rate during cycle 62
role in endometrial receptivity
63–4
endpoints, child outcome studies
269–71
eosinophils, uterine, in LIF-null mice

190, 191–2
EP2 receptors 8–9, 11
EP4 receptors 8
epiblast 129
epidemiological studies 286
epidermal growth factor (EGF) 6, 50,
91, 110
epidermal growth factor receptor
(EGFR; ErbB1) 91, 93
epigenetic modification 141–54
cloned embryos 146–8
effects of ART 155, 161–3
factors associated with 142–4
research needs 284
see also genomic imprinting
EP receptors 6
ErbB1 *see* epidermal growth factor
receptor
ErbB4 53, 93
ERKO (ERα knockout) mice 109
ETS proteins 74
European Society of Human
Reproduction and Embryology
(ESHRE) 176
expectant treatment, miscarriage
225–6
extracellular matrix (ECM),
endometrial
decidualisation changes 70
embryo attachment 53–4
in vitro models of embryo
interactions 93–7
MMP-mediated degradation 71
regulation of turnover 40–3, 44
vascular stabilisation role 32, 40
extravillous trophoblast 19

factor V Leiden (FVL) 234, 235
factor VIIa 34
fallopian tube *see* uterine tube
FAS/FAS ligand (FASL) 11
fertilisation 124–5
guidance of sperm to site of 124
sperm functional demands 119,
120

fertility
  ART-conceived adults 271
  see also infertility
fetal loss 219–20
  late 220
  spontaneous second-trimester 220
fetal–maternal interface, tissue
  remodelling at 70–8
fetal period 219
fetal reduction, selective 257
FGF4 136
fibrin 37
fibrinolytic activity 230
fibronectin 50, 53, 93
fibulins 52, 54
financial arrangements, single-embryo
  transfer 264
FLT1 64
fluorescence *in situ* hybridisation
  (FISH)
    miscarried tissue 221, 222
    pre-implantation genetic testing
      172–3, 176, 177, 178
follicles (ovarian)
    gonadotrophin and steroid actions
      108–10
    growth and development 103–4
    in vitro systems 111–13
    oocyte regulation of development
      107
follicle-stimulating hormone (FSH)
    action within ovary 108–9
    receptors 109
follistatin 110
Fos 72–3
FP receptors 6, 8

galectin-1 245
gamete biology, research needs 284
gap junctions, oocyte 105, 107
gelatinases 40, 71
    see also matrix metalloproteinase 2;
      matrix metalloproteinase 9
gene arrays *see* DNA microarrays
gene expression profiling 54–5, 85–7,

92, 203
    see also DNA microarrays
genes, involved in implantation 5–6,
  53–5, 85–7, 91–2
genetic counselling 171
genetic testing, pre-implantation *see*
  pre-implantation genetic testing
genomic imprinting 143
    ART-conceived children 276–7
    effects of ART 155, 161–3
    oocyte maturation and 111
    see also epigenetic modification
glutathione peroxidase 246
glutathione peroxidase 3 (GPX3) 86,
  210
glycam 1 52
glycans 52, 55, 192
glycocalyx, uterine 50–1, 192, 193
glycodelin (PP14) 4, 245
gonadotrophin-releasing hormone
    (GnRH) agonists 247
gonadotrophins
    action within ovary 108–10
    superovulation induction 103,
      157–8
gp130 6, 186
    knockout mice 186, 195–6
    uterine expression 188, 189
G-protein-coupled receptors
    (GPCRs) 6, 80
granulocyte macrophage colony-
    stimulating factor (GM-CSF) 50
granulosa cells 105
    gonadotrophin and steroid actions
      108–10
    oocyte-mediated regulation 107
growth, ART-conceived children 275
growth differentiation factor 9
    (GDF9) 107, 110, 158

H19 gene 162
haemorrhage, decidual 33
haemostasis
    endometrial, role of
decidualisation 33–9, 43

reproductive 230
haemostatic abnormalities
    global markers 235–6
    see also thrombophilic defects
hatching, embryo 50
health policy/education, consensus
    views 285–6
hedgehog proteins 66
heparan sulphate proteoglycan 53, 70,
    233
heparin
        in antiphospholipid syndrome
        232, 233
        immunological effects 233, 247
heparin-binding EGF-like growth
    factor (HB-EGF) 52, 53, 91
        in LIF-null mice 195
        in solid-phase assays 93, 94
HESCs *see* human endometrial
stromal cells
histone H1, in cloned embryos 145
histone H4, acetylation 143–4, 147
histones
    core 141–2
    post-translational modifications
        143–4, 147
HLA
    trophoblast expression 18, 19–21
    typing, pre-implantation 179
HLA-A 20
HLA-B 20
HLA-C 20
    NK cell recognition 25, 26, 27
    pre-eclampsia and 27–8
HLA class I molecules
    expression by trophoblast 20
    NK cell recognition 25, 26–8
HLA class II molecules 20
HLA-E 20
    NK cell recognition 25, 27
HLA-F 20
HLA-G 20
    macrophage recognition 22
    NK cell recognition 25, 26–7
HoxA10/HoxaA10 6, 192, 207

HoxA11 6, 189
H-type-1 antigen 192–4
human chorionic gonadotrophin
    (hCG)
        regulation of LIF 186, 196
        secretion by blastocysts 93, 95
human endometrial stromal cells
    (HESCs), decidualised
        endometrial haemostasis and
        33–9
        endometrial vascular stability and
        33, 40–3
        prevention of endometrial
        bleeding 33
Human Fertilisation and Embryology
    Authority (HFEA) 171, 176, 178
    database linkage 271, 286
human leucocyte antigen *see* HLA
12-hydroxy-eicosatetraenoic acid (12-
    HETE) 208
15-hydroxyprostaglandin
    dehydrogenase (PGDH) 4
17β-hydroxysteroid dehydrogenase
    (17β-HSD type 2) 4
hyperhomocysteinaemia 234
hypertension, pregnancy-induced 243
hypoblast 129
hysterosalpingography 247

ICSI *see* intracytoplasmic sperm
    injection
ICSI-CFO study 271–4
Igf2 gene 162
ILT 24, 26
ILT2/4 22, 25, 27
immune response gene 1 (IRG1) 54,
    207–9
immunoglobulins, intravenous 232,
    247, 284
immunological models 16–18
immunology 16–31
    pre-eclampsia 27–8
    trophoblast 19–20
implantation
    adhesion molecules and 9, 49–60

embryo interactions 79–89
endocrine and paracrine signalling 3–15
endometrial haemostasis and vascular stability 32–48
experimental models in human 92–7
failure 49, 55–6, 90
genes involved 5–6, 53–5, 85–7, 91–2
immunology 16–31
maternal barrier 50–1
role of LIF 185–202
stages 90–1
window (timing) 49, 71, 205–6
imprinting, genomic see genomic imprinting
indoleamine 2,3-dioxygenase (IDO) 245
infectious nonself model 16–18
infertility 240
assisted reproductive technology see assisted reproductive technology
endometrial receptivity studies 55, 209
in endometriosis 212
implantation failure see implantation, failure
obesity and 82
pregnancy outcome and 157, 241–2
unexplained 90, 242
see also subfecundity
inflammatory response, endometrial 246, 247
inhibins 110
inner cell mass (ICM) 129
embryo axis determination and 137
epigenetic regulation 143, 144
immunosurgery isolation method 134–6
lineage, establishment 130–3
transcription factors regulating 136–7

insulin-like growth factor binding proteins (IGFBPs) 110–11
insulin-like growth factor receptor type 2 (IGFR2) gene 155, 161–3
insulin-like growth factors (IGF) 110–11, 186
integrin $\alpha_4\beta_1$ 53
integrin $\alpha_5\beta_1$ 50
integrin $\alpha_v\beta_3$ 51–3, 209
integrin β_1 6, 53–4
integrins 9, 52
interferon γ 233, 247
interleukin 1 (IL1)
LIF and 189
MMP9 gene regulation 74
interleukin 1β (IL1β) 50
LIF and 186, 188
microarray study 204, 206
interleukin 11 (IL11) 44, 91
receptor 6, 91
intervillous space 19
intracytoplasmic sperm injection (ICSI)
defining good sperm 126
genomic imprinting changes 162
paediatric outcome 270, 271–7
pregnancy outcomes 159–60, 241–2
pre-implantation genetic testing 172, 177
sperm functional demands 119, 120
intrauterine growth restriction, placental bed arterial remodelling and 243, 244
intrauterine insemination (IUI) 124
sperm functional demands 119, 120
intravenous immunoglobulins 232, 247, 284
in vitro culture (IVC)
genomic imprinting changes 162
perinatal outcomes 155, 159–60
in vitro fertilisation (IVF) 103
defining good sperm 126

defining success 263
embryo transfer *see* embryo
transfer
genomic imprinting changes 162
implantation failure problem 90
paediatric outcome 270, 271–7
pregnancy outcomes 159–60,
241–2
pre-implantation genetic testing
172, 176, 177
sperm DNA damage 126
sperm–egg recognition 124–5
sperm functional demands 119,
120
in vitro maturation (IVM) 113
consensus views 284, 285
pregnancy outcomes 158
IP receptors 6
ISP1/ISP2 50

JAK/STAT pathway 82, 188
JAM-1 132, 133, 134
Janus kinases (JAKs) 82
Jun 72–3

karyotype abnormalities *see*
chromosomal abnormalities
karyotyping, miscarried tissue 221
KCNQ1 gene 163
KIR 24–6, 27–8
KIR2DL1/2/3 25, 26
KIR2DL4 25, 26
kit ligand 107

labour, initiation of 8
laminins 52, 54
lamins, nuclear
in cloned embryos 145
oocyte/egg cytoplasmic extracts
and 150
large offspring syndrome (LOS) 155,
160, 161–2
laser capture microdissection (LCM)
213
lectins 192

leptin
endometrial role 82–4, 188
in oocyte development 107
receptors (OB-R) 82–4
leucocytes
chemokine-mediated regulation
79
infusions, paternal 247, 284
uterine mucosal 21–7
in LIF-null mice 190, 191–2
see also macrophages; natural killer
(NK) cells
leukaemia inhibitory factor (LIF) 6,
54, 185–202
function in humans 91, 186–8
knockout (null) mice 53, 186,
187, 195–6, 197
uterine cellular changes 189,
190–2
uterine molecular changes
192–4
uterine ultrastructural changes
192, 193
molecular responses in stroma
195
peri-implantation embryonic
development and 195–7
regulation 188
uterine cellular targets 188–92
leukaemia inhibitory factor receptor β
(LIFRβ) 186
knockout mice 186, 195–6
leukaemia inhibitory factor receptors
(LIFR) 186
regulation 188
uterine expression 188, 189
LGR7 84–5
LGR8 85
12/15-lipoxygenase *(Alox15)* 207–9
live birth rates
defining success in IVF 263
one- *versus* two-embryo transfer
259, 260–1
longitudinal studies, practical
difficulties 269

L-selectin 92
luminal epithelium (LE), endometrial
    see endometrial luminal epithelium
lupus anticoagulant (LA) 232
luteinising hormone (LH)
    action within ovary 108–9
    receptors 109
lymphocytes, uterine mucosal 21–4

macrophages, uterine 21–2
    in LIF-null mice 190, 191
    in pre-eclampsia 246
male-factor infertility
    pre-implantation genetic diagnosis
        177
    sperm DNA damage 126
    sperm–zona interaction 125
    see also intracytoplasmic sperm
        injection; sperm
manganese superoxide dismutase 210,
    246
Mater gene 106
maternal-effect genes 106
Matrigel, three-dimensional co-
    cultures 97, 98
matrix metalloproteinase 1 (MMP1)
    40–3, 44
matrix metalloproteinase 2 (MMP2)
    40, 41, 42, 43, 71
matrix metalloproteinase 3 (MMP3)
    40–3, 44
matrix metalloproteinase 7 (MMP7)
    92
matrix metalloproteinase 9 (MMP9)
    71
    gene *see MMP9* gene
    LIF-mediated regulation 196
    regulation of transcription 72–5
    in trophoblast invasion 72
matrix metalloproteinases (MMPs)
    32, 71–2, 91
    LIF and 195
    prostanoid-mediated regulation 9
    uPA and PAI-1 interactions 40–3
maturation-promoting factor (MPF)

145, 146, 148
Matzinger's danger model 17, 18
maximal clot amplitude (MA) 236
medical service use, ART-conceived
    children 274
medical treatment, miscarriage 225
medroxyprogesterone acetate (MPA)-
    induced decidualisation 34–43
membrane-type matrix
    metalloproteinases (MT-MMPs)
    51, 71
menstrual cycle
    chemokine receptors 81
    endocrine signalling in
    endometrium 4–5
    gene expression profiling 54, 86,
        209, 210–11
    LIF expression 186
    relaxin receptor LGR7 85
    structural vascular changes 62–3
    see also endometrial receptivity
menstruation 61, 62, 63
metallothioneins 210
methylene tetrahydrofolate reductase
    (MTHFR) C667T variant 234
MHC *see* HLA
microarrays *see* DNA microarrays
mifepristone
    microarray studies 207, 208,
        211–12
    in miscarriage 225
miscarriage 229
    aetiology 221–3
    diagnosis 223
    first-trimester 219–20
        protective factors 254, 255
        risk factors 253–5
    missed 219, 220
    one- *versus* two-embryo transfer
        259, 261
    patient examination 223–4
    preventive treatment 247
    recurrent *see* recurrent miscarriage
    research needs 284
    second-trimester 220, 221

subfecundity and 241
terminology 219–21
treatment 224–6
misoprostol, in miscarriage 225
missed miscarriage 219, 220
'missing self' hypothesis 17, 18
mitochondrial DNA (mtDNA)
158–9
mitogen-activated protein kinase
(MAPK) 6, 146, 148
MMP9 gene 72, 73
p53-mediated regulation 73, 74–5
regulation by transcription factors
72–4
see also matrix metalloproteinase 9
morula 130
mouse genetic models 5–6, 91
adhesion molecules 53–4
LIF 186
MSX1 194
MUC1 9, 51, 52, 192
MUC4 51, 52
mucins 9, 51, 52
multiple pregnancy 156
adverse effects 256
after ART 256, 269–70, 286
after PGD 176
one- *versus* two-embryo transfer
259, 260–1
paediatric outcome 268
prevention strategies 257
see also twin pregnancy

Na,K-ATPase 129, 133, 134
Nanog 136–7
National Women's Health Study
253–5
natural killer (NK) cells 18
HLA expression and 20–1
in peripheral blood 284
receptors 24–6
uterine (uNK cells) 20–1, 24–7,
244
angiogenic growth factors 65
functions 24, 29, 43–4

gene expression studies 245
in LIF-null mice 190, 191–2
pre-eclampsia and 27–8
trophoblast HLA recognition
25, 26–7
neonatal service use, ART-conceived
children 274
neurological outcomes, ART-
conceived children 276
neuropilin 66
NKG2 26
see also CD94/NKG2A
NKG5 24
NKT cells 21
Notch/jagged proteins 66
nuclear factor kappa B (NFκB) 74,
246
nuclear reprogramming 141–54
in cloned embryos 144–8
defined 144
experimental induction 148–50
nuclear transfer (NT)
cloning by 142
nuclear remodelling after 144–8
see also somatic cell nuclear
transfer
nucleolar disassembly, in cloned
embryos 145
nucleosome 141–2

obesity 82
occludin 134, 136
OCT4/*Oct4* 136–7, 149, 150
oestradiol (E$_2$)
chemokine receptor up-regulation
81
endometrial effects 3, 4–5
plus progestin-induced
decidualisation 34–43
oestrogen receptors (ER) 6
alpha (ERα) 5, 109
beta (ERβ) 5, 109
endometrial 4–5
ovarian 109
oestrogens

action within ovary 108–10
regulation of LIF 188
olfactomedin 86
olfactory receptor (hOR17–4) 124
oncostatin M (OSM) 195, 196
oocytes 103–18
cryopreservation 161
cytoplasmic extracts for nuclear
reprogramming 150
development 103–4
genomic imprinting 111
growth and maturation 105–8
in vitro maturation *see in vitro*
maturation
nuclear transfer *see* nuclear transfer
other factors affecting competence
110–11
research needs 284
steroid actions 109–10
see also eggs
osteopontin 53, 54, 86
ovarian follicles *see* follicles
ovary
gonadotrophin and steroid actions
108–10
in vitro culture systems 111, 112
ovulation 105
oxidative stress 244, 246

p53 protein
gatekeeper function 75
MMP9 gene regulation 73, 74–5,
76
paediatric outcome
ART 268–79, 285
literature review 271–7
methodological difficulties
268–71
twin pregnancy 256, 271
paracrine regulation, implantation
process 3, 6–11
paternal leucocyte immunisation 247,
284
pathogen-associated molecular
patterns (PAMPs) 16–18

periconceptual manipulation, uterine
milieu 246–7
pericytes 62
perinatal outcomes *see* pregnancy
outcomes
perlecan 52
peroxisomal proliferator activator
receptors (PPARs) 6–7, 208
phospholipase A_2 (PLA$_2$) 6, 7
pifithrin alpha (PFT) 75, 76
pinopods 186, 192
placenta 16
placental growth factor (PGF; PlGF)
24, 65
placental infarction, in thrombophilias
233, 234
placental protein 14 (PP14;
glycodelin) 4, 245
placentation 70
defective deep, pregnancy
outcome 242–5
early 19
plasmin 32, 37, 40, 71
plasminogen activator inhibitor 1
(PAI-1) 32, 37–9, 40–3, 195, 230
plasminogen activator inhibitor 2
(PAI-2) 230
plasminogen activators 230
plurality at birth, ART-conceived
babies 269–70
pluripotent cells, somatic cell de-
differentiation into 149
podosome-like structures 95, 96
polar body biopsy 169, 176
polycystic ovary syndrome (PCOS)
158, 246
polymerase chain reaction (PCR),
pre-implantation genetic diagnosis
172, 174–5
pre-decidualisation 21
pre-eclampsia
defective deep placentation 243,
244
immunology 27–8, 245
inter-pregnancy interval and 241

oxidative stress 246
pregnancy
    early loss *see* early pregnancy loss
    prothrombotic state 230
    termination 170, 171
    time to (TTP), pregnancy
        outcome and 241
pregnancy outcomes 240–52
    ART 156–61, 241–2
    defective deep placentation and
        242–5
    pre-implantation genetic testing
        172, 176, 178
    prothrombotic disorders 231
    reproductive disorders 242
    single-embryo transfer 258–61
    subfecundity 240
    twin pregnancy 256
pre-implantation genetic diagnosis
    (PGD) 169, 170–6
    clinical considerations 171–2
    clinical procedures and
    embryology 172
        funding 286
        HLA typing and 179
        indications 172–5
        outcomes 176, 271
        regulation 176
Pre-implantation Genetic Diagnosis
    International Society (PGDIS) 176
pre-implantation genetic screening
    (PGS) 169, 176–8
        funding 286
        indications 177
        limitations and drawbacks 177–8
        research needs 285
pre-implantation genetic testing
    (PGT) 169–82
        advances 176–9
        consensus view 285
        embryo biopsy 169–70
        future developments 179–80
        social sex selection 178
pre-implantation HLA typing 179
prenatal diagnosis (PND) 170

preterm labour, preventive therapy
    247
primates, non-human 91
progesterone
    endometrial haemostasis and 34,
        35, 37
    endometrial responses 3–5, 245–6
    endometrial vascular changes and
        62–3
    LIF regulation 188
    periconceptual therapy 247
    regulated endometrial genes
        207–9, 212
    relative insensitivity in
        endometriosis 246
progesterone receptors (PR) 4–5, 6,
    44, 207, 209
progestin-induced decidualisation
    32–48
programmed cell death, in
    implantation 11
prolactin (PRL) 44
prospective studies, practical
    difficulties 269
prostacyclin (PGI$_2$) 6, 7
    role in implantation 9, 11
prostaglandin D$_2$ (PGD$_2$) 6, 7
prostaglandin E$_2$ (PGE$_2$) 6, 7
    regulation by LIF 189
    role in implantation 9, 11
prostaglandin F$_{2\alpha}$ (PGF$_{2\alpha}$) 6, 7, 8, 50
prostaglandins (prostanoids)
    LIF-mediated regulation 189, 195
    receptors 6
    regulation of implantation 6–11,
        50
proteases
    in trophoblast invasion 71
    see also matrix metalloproteinases
protein kinase A (PKA) 109
protein kinase C (PKC) 54, 130
    atypical 132, 133
    in trophectoderm differentiation
        134, 135, 136
protein S 230

prothrombin G20210A 234
prothrombotic disorders
    adverse pregnancy outcomes 231
    global markers 235–6
    role in recurrent miscarriage
        231–6
    prothrombotic state of pregnancy
        230

RAB13 134, 136
recurrent miscarriage (RM) 229–39
    aetiology 230
    defective deep placentation and
        243–4
    defined 229
    karyotypical abnormalities 221
    pre-implantation genetic testing
        174, 177
    preventive therapy 232, 247, 284
    research needs 284
    role of prothrombotic disorders
        231–6
relaxin 84–5
relaxin receptor LGR7 84–5
reproductive disorders
    adverse uterine milieu 245–6
    manipulation of uterine milieu
        246–7
    and pregnancy outcome 242
research, future, consensus views
    283–5
retinoblastoma 270
retinopathy of prematurity 275
RGD adhesion sequence 123
risk perception, single-embryo transfer
    and 263–4
Ron 50

S100E gene 212–13
selectins 52, 53
self/nonself model 16, 17
semaphorins 66
semen analysis 119–20
sex determination, embryo 170,
    172–3

sex selection
    social 178
    in X-linked disorders 172–3
sex steroids
    action within ovary 108–10
    endometrial preparation for
        implantation 3–5
    see also androgens; oestradiol;
        progesterone
sexual maturation, ART-conceived
    children 271
single-embryo transfer (SET) 256–67
    consensus view 285
    consumer choice and risk
        perception 263–4
    defining success 263
    elective (eSET) 257
    evidence for 258–61
    financial aspects 264
    implementation 261–4
    policy setting 263
    rationale 256–7
    regulation 264
single-gene disorders, pre-
    implantation diagnosis 173, 174–5
smooth muscle cells, vascular 62, 63
sodium butyrate 148
solid-phase assays, blastocyst
    attachment and trophoblast
    outgrowth 93, 94
solute carrier family 1 member 1
    (SLCA1) 86
somatic cell nuclear transfer (SCNT)
    chromatin condensation after 146
    cloning by 142
    epigenetic remodelling after
        146–8
    nuclear architecture after 145
    nuclear reprogramming after
        144–8
somatic cells
    de-differentiation 149
    differentiation potential 148
    nuclear reprogramming with
        cytoplasmic extracts 149–50

SOX2 136
SPARC/osteonectin 52
specificity protein 1 (SP1) 34–6, 74
sperm 119–28
    capacitation 123
    cryopreservation 160–1
    defining 'good' 119–26
    DNA quality 125–6
    functional demands 119, 120
    function tests 120, 121
    hyperactivation 121–3
    research needs 284
    sorting into X and Y 170, 173
    survival 123
    transport 121–3
sperm–egg recognition 124–5
sperm–epithelial contact, in uterine
    tube 121, 123–4
spiral arterioles 62
    cyclical changes 62, 63
    physiological transformation 243
        failure 243–5
    trophoblast invasion 19, 33, 242–3
STAT1 246
STAT3 83, 188–9
STATs 82
stem cells
    adult, differentiation potential 148
    in LIF-null mice 197
    see also embryonic stem (ES) cells
steroidogenesis, ovarian 108
steroid therapy 232, 247, 284
stromelysins 40, 71
    see also matrix metalloproteinase 3
structural abnormalities, miscarried
    pregnancies 222–3
subfecundity 240
    adverse pregnancy outcome and
        241
    adverse uterine milieu 246
superovulation 103
    pregnancy outcomes after 157–8
superoxide dismutase, manganese
    210, 246
suppressor of cytokine signalling

protein 3 (SOCS3) 188
surgical evacuation of uterus, in
    miscarriage 224–5
surrogates, embryo transfer to 157
syncytiotrophoblast 19, 20
systemic lupus erythematosus (SLE)
    232

tenascins 52, 195
termination of pregnancy 170, 171
Th2/Th2 responses 22
thermotaxis, in sperm guidance 124
three-dimensional co-cultures,
    endometrial cells and blastocysts
    97, 98
thrombin 34, 230
thrombin–antithrombin (TAT)
    complexes 230, 235
thromboelastography (TEG) 235–6
thrombophilic defects 229, 231–5
    acquired 231–3
    inherited 233–5
thromboprophylaxis, in
    antiphospholipid syndrome 232, 233
thrombospondins 52
thromboxane (TXA$_2$) 6, 7
tight junctions (TJ), early embryo
    133–4, 135, 136
time to pregnancy (TTP), adverse
    pregnancy outcome and 241
tissue factor (TF) 32, 33–6, 37, 43
tissue inhibitors of matrix
    metalloproteinase 1 (TIMP1) 41,
    42, 43, 195
tissue inhibitors of matrix
    metalloproteinases (TIMPs) 40, 71,
    91
tissue-type plasminogen activator
    (tPA) 37–9
T lymphocytes 16
    decidual 22–4, 28
TPA (phorbol ester) 72, 130
TP receptors 6
transcription factors
    in embryonic cell lineage

diversification 136–7
MMP9 gene regulation 72–4
trans-differentiation 148, 149
transforming growth factor-α (TGF-α) 110
transforming growth factor-β (TGF-β) 110, 186
transplantation immunology 16, 22, 23
T regulatory (Treg) cells 24
trichostatin A 148
triplets 270
trisomies
    maternal age-related 156–7
    pre-implantation screening 177
trophectoderm 129
    differentiation 133–4
    epigenetic regulation 144
    from isolated inner cell mass cells 136
    lineage, establishment 130–3
    transcription factors regulating 136–7
trophinin 52, 53
trophoblast
    differentiation 19
    endovascular 19, 20, 32
    extravillous 19
    HLA expression 18, 19–21
    immunological response 19–24
    interstitial 20–1
    outgrowth, solid-phase assays 93, 94
    recognition by uterine NK cells 26–7
    villous 19, 20
trophoblast invasion 19, 71
    defective 243–5
    endometrial cell–blastocyst co-cultures 95–7
    endovascular 19, 32, 33, 242–3
    excessive 19
    immunology 28–9
    interstitial 242
    regulatory factors 72

role of COX2 and prostanoids 9
role of MMPs 71–2
tryptophan 245
tube *see* uterine tube
tumour necrosis factor (TNF) 74
tumour necrosis factor α converting enzyme (TACE) 51
Turner syndrome 159
twin pregnancy
    adverse effects 256
    consumer perceptions 263–4
    paediatric outcome 271
    prevention strategies 257
    see also multiple pregnancy
twins, monozygotic 160
two-embryo transfer *see* double-embryo transfer

ultrasonography, in early pregnancy problems 222, 224
urokinase plasminogen activator (uPA) 32, 38, 40–3, 196
uterine glands, in LIF-null mice 189, 190
uterine milieu
    adverse 245–6
    periconceptual manipulation 246–7
uterine receptivity *see* endometrial receptivity
uterine (fallopian) tube
    implantation 92
    sperm behaviour and functions 122
    sperm–egg recognition and fertilisation 124–5
    sperm–epithelial contact 121, 123–4
    sperm transport 121–3
uterodomes 186, 192

vaginal examination, in early pregnancy bleeding 223–4
vascular cell adhesion molecule 1 (VCAM-1) 53

vascular endothelial growth factor
(VEGF) 10–11, 63, 65–6
vascular endothelial growth factor A
(VEGF A) 61, 64, 65–6
vascular endothelial growth factor C
(VEGF C) 24
vascular smooth muscle cells 62, 63
vasculature, endometrial 61–9
   cyclical changes in structure 62–3
   endometrial receptivity and 63–4
   key factors regulating 64–5
   regulation of stability by
    decidualised HESCs 33, 40–3
   research needs 283
   see also angiogenesis; endothelial
    cells, endometrial

white cells *see* leucocytes
Wilms tumour 276
Wnt7a 189–91
WNT proteins 66, 211

Xenopus oocytes/eggs, cytoplasmic
   extracts 149–50
X-linked genetic disorders
   pre-implantation diagnosis 170,
    172–3
   sperm sorting 170

Zar1 gene 106
ZO-1 136
ZO-1α 134, 135
ZO-2 134
zona pellucida, sperm interaction
   124, 125
zygotes, *in vitro* culture *see in vitro*
   culture